Pediatric Respiratory Therapy

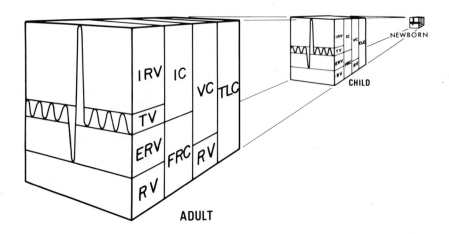

ADULT   CHILD   NEWBORN

The tremendous changes that occur with growth must be appreciated in order for the principles of respiratory care developed for the adult to be applied successfully to the child or the infant.

Pediatric Respiratory Therapy

THIRD EDITION

Marvin D. Lough, R.R.T

Technical Director of Pediatric Respiratory Therapy and Pulmonary Function Laboratory, Rainbow Babies and Childrens Hospital; Clinical Instructor, School of Respiratory Therapy, Cuyahoga Community College, Cleveland, Ohio

Carl F. Doershuk, M.D.

Professor of Pediatrics, Case Western Reserve University School of Medicine; Director, Cystic Fibrosis Center and Respiratory Therapy, Rainbow Babies and Childrens Hospital Cleveland, Ohio

Robert C. Stern, M.D.

Professor of Pediatrics, Case Western Reserve University School of Medicine; Associate Pediatrician and Director, Pulmonary Clinic, Rainbow Babies and Childrens Hospital, Cleveland, Ohio

YEAR BOOK MEDICAL PUBLISHERS, INC.
CHICAGO

0   9   8   7   6   5   4   3   2   1

Library of Congress Cataloging in Publication Data
Main entry under title:

Pediatric respiratory therapy.

   Includes bibliographies and index.
   1. Pediatric respiratory diseases.   2. Respiratory
therapy for children.   I. Lough, Marvin D.   II. Doershuk,
Carl F., 1930-   .   III. Stern, Robert C., 1938-   .
[DNLM: 1. Respiratory Therapy—in infancy & childhood.
2. Respiratory Tract Diseases—in infancy & childhood.
3. Respiratory Tract Diseases—therapy. WS 280 P368]
RJ431.P418   1985   618.92'22   85-2500
ISBN 0-8151-5639-1

Sponsoring Editor: Diana L. McAninch
Manager, Copyediting Services: Frances M. Perveiler
Production Project Manager: Sharon W. Pepping

82427

Contributors

Gordon Borkat, M.D.
Assistant Clinical Professor of Pediatrics, Case Western Reserve University School of Medicine, Chairman, Department of Pediatrics, Fairview General Medical Center, Cleveland, Ohio

Waldemar, A. Carlo, M.D.
Assistant Professor of Pediatrics, Case Western Reserve University, Assistant Pediatrician, Rainbow Babies and Childrens Hospital, Cleveland, Ohio

Robert C. Chatburn, R.R.T.
Clinical Research Therapist, Department of Respiratory Therapy, Rainbow Babies and Childrens Hospital, Cleveland, Ohio

Carl F. Doershuk, M.D.
Professor of Pediatrics, Case Western Reserve University School of Medicine, Director, Cystic Fibrosis Center and Respiratory Therapy, Rainbow Babies and Childrens Hospital, Cleveland, Ohio

Avroy A. Fanaroff, M.B. (Rand), M.R.,C.P.E., D.C.H.
Professor of Pediatrics, Case Western Reserve University School of Medicine, Associate Pediatrician and Director of the Newborn Nurseries, Rainbow Babies and Childrens Hospital, Co-Director of the Cleveland Regional Perinatal Network, Cleveland, Ohio

Robert J. Fink, M.D.
Assistant Professor of Child Health and Development, George Washington University, Director, Division of Pulmonary Medicine and Cystic Fibrosis Center, Children's Hospital National Medical Center, Washington, D.C.

Christopher C. Green, M.D.
Assistant Professor of Pediatrics, University of Wisconsin School of Medicine, Madison, Wisconsin

Carolyn M. Kercsmar, M.D.
Assistant Professor of Pediatrics, Case Western Reserve University, Director, Asthma Center, Rainbow Babies and Childrens Hospital, Cleveland, Ohio

Jerome Liebman, M.D.
Professor of Pediatrics, Case Western Reserve University School of Medicine, Associate Pediatrician, Rainbow Babies and Childrens Hospital, Cleveland, Ohio

Marvin D. Lough, R.R.T.
Technical Director of Pediatric Respiratory Therapy and Pulmonary Function Laboratory, Rainbow Babies and Childrens Hospital, Clinical Instructor, School of Respiratory Therapy, Cuyahoga Community College, Cleveland, Ohio

Richard J. Martin, M.B., F.R.C.P.(C)
Associate Professor of Pediatrics, Case Western Reserve University School of Medicine, Assistant Pediatrician, Division of Neonatology, Rainbow Babies and Childrens Hospital, Cleveland, Ohio

David M. Orenstein, M.D.
Associate Professor of Pediatrics, University of Pittsburgh School of Medicine, Chief, Pediatric Pulmonary Division, Children's Hospital of Pittsburgh, Pittsburgh, Pennsylvania

Robert C. Stern, M.D.
Professor of Pediatrics, Case Western Reserve University School of Medicine, Associate Pediatrician and Director, Pulmonary Clinic, Rainbow Babies and Childrens Hospital, Cleveland, Ohio

Jan S. Tecklin, M.S., L.P.T.
Assistant Professor, Department of Physical Therapy, Beaver College, Glenside, Pennsylvania

Robert E. Wood, Ph.D., M.D.
Associate Professor of Pediatrics, University of North Carolina School of Medicine, Chief, Pediatric Pulmonary Division, University Hospitals of North Carolina, Chapel Hill, North Carolina

Preface to the Third Edition

Continued increases in knowledge of pediatric pulmonary physiology and disease have led to improved care techniques, respiratory support, and monitoring. This third edition of *Pediatric Respiratory Therapy* provides current information related to pediatric respiratory disease in a single practical reference not only for respiratory therapists and pulmonary physicians, but also for physical therapists, nursing personnel, social workers, and primary care physicians who are interested in pulmonary disease and who work with infants and children requiring respiratory care.

The chapters on Evaluation and Care of the Newborn Infant, Respiratory Diseases and Treatment, Respiratory Therapy, and Mechanical Ventilation have been extensively revised. The chapter on Bronchial Hygiene is by a new author. Other new authors and new information have been added to other chapters.

This text was developed to provide a useful source of practical information and to contribute substantially to the understanding of pediatric disease and the effective delivery of respiratory care to pediatric patients.

The knowledge and experience detailed in this edition were acquired in part during a period of clinical research and training supported by NIH Grants HL07415 and AM27651, The Reinberger Foundation and Cystic Fibrosis Foundation, and United Way Services of Cleveland.

MARVIN D. LOUGH, R.R.T.
CARL F. DOERSHUK, M.D.
ROBERT C. STERN, M.D.

Preface to the First Edition

This book is intended for students and postgraduate health personnel—including respiratory therapists, physical therapists, nurses and nursing staff and physicians—interested in pulmonary disease or respiratory care in infants and children. Several textbooks are available that cover in detail the many aspects of adult inhalation therapy; however, this book represents the first comprehensive attempt to provide specific information about respiratory therapy in the pediatric age group.

A recent survey conducted by the United States Government concluded that one of every ten children is handicapped by asthma, bronchitis, bronchiectasis, cystic fibrosis, emphysema or other pulmonary disorders. These conditions are responsible for 55% of all childhood chronic diseases. Hospital statistics show that a respiratory condition is the primary cause for admission of 42% of hospitalized children. This text was developed to provide a useful source of practical information and to contribute substantially to the understanding of pediatric diseases and the effective delivery of respiratory care to pediatric patients.

The information covering the development of the lung and respiratory defense as related to health and disease has been brought together in a concise and useful way. The methods and techniques described for inhalation therapy, mechanical ventilation, newborn care and the respiratory distress syndrome, pulmonary function testing, respiratory physical therapy and care of equipment are those with which the authors are personally familiar and, in most cases, are those used in Rainbow Babies and Childrens Hospital. The section covering disease is oriented to a description of the problems requiring respiratory care measures.

All of the information is based on a broad experience of over 15 years with pediatric respiratory care. It is increasingly clear that children simply are not small adults, either in their reaction to disease or in their response to various methods of treatment. The high incidence of pulmonary disease in children further highlights their need for effective specific respiratory therapy as outlined in this book.

The knowledge and experience detailed in this book were acquired in part during a period of clinical research support by Grant HE 13885 from the National Heart and Lung Institute, The Cleveland Chapter of the National Cystic Fibrosis Research Foundation and The Health Fund of Greater Cleveland.

Marsha Culp, Ruth Fagan and Florence Ledwell provided invaluable secretarial assistance, Nelson Egleton provided graphic illustrations, Jack Hardesty produced many of the photographs and Ann Taylor, Elaine Burton and Laura Levinthal provided original medical illustrations.

Over the years the dedicated members of the respiratory therapy division, the pulmonary function laboratory, the physical therapy department, the laboratory services, the house and nursing staffs, and Assistant Director Dalia Zemaityte, R.N., of Rainbow Babies and Childrens Hospital have contributed enormously to the pulmonary program.

We especially wish to thank all members of our families for their many sacrifices and gratefully acknowledge their understanding, support and encouragement, without which this book could not have been completed.

Cleveland, Ohio, 1973   MARVIN D. LOUGH
                                           CARL F. DOERSHUK
                                           ROBERT C, STERN

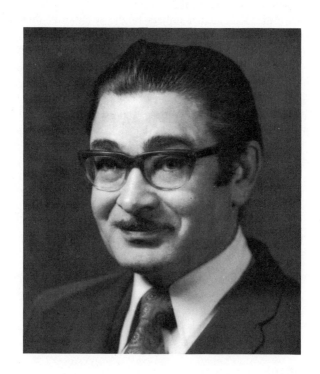

Dr. LeRoy W. Matthews

Dedication

This pediatric respiratory therapy textbook was the first of its kind in a field that is growing rapidly. The stimulus for this book was the improved evaluation and care of pediatric pulmonary patients initiated in 1957 by LeRoy W. Matthews, M.D.

Lee recognized the need for a specialized center for comprehensive care of patients with cystic fibrosis. He subsequently developed the nation's first pediatric pulmonary center when he recognized that children with a variety of other pulmonary disorders would also benefit from improved diagnostic evaluation and specialized care. Both clinical and basic research was an integral part of the new center. In developing a strong pulmonary program he has had a major influence on the education and training of most of the contributors to this book.

In addition to comprehensive care, he proposed the use of measures to prevent, or at least delay, the onset of significant pulmonary disease in those at greatest risk, such as patients with cystic fibrosis. This concept has dramatically improved survival.

Lee received his M.D. degree from the Harvard Medical School in 1949. He came to Cleveland as an intern in pediatrics in that year and then stayed at University Hospitals of Cleveland, Rainbow Babies and Childrens Hospital, and Case Western Reserve University School of Medicine. He was named Professor of Pediatrics in 1967 and served as Chairman of the Department of Pediatrics from 1970–1976. His wife, Blanche, has provided continuing support throughout his career.

Through his teaching and his personal example of devoted patient care, Lee has benefited patients of all ages. His selfless hard work, his enthusiasm, his unflagging determination, his leadership, and his compassion for his patients and their families provided the inspiration for the development of this book.

CONTENTS

Development of the Respiratory System

CHRISTOPHER C. GREEN, M.D.
CARL F. DOERSHUK, M.D.

1

THE ANATOMIC AND FUNCTIONAL DEVELOPMENT of human organ systems is an ongoing process that begins with fertilization and continues into adult life. In the complex respiratory system, significant development continues after birth and is related to the manifestations of pulmonary disease. The respiratory system should be viewed as an anatomical and biochemical continuum, from the nose to the alveoli, which is reflected in changing pulmonary physiology and manifestations of respiratory disease in infants and children.

In utero, the development of the upper respiratory tract parallels the differentiation of the facial structures and the branchial clefts, while the conducting airways and respiratory portions of the lung follow a very different developmental timetable. The conducting airways begin to develop early in embryonic life, and the number of these airways present by the 16th week of gestation remains unchanged throughout life. The other respiratory structures begin to develop soon after completion of the conducting airways, including development of a rich vascular supply from the 24th week until birth.

While sufficient respiratory surface is present to support life after the 28th week, there is a marked difference between the number and size of the respiratory structures present at birth and those in adult lungs. The development of the surfactant system parallels alveolar development.

This chapter describes the pre- and postnatal development of the human lung and the changes that occur with the onset of respiration. Several reviews are available for more complete details.[6, 13, 14, 17]

ANATOMY

The lung can be divided into respiratory and nonrespiratory structures. The nonrespiratory structures, or conducting airways, consist of the trachea, right and left main-stem bronchi, segmental and subsegmental bronchi, varying gen-

1

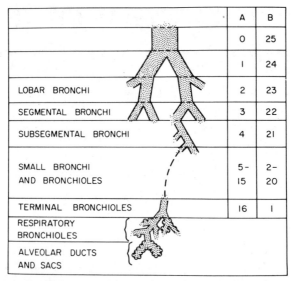

	A	B
	0	25
	1	24
LOBAR BRONCHI	2	23
SEGMENTAL BRONCHI	3	22
SUBSEGMENTAL BRONCHI	4	21
SMALL BRONCHI AND BRONCHIOLES	5 – 15	2 – 20
TERMINAL BRONCHIOLES	16	1
RESPIRATORY BRONCHIOLES		
ALVEOLAR DUCTS AND SACS		

Fig 1–1.—Two systems of numbering the conducting airways: **A,** counting starts with upper airways and progresses downward; **B,** counting begins with last fully epithelialized generation and progresses upward. The numbers given represent mean counts. The respiratory bronchioles, alveolar ducts, and alveolar sacs comprise the acinus. (From Charnock, E.L., and Doershuk, C.F.: Developmental aspects of the human lung, Pediatr. Clin. North Am. 20:275, 1973.)

erations of smaller bronchi and bronchioles, and a generation of terminal bronchioles (Fig 1–1).

In the developed lung, each lobe possesses a characteristic pattern of asymmetric dichotomous branching airways, with none of the lobes having the same pattern (Fig 1–2). From lobe to lobe, the number of airways varies, as do the path lengths of different segments. Lungs of similar age and size tend to show a uniform pattern of airways, although minor variations occur. The functional significance of airway branching is to increase the number of terminal bronchioles from which the respiratory portions of the lung grow. The respiratory or acinar portion of the lungs consists of respiratory bronchioles, alveolar ducts, alveolar sacs and alveoli. It is important to remember that new structures continue to develop in this area well past birth, with major changes observed as early as the first 2 months. Only 10% of the adult complement of gas exchange units is present in infants at the time of full-term delivery (see Table 9–2).

A basic understanding of this developmental continuum is necessary for those who treat the respiratory problems of children, since changes are occurring not only in anatomy but also in the physiologic parameters of the lungs.

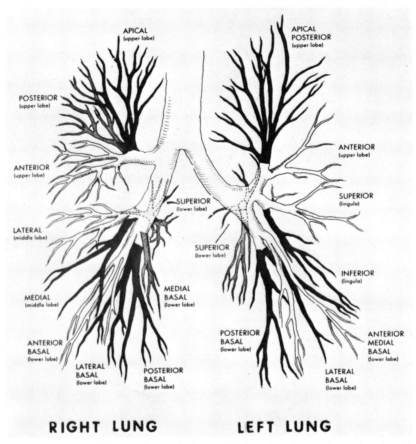

Fig 1–2.—Branching pattern of airways in the developed lung showing the major bronchial segments.

INTRAUTERINE DEVELOPMENT

Soon after fertilization, the developing embryo, by a process of cellular differentiation, forms three primary germ layers: the ectoderm, mesoderm, and endoderm. By the time of the first appearance of the respiratory system at 24 days gestation, these germ layers are well established, and the endoderm exists as a longitudinal tube. Only the endoderm and mesoderm (both cellular and noncellular) will form the respiratory structures, and there is no contribution from the ectoderm.

The earliest evidence of embryonic respiratory structures begins with the appearance of a ventral groove in the cervical region of the endodermal tube in the 24-day embryo. This groove develops into a ventral pouch to form the primitive lung bud, which grows into and develops within the median mass of mesoderm. The endoderm and mesoderm are interdependent and it is likely that the mesoderm directs the development of the endodermal structures.

Lung Development

At 26 to 28 days, a series of asymmetric dichotomous branchings of the primitive lung bud initiate the development of the bronchial tree (Fig 1–3). The right and left lung buds branch out laterally into their respective pleural cavities, carrying with them the mesodermal tissue, which continues to adapt itself to the shape of the developing bronchial tree. Gradually, the lobes of the lungs take form. The endoderm eventually forms the respiratory epithelium. The cellular mesoderm surrounding the bronchial tree ultimately differentiates into the muscle, connective tissue, and cartilaginous plates of the airways and the supporting tissues of the alveolar walls. The elastic and collagen tissues of the

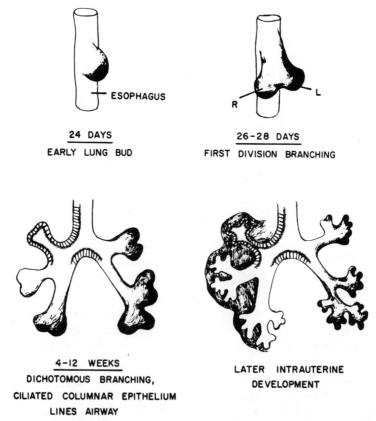

Fig 1–3.—Development of the lung. (Modified from Avery, M.E.: *Lung Development: The Lung and Its Disorders in the Newborn Infant* [Philadelphia: W.B. Saunders Co., 1968].)

airways, pleura, septa, and lung are formed from noncellular mesoderm, the mesenchyma.

Fetal lung development has been described as occurring in four phases. The *embryonic period* has been described as the first 5 weeks following ovulation and includes the earliest phases of lung development. The next phase is characterized by a glandular appearance of the developing airways, which are lined by columnar epithelium and separated from each other by poorly differentiated mesenchyma. This phase, previously described as the *glandular phase,* ends at approximately the 16th week and is termed the *pseudoglandular period.* The *canalicular phase* extends from the 16th to the 26th week and is characterized by flattening of the epithelium that lines the airways and an accompanying proliferation of the mesenchyma with the development of a rich capillary plexus within it. Structural and biochemical changes occur in the epithelial cells, while capillaries begin to protrude into the epithelium. Late in this period, initiation of the development of gas exchange units of the lung is accompanied by the appearance of Type I and Type II alveolar lining cells.[16]

Further intrauterine development of these respiratory structures occurs during the *terminal sac period,* which extends from the 26th week until after full-term birth. This period, previously termed the *alveolar period,* is characterized by the development of terminal sacculations at the distal ends of the terminal airway generations. It is during this phase of lung development that pulmonary surfactant first appears in the tracheal and amniotic fluids.

Airways and Bronchial Structures

By the 6th week of gestation the segmental bronchi are formed. This branching and formation of new conducting airways continues until the 16th week. Sixty-five to 75% of the branching occurs in a burst of activity between the 10th and 14th weeks. After 16 weeks the conducting airways lengthen by longitudinal growth. Ultimately, 8 to 18 bronchial divisions are found in the upper lobes. The longer conducting airways of the lingula, middle lobe, and anterior and posterior basal segments contain 20 to 32 generations.

The ductular nature of the developing bronchi is established early, with a ciliated columnar epithelium present at 13 weeks. As branching progresses, this columnar epithelium extends peripherally. At the level of the bronchioles, there is a gradual transition from columnar to a cuboidal epithelium.

The respiratory bronchioles begin development during the 14th to 16th weeks. Primitive alveolar structures appear at the 26th week. These acinar structures continue to develop through the rest of gestation. However, a major portion of the acinar development occurs after birth.

DIAPHRAGM.—The diaphragm is the major motor structure responsible for the ventilation of the lung after birth. It is a muscular organ whose simple shape and design do not indicate its complex origins. Failure in its development can result in life-threatening malformations. It is considered to be the most efficient organ in that it has the lowest oxygen consumption per unit of work.

Prior to the 7th week of gestation, the pleural cavities are continuous with the peritoneal cavity via the pleuroperitoneal canals. Early in the 7th week, the enlarging abdominal organs develop a ventral mesodermal fold called the *septum transversum*. This septum forms the major portion of the diaphragm. From above, the pleuroperitoneal membranes are developed from the lateral thoracic wall. These membranes close the pleuroperitonel canals and, with contributions from the thoracic muscles, form the lateral portions of the diaphragm. Minor contributions are derived from the mesentery of the gastrointestinal tract, the periaortic tissues, and the mesenchyma behind the upper abdominal organs. Embryologic differentiation of the diagram is complete by the end of the 7th week.

Bronchial Wall and Trachea

Knowledge of the development of the epithelium, mucous glands, goblet cells, cartilage, and muscle tissue is important to understanding pathophysiologic pulmonary events. Scanning electron miscroscopy permits visualization of the surface epithelium of an airway (Fig 1–4).

EPITHELIUM AND CILIA.—Epithelial and cilial development parallels the development of the conductive airways, and by the 10th week of gestation the epithelium in developed bronchi consists of a superficial layer of columnar cells and deeper basal layers of irregularly appearing cells resting on a well-defined basement membrane. The basement membrane at 10 weeks appears as an interrupted layer of PAS-positive* material and by the 12th week is well developed and complete. Cilia, which have been observed on the epithelial surfaces as early as the 7th week, are found extending throughout the conducting airways by the 13th week.

Epithelial development proceeds peripherally with the generation of new bronchial segments, but in the peripheral airways the epithelium changes to a single layer of columnar cells that gradually diminish in height until the epithelium becomes cuboidal in the smaller bronchioles.

MUCOUS GLANDS.—The anlage of mucous glands appears in the 12th week as groups of well-defined clusters of cells at the base of epithelial folds. These clusters penetrate to the basement membrane and form tubules. By the 14th week the proximal glands consist of tubular and acinar structures, while peripherally the glands are still only tubular in structure. New glands continue to appear until the 25th or 26th weeks, after which development apparently proceeds only by growth of individual glands. When fully developed, the secretory portions of the mucous glands are found both in the submucosa and beneath the cartilage.

Early in development, the mucous gland consists of only mucous cells. Beyond the 25th week, serous cells begin to appear. In the newborn, the mucous

---

*PAS—Periodic Acid Schiff.

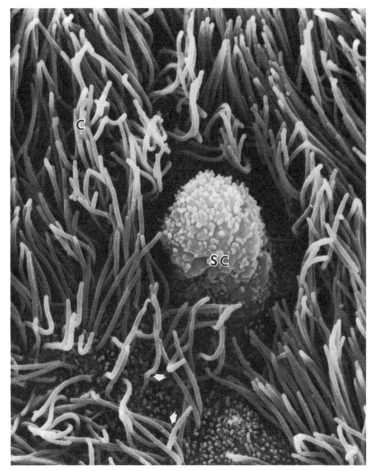

Fig 1–4.—Scanning electron microscope view of the surface epithelium of a bronchiole from a young adult monkey shows ciliated cells with cilia *(c)* and one secretory cell *(sc).* Arrows indicate microvilli. 14 mm = 1 μm. (Courtesy of the California Primate Research Center, M.E. Brummer and L.W. Schwartz.)

gland produces a pattern of secretions different from that produced in the adult. This difference persists over the first few months of life, but its significance is unknown.

With successive bronchial generations there is a stepwise decrease in gland density. Glands do not extend as far peripherally as cartilage and are found in only one third to one half of the bronchial generations in any one pathway. In segmental bronchi of a 14-week fetus, the concentration of mucous glands is approximately 50 glands/sq mm, while at birth, the concentration drops to 17 glands/sq mm in the same area. In the adult, lung density of mucous glands is approximately 1 gland/sq mm, and the total number of glands has been estimated at 6,000. This represents a considerable decrease in the number of glands per square millimeter of epithelial surface from that found in the infant, presumably the result of continued longitudinal growth of bronchi with no absolute increase in the number of glands.

One characteristic of mucous glands is their increase in size in patients with pulmonary disease. Histologic studies of bronchial and bronchiolar walls of normal infants, children, and adults compared with those of children with cystic fibrosis and bronchiolitis have demonstrated hypertrophy of mucous glands. Extreme mucous gland hypertrophy is noted in the lungs of children dying from pulmonary disease due to cystic fibrosis. The Reid index provides a measure of mucous gland hypertrophy.[15]

GOBLET CELLS.—Goblet cells first appear in the trachea and large bronchi at 10 weeks gestation as vacuolated cells in the crypts of the epithelial folds. By the 16th week, the goblet cells are well established, but even as late as 24 weeks, they are present only in the proximal intrasegmental bronchi. Beyond 32 weeks, the goblet cells are found in a pattern similar to that of the mucous glands and only occasionally are found distal to them. Estimates of goblet cell density have varied between 1 to 30 and 1 to 100 epithelial cells, and their volume is reported to be only one fortieth of that of the mucous glands. The number of goblet cells increases as a consequence of irritation and infection and, in patients with cystic fibrosis, have been found extending into the bronchioles even in infants. The mucous glands and goblet cells are the principal sources of the tracheobronchial secretions.

SMOOTH MUSCLE.—Smooth muscle fibers are found as components of blood vessels and lymphatics, around the bronchi and bronchioles, and scattered throughout the lung. In the developing fetus, muscle fibers are found in airway walls only in the last few weeks of gestation. Immature smooth muscle cells appear in the pulmonary arteries by the 12th week of gestation and gradually mature during the next 12 weeks.[10] In the lungs of newborns, smooth muscle cells extend into the terminal bronchioles and the free edges of septa. These septa form the entrance to the saccular structure and are thin and poorly developed. Apparently only in children over 3 years of age is there a significant increase in the muscle. In the mature bronchioles, the ratio of muscle to wall thickness is usually 1:3. There reportedly is no further increase in the ratio of smooth muscle mass to the bronchial wall thickness with increasing age. Lungs of children who die from obstructive respiratory diseases show an accelerated development of bronchiolar smooth muscle. Presumably, this muscular hypertrophy contributes to the airway obstruction.

CARTILAGE.—Cartilage begins to differentiate from the mesodermal tissues surrounding the developing tracheobronchial tree during the 4th week of gestation. As early as the 6th week, a network of fibrils identical to those of connective tissue is present. By the 7th week, rings of cartilage are visible in the trachea, and as development proceeds, a peripheral spread is observed. By the 11th week, cartilage is present in lobar bronchi. There is no burst of activity in the development of cartilage as is seen in bronchial development, and it is only after the 16th week that the number of airways with cartilage begins to approach the number in the mature lung. After the 24th week, the number of generations that contain cartilage remains constant; however, the cartilage continues to mature even after birth.

Cartilage is distributed along the developing bronchial tree in a uniform and predictable manner. In the adult lung, the cartilage in the trachea, mainstem bronchi, and lobar bronchi exists as rings and gives circumferential support to the airway. More peripherally, single plates of cartilage are seen in another four to six generations. In a pattern similar to that of glands, cartilage is most prominent in the regions of bifurcations of the bronchi, and the last visible cartilage plate is found at the bifurcation of bronchi about 1 mm in diameter. Airways proximal to the last cartilage are called *bronchi*, while those distal to it are called *bronchioles*.

TRACHEA.—The trachea (Fig 1–5) is a thin-walled, fairly rigid tube that in the adult is about 11 cm long and 2.0 to 2.5 cm in diameter. Its most charac-

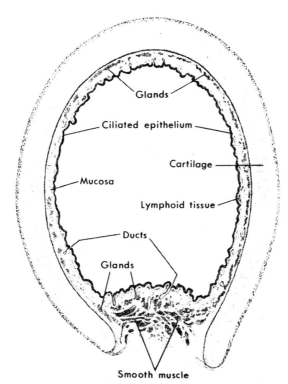

Fig 1–5.—Cross-section through the trachea. (From Bloom, W., and Fawcett, D.W.: *A Textbook of Histology* [Philadelphia: W.B. Saunders Co., 1975], p. 748.)

teristic feature is the framework of 16 to 20 cartilages that encircle the trachea, except in its posterior aspect, which is membranous and contains smooth muscle. The epithelium is of the ciliated pseudostratified columnar type and rests on a distinct basement membrane. Goblet cells are scattered throughout the epithelium, and there are elastic fibers and submucosal glands within its wall.

Development of Other Tissues

CONNECTIVE TISSUE.—Connective tissue—including collagen, elastic fibers and ground substance (the proteoglycans)—comprises approximately 25% of the mass of the adult human lung and is vital to the development, structure, and function of the lung.[5] The importance of the connective tissues is in the formation of a network that will become the supportive structure for the airways, vascular tree, and gas exchange units.

Collagen is a structurally important component of the tracheobronchial tree, vascular tree, parenchyma, and pleura. The elastic properties of the lungs have been attributed to the presence of these fibers in lung parenchyma, airways, and pleura.

Biochemical studies have demonstrated that elastin appears before the 14th week and that there is an increase in the elastin–amino acid ratio after the 36th week. This ratio is an indicator of elastin maturity and is the same in the full-term newborn as it is in the adult.

In patients with idiopathic respiratory distress syndrome, congenital pulmonary atelectasis, or neonatal pulmonary hemorrhage, the lung elastin—amino acid ratios are significantly lower than those found in normal newborns' lungs.[3, 18] This abnormal ratio may be a reflection of pulmonary immaturity or a predisposing factor in neonatal lung disease. Elastic tissue abnormalities have also been reported in persons with other pulmonary diseases such as adult emphysema.

All organ systems contain an amorphous, acellular, poorly described material termed *ground substance,* which is composed of electrolytes, proteins, glucose, urea, and other chemical constituents. This amorphous matrix generally occupies the extracellular space surrounding other connective tissue elements.

In the early fetal lung, collagen constitutes the principal connective tissue element and, at term, is the dominant connective tissue around the airways, in the blood vesels, and in the pleura and septa. The septal pattern in the fetus is similar to that in the adult lung. The exact role of the connective tissue septa remains to be determined, but it is generally accepted that they form a framework insuring even distribution of pressure within the lobes. The septa are irregularly distributed, so collateral ventilation occurs less effectively in some areas of lung than in others.

Elastic tissue is the predominant connective tissue in the respiratory portion of the lung. It is present around the primitive alveoli at 20 weeks, and by 26 weeks it is found at the opening of the alveolar saccules. The presence of elastic tissues at the opening of alveolar sacs may play a role in the distribution of ventilation postnatally.

A change in the relationship of the relative amounts of collagen and elastic tissue during postnatal growth has been observed. From childhood to adult life there appears to be no change in the amount of collagen tissue, but the amount of elastic tissue increases significantly. By age 18 years, elastic fibers surround the mouths of alveoli and branch extensively throughout the alveolar walls.

An interesting theory of lung development suggests that elastic tissue fibers in the respiratory portion of the lung exert a constant inward force and act as a fishnet through which the alveolar structures develop. If elastic tissue is important in the development of the respiratory portions of the lung, interference with its formation could affect profoundly the eventual number and size of alveoli. Inflammation involving the pulmonary connective tissues early in life might also adversely affect subsequent lung development.

LYMPHATICS.—The formation and function of the lymphatics in the fetal and newborn lung have received relatively little attention. Lymph channels appear during the 20th week of gestation, are well developed by the newborn period, and are easily demonstrated in inflated lungs along with groups of cellular elements scattered throughout the lungs. The lymphatic channels assist in the clearance of amniotic fluid from the lung. They also serve to regulate the amount of interstitial fluid and serve as a modulator of pulmonary vascular volume.

NEUROEPITHELIAL BODIES.—Recent studies have shown specialized areas of epithelium scattered throughout the intrapulmonary bronchi, bronchioles, and alveoli.[9] These structures, termed *neuroepithelial bodies,* are found in fetal, infant, and adult lungs. They contain afferent and efferent nerve endings and are closely related to capillary structures.

The neuroepithelial bodies probably possess various secretory functions, modulating not only vasomotor functions, but also other bronchial and bronchiolar functions such as mucous secretion, smooth muscle tone, and integration of the activities of the pulmonary unit lobules. Their function as secretory chemoreceptors in the fetal lung may partially explain the active pulmonary vasoconstriction seen during fetal life, the rapid vasodilation upon aeration, and even the pulmonary hypoperfusion during the idiopathic respiratory distress syndrome. They have also been implicated in the pathogenesis of both bronchial asthma and pulmonary edema induced by the central nervous system. Since they share several ultrastructural features with oat-cell carcinomas and bronchial carcinoids, it is possible that they too could secrete bradykinin or allied substances. By virtue of their position and structure, the neuroepithelial bodies may serve stretch and/or tactile neuroreceptor functions as well.

It may be that the serotonin secreted by the neuroepithelial bodies during hypoxia contributes to a vasoconstrictor response resulting in blood being shunted from the poor to the better oxygenated and ventilated portions of the lung, providing an intrapulmonary chemoreceptor system that finely modulates ventilation–perfusion ($\dot{V}/\dot{Q}$) ratios. The fetal age at which these bodies first appear is not clear, and further study is needed to define their full functional significance.

THE GAS EXCHANGE UNIT

Previous sections of this chapter have described the anatomic and functional development of the respiratory system as it prepares to act as the organ of gas exchange. Gas exchange is composed of three interrelated functions: ventilation of the respiratory tissues, diffusion of gas, and adequate perfusion of the pulmonary capillaries. The integrated functioning of all these components is essential to the maintenance of extrauterine life. For the purposes of this chapter, the gas exchange unit is composed of respiratory bronchioles, alveolar ducts, alveolar saccules, and alveoli together with the tissues that form their boundaries and the pulmonary capillaries (Fig 1–6). A discussion of the development of the gas exchange unit must encompass both the pre- and postnatal periods since this development continues into mid-childhood.

In the canalicular phase of pulmonary development, a thinning of the epithelium at the distal ends of the conducting airways is observed at 20 weeks. Capillaries are present, but the number actually in contact with potential air spaces is minimal. By 22 weeks, evagination of the thinner areas of epithelium is observed, and capillary buds are found in more intimate contact with the epithelium.

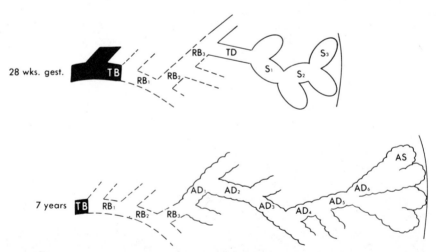

Fig 1–6.—Diagrammatic representation of the acinus at 28 weeks gestation and at 7 years. At each age, airway generations are drawn the same length so that an increase in length represents an increase in generations. See text for discussion. Abbreviations: *TB*, terminal bronchiole; *RB*, respiratory bronchiole; *TD*, transitional duct; *S*, saccule; *AD*, alveolar duct; *AS*, alveolar sac. (From Meyrick, B., and Reid, L.: The alveolar wall, Br. J. Dis. Chest 64:121, 1970.)

At 24 weeks, capillary invasion is more advanced, and cellular differentiation into Type I and Type II alveolar cells is noted. However, the air spaces are poorly developed, and the potential air–blood interface is not well defined. In the 26th week, the onset of the terminal saccule phase is characterized by further development of the alveolar saccules, development of the intersaccular septa, and marked proliferation of the pulmonary capillary bed. This capillary bed gradually becomes contiguous with the developing pulmonary arterioles.

By 28 weeks, alveolar saccules are still lined with a cuboidal epithelium, but alveolar ducts and respiratory bronchioles are distinguishable. Capillaries are numerous, and the functional differentiation of Type II alveolar cells is occurring with proliferation of lamellar bodies. These bodies are believed to be the location of synthesis of the pulmonary surfactant.

At 30 weeks, partial alveolarization has occurred with thinning of the saccular epithelium. The intersaccular septa, with prominent elastic tissue fibers, are now identifiable. At 34 weeks, the potential gas exchange unit is well developed with respiratory bronchioles, alveolar ducts, and the primitive saccular structures. Capillary invasion is pronounced, and the Type I alveolar cells are developed as thin lining cells. The thin walls of these cells will facilitate diffusion of gas from the alveoli to the capillary spaces. The metabolically active Type II cells are seen in the septa and at the mouths of the saccular structures.

Toward the end of full-term gestation, the intersaccular septa bear numerous shallow, saucer-shaped depressions, which are the "alveoli" of the newborn lung. At birth, the respiratory unit of the lung consists of three orders of respiratory bronchioles, a generation of transitional (alveolar) ducts, and terminal clusters of alveolar saccules and primitive alveoli. The alveoli in newborns are smaller and less deep than those observed in infants at 37 days and 2 months of age, suggesting that development continues in extrauterine life. Thinning of the intersaccular septa occurs as intrauterine maturation progresses, but these septa are obviously broader in infants at term than the typical interalveolar septa seen in the mature lung.

Type I cells are characterized by a small perinuclear body with cytoplasmic extensions lining a relatively large part of the alveolar surface. Type II alveolar cells are larger and rounded, without extensions, and contain lamellar inclusion structures termed *osmiophilic bodies* by most observers. These inclusions, which are characteristic of Type II alveolar cells, are comparable in fetal, neonatal, and adult lungs. The "alveolar" portion of the fetal lung is characterized by thick interalveolar septa, relatively few capillaries in contact with fluid spaces, many Type II alveolar epithelial cells, and fewer Type I cells. Type I cells are more numerous in respiratory bronchioles and alveolar ducts. In the lungs of neonates dying from nonpulmonary causes, this portion of the lung is different in that the septa are thin and there are relatively few Type II cells and a greatly increased blood–air barrier. In late fetal life, the number of alveolus-like structures is reported to increase to 42 alveoli per terminal lung unit at 32 weeks and to 340 alveoli per terminal lung unit at 40 weeks (Table 1–1).

At birth, about 24 million of these primitive alveoli are present. The acinus

TABLE 1–1.—ALVEOLAR COUNTS AT
VARIOUS STAGES OF DEVELOPMENT*

AGE GROUP	ESTIMATED NUMBER OF ALVEOLI PER TERMINAL LUNG UNIT
Gestational period	
24–27 weeks	42
32–35 weeks	130
Birth (40 weeks)	340
1 year	1,370
2–3 years	1,556
4–5 years	1,715
7–8 years	2,200
9–10 years	2,630
11–12 years	3,200

*From Emery, J.L., and Mithal, A.: The number of alveoli in the terminal respiratory unit of man during late intrauterine life and childhood, Arch. Dis. Child. 35:544, 1960.

or gas exchanging portion includes three orders of respiratory bronchioles, a generation of transitional (alveolar) ducts, and terminal clusters of alveolar sacs with relatively few narrow and shallow alveoli, as shown in Figure 1–6. The alveolar structures become larger and more numerous in the 37-day-old and 2-month-old infant lungs, suggesting that their development continues in the early postnatal period.

A section through a respiratory bronchiole and the alveolar ducts of an adult is shown in Figure 1–7. Use of the scanning electron microscope permits a different visualization of the peripheral airways and surrounding alveoli (Fig 1–8).

LUNG FLUID AND THE SURFACTANT SYSTEM

The fetal lung is a metabolically active organ secreting fluid that reaches the amniotic fluid. This is demonstrated indirectly by the fact that if the trachea of a fetal animal is ligated, distention of the lung occurs. In comparison with amniotic fluid, the fluid from the lungs is more acidic (pH 6.4 compared to 7.07) and differs in total osmolality and in protein, urea, and bicarbonate concentrations. Sodium and potassium concentrations are similar for lung fluid, fetal plasma, and lymph fluid; however, there are higher concentrations of hydrogen and chloride ions and less bicarbonate ion in lung fluid. These differences cannot be explained by simple membrane difffusion and indicate that the lung actively secretes its fluid.

Although the origin of the fluid is obscure, its presence and significance cannot be denied. In assessing the lungs of stillborn babies and neonates, it must be remembered that, in its intrauterine state, the lung contains an estimated 10 to 20 ml of fluid per kilogram in mature fetal lambs, which is ap-

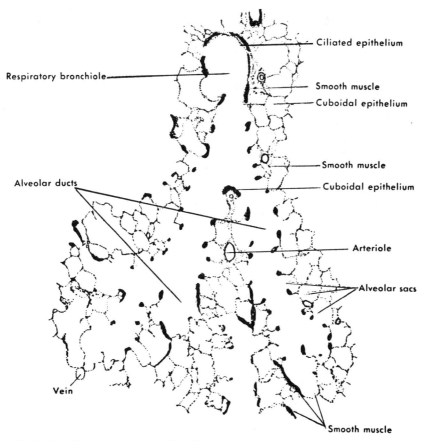

Fig 1–7.—Drawing of a section through a respiratory bronchiole and two alveolar ducts of adult human lung. Note the smooth muscle in the walls of the alveolar ducts. (From Bloom, W., and Fawcett, D.W.: *A Textbook of Histology* [Philadelphia: W.B. Saunders Co., 1975], p. 748.)

proximately equal to the functional residual capacity. Therefore, the aeration of the lung with the first breaths is not the inflation of a collapsed empty organ but the rapid replacement of intra-airway and alveolar fluid by air. It is felt now that collapsed areas in the postnatal lung should be considered pathologic rather than simply unexpanded.

While the origin of the tracheal fluid remains unknown, there seems to be little doubt regarding the origin of the surface-active material (surfactant) found in both the lung and amniotic fluids. Concomitant with the appearance of surfactant in the fetal lung, an increase in the osmiophilic bodies in Type II alveolar cells has been observed. Surfactant lines the alveolar walls and serves to maintain the stability of the alveolar structures by lowering surface tension. The formation, composition, and clinical importance of surfactant have been reported.[4, 7, 16]

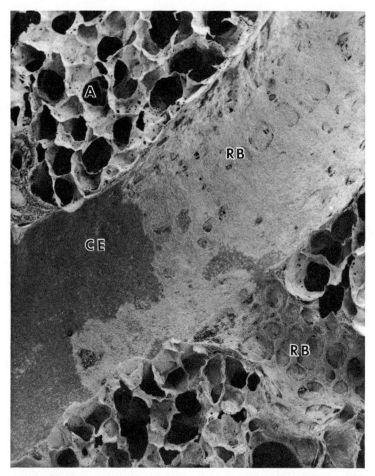

Fig 1–8.—Electron microscope view of a terminal bronchiole, respiratory bronchioles **(RB)**, and alveoli **(A)** from a young adult monkey. The bronchiole leads to the respiratory bronchioles and then to the alveolar ducts and alveoli. *CE* = ciliated epithelium. 13 mm = 100 μm. (Courtesy of the California Primate Research Center, M.E. Brummer and L.W. Schwartz.)

Surfactant consists of lipids—mainly lecithin—along with proteins and carbohydrates. It first appears in the 22nd to 24th weeks, corresponding to the time at which the methyltransferase enzyme system becomes active. This system produces lecithin and makes extrauterine life possible; however, this enzyme system is most adversely affected by acidosis, hypothermia, and hypoxia. In the 35th week, a second, more important, lecithin-producing enzyme system appears. The maturation of this system, the phosphocholine transferase system, parallels late fetal development of the respiratory portion of the lungs.

The significance of concentrations of various components of surfactant in amniotic fluid has been reported.[4] Use of starch-gel electrophoresis to analyze for lecithin and sphingomyelin has provided a means for estimating pulmonary maturity. A changing ratio of lecithin to sphingomyelin (L/S ratio) has been observed beyond the 35th week. When the ratio reaches 2:1, pulmonary maturity is felt to be sufficient to sustain extrauterine life. The test is reported to be significant in the management of complicated pregnancies in high-risk mothers.

The rate of phospholipid synthesis, which reaches a maximum at term or shortly after birth, has been shown in animal lungs to decline rapidly thereafter to the levels observed in the adult lung. Administration of adrenal corticosteroids has accelerated pulmonary maturity in fetal rabbits, and decreased respiratory distress has been noted in steroid-treated, premature rabbits. Prematurely born human infants whose mothers received steroids prenatally have lower incidence of respiratory distress than do infants whose mothers had not received this treatment. These experimental biomedical and physiologic studies suggest that this effect may be due to acceleration of the surfactant-producing enzyme systems.

With an L/S ratio of 1:1, the risk of development of hyaline membrane disease is greater than 90%. However, when the L/S ratio is greater than 2:1, the risk of hyaline membrane disease becomes less than 5%. With an L/S ratio of 1.5:1 (called a *transitional* L/S ratio), the risk of hyaline membrane disease is approximately 50%. The factors associated with fetal lung maturation are shown in Table 1–2.

TABLE 1–2.—FACTORS ASSOCIATED WITH FETAL
LUNG MATURATION

Accelerated maturation
    1. Maternal hypertensive syndromes
       a. Renal
       b. Cardiovascular
       c. Severe "chronic" toxemia
    2. Hemoglobinopathy—sickle C disease
    3. Narcotic addiction (heroin, morphine)
    4. Infection
       a. Chorioamnionitis
       b. Viral
    5. Placental conditions
       a. Smaller parabiotic twin
       b. Circumvallate placenta
       c. Chronic abruptio placentae
       d. Placental infarction (placental insufficiency)
       e. Prolonged rupture of membranes
    6. Corticosteroids
Delayed maturation
    1. Maternal diabetes mellitus
    2. Hydrops fetalis

BIRTH AND THE ONSET OF RESPIRATION

At birth the newborn infant enters an uncontrolled environment and must initiate respiration, readjust the circulation, maintain body temperature, and adjust the acid-base balance. These functions must be performed rapidly, for failure in any one system will have a profound influence on the others. The initiation of respiration must precede all of these functions and perhaps consumes the most energy of the perinatal changes. Initial respiratory forces are directed toward removing the lung fluid, overcoming the surface tension encountered in the respiratory portions of the lung, and reshaping the nonrespiratory pulmonary tissues.

The lungs and pulmonary circulation develop both morphologically and biochemically in utero in preparation for birth and the onset of their major role of gas exchange. In order for the lungs to assume this function, there has to be a rapid transformation from a fluid-filled to an air-filled lung with end-expiratory stability at birth.[11] The processes pertinent to this transformation include the type of delivery, the establishment of an effective pulmonary circulation, the initiation and maintenance of the mechanisms of breathing, and pulmonary gas exchange.

Birth normally occurs with a vertex presentation through the vagina. During passage of the fetus through the birth canal, the fetal chest is compressed by the cervix and a quantity of pulmonary fluid is forced out through the fetal mouth. After the chest passes through the cervix, the elastic chest wall of the fetus regains its expanded shape, a relative intrapulmonary vacuum develops, air is drawn into the lungs and the beginning of the pulmonary gas volume is rapidly established.

In the newborn infant, pulmonary fluid volume and initial functional residual capacity are comparable, ranging between 25 and 35 ml/kg body weight. It is estimated that 10 to 15% of the pulmonary fluid is removed by cervical chest compression. The remainder is removed from the lung by the pulmonary circulation and the pulmonary lymphatic circulation during the first few days of life. This clearance of lung fluid is facilitated by the Valsalva effect and the relatively low oncotic pressure of lung fluid. There is a relationship between the onset of ventilation, the decrease in alveolar fluid, and the steady increase in lymphatic flow.[12]

If the baby is delivered breech or by a casarean section, the expulsion of fluid caused by cervical chest compression does not occur, and there is more fluid to be removed via the pulmonary lymphatics and circulation. Many reports have shown that there is an increased incidence of respiratory distress in these infants, presumably because of slower and less effective transformation from a fluid-filled to an air-filled lung.

The First Breath

The first breath of extrauterine life is the result of respiratory muscle contraction. Chest wall recoil after escape from the vagina is not a factor in the first breath.[11] There is variation in the volume of the first breath, ranging between 15 and 80 ml in a full-term infant, a volume between tidal volume and crying vital capacity. The negative intrathoracic pressure during the first breath ranges between -30 and -90 cm H_2O pressure to overcome all of the opposing forces and to establish a gas–liquid interface. The inspiratory pressure rapidly decreases to less than -20 cm H_2O within a few breaths. Although surfactant is present prenatally, it does not lower surface tension until the air–liquid interface is established. Increases in compliance and changes in airway resistance, residual volume, and functional residual capacity continue over a period of days. Expiratory tidal volume is less than inspiratory volume during the first few breaths while the residual volume is being established.

Multiple stimuli have been implicated as being important to the initiation and maintenance of sustained respiration, including the sensory stimuli associated with delivery, the change in temperature from the intrauterine to extrauterine environment, the change from dark to light environment, and the change from suspension in amniotic fluid. In both animal and human studies, it has been shown that there are rhythmic intrauterine breathing movements from as early as 10 to 12 weeks of gestation.[1, 11] It is suggested that the fetal intrauterine breathing movements strengthen the muscles of respiration and prepare the fetus for extrauterine respiration.

Vascular Changes

Coincident with the filling of the lungs with air, the newborn PaO_2 increases dramatically and there is a rapid, marked decrease in pulmonary vascular resistance and a rapid increase in pulmonary blood flow. The increase in pulmonary blood flow along with the establishment of effective ventilation permits the lung to begin its major function as the organ of extrauterine gas exchange.

In utero studies of pulmonary vascular physiology have shown a gradual and sustained increase in pulmonary vascular resistance during gestation, presumably due to a gradual increase in the mass of the pulmonary arteriolar smooth muscle as well as muscle spasm resulting from the relative hypoxemia of intrauterine life. After birth, the increase in PaO_2 following the first breaths alleviates hypoxic stimulation to spasm of the pulmonary arteriolar smooth muscle and a rapid 65 to 75% decrease in pulmonary vascular resistance. The remaining decrease of pulmonary vascular resistance to adult levels normally occurs during the 4 to 6 weeks following delivery, paralleling an active involution of the pulmonary arteriolar smooth muscle.

During intrauterine life, gas exchange between the fetus and mother occurs across the placenta. There is a capillary interface separating the maternal and fetal placental circulations. Under normal physiologic conditions, there is essentially no mixing of these two circulations. The maternal placental arterial system has a PO_2 of 90 to 100 mm Hg at sea level. Oxygen diffuses to the fetal placental circulation, which has a lower PO_2 so that the O_2 gradient favors diffusion of oxygen from the mother to the fetus. The relatively higher PCO_2

of fetal placental arterial blood creates a CO_2 diffusion gradient into the maternal placental circulation, and the fetal placental venous P_{CO_2} is slightly higher than that of the mother.

BIRTH

A schematic diagram of the fetal circulation is shown in Figure 1–9. Placental venous blood returning from the fetal placental circulation to the inferior vena cava via the umbilical vein and ductus venosus has the highest P_{O_2} in the fetus (average 32 to 33 mm Hg). This blood mixes with systemic venous blood returning to the heart from the lower body of the fetus via the inferior vena cava, producing a slight decrease in the P_{O_2} of the placental venous blood. This mixture of blood then enters the right atrium. Systemic venous blood from the upper half of the fetus returns to the right atrium via the superior vena cava. The flow characteristics of the right atrium are such that most of the least oxygenated blood returning to the right atrium from the superior vena cava is preferentially directed across the tricuspid valve into the right ventricle. At the same time, the most oxygenated blood, returning to the right atrium from the

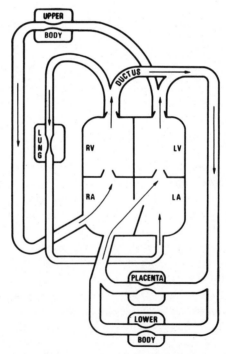

Fig 1–9.—Schematic diagram of the fetal circulation. The foramen ovale is between the right and left atria. **RV,** right ventricle; **LV,** left ventricle; **RA,** right atrium; **LA,** left atrium.

inferior vena cava, is preferentially directed through an opening in the atrial wall (the foramen ovale) and into the left atrium.

The blood that enters the right ventricle is then ejected into the main pulmonary artery, from which there are two possible exits. About 20% of this blood goes to the lungs, and 80% goes through the large ductus arteriosus, which has about the same caliber and resistance as does the aorta. As noted earlier, the intrauterine pulmonary vascular resistance is very high, probably primarily due to the relatively low Po_2 of the pulmonary arterial blood and vasoconstriction of the muscular pulmonary arterioles. These so-called resistance vessels of the lung produce most of the pulmonary vascular resistance present in utero. The very large patent ductus arteriosus offers less vascular resistance than the pulmonary vascular bed because the ductus connects to the aorta and the lower-resistance placental circulation. This vascular arrangement produces a fetal systemic vascular resistance lower than fetal pulmonary vascular resistance, thereby favoring a right-to-left shunt of blood across the ductus arteriosus.

Blood from the left atrium enters the left ventricle and is then ejected into the ascending aorta. The three vessels coming off the aortic arch of the ascending aorta before the ductus arteriosus supply the most oxygenated blood to the head, brain, and upper extremities of the fetus. The rest of the blood ejected from the left ventricle mixes with blood being shunted right to left across the ductus arteriosus, thereby providing a slightly lower Po_2 to the fetal structures below the ductus arteriosus. A portion of the descending aorta blood flow reenters the placental circulation to be reoxygenated.

Following delivery, the umbilical cord is clamped, and the placental circulation is excluded from the baby's circulation. This causes the systemic vascular resistance to rise. At the same time, with the marked decrease in pulmonary vascular resistance following the onset of ventilation, there is a reversal of the ratio of systemic-to-pulmonary vascular resistance that reverses the direction of ductal blood flow, another factor that serves to increase the pulmonary blood flow. The increase in arterial Po_2 also stimulates the ductus arteriosus to constrict, and it normally becomes progressively restricted with an increased intrinsic resistance. With the higher pressure and resistance in the aorta as compared to those in the pulmonary artery, the left atrial pressure becomes greater than the right atrial pressure and serves to functionally close the foramen ovale. These changes that occur shortly after birth are called *transitional changes,* and the circulation during this time is called the *transitional circulation* (Fig 1–10).

Within the first 12 hours after birth of the full-term neonate, the ductus arteriosus normally closes, and there is no longer a left-to-right shunt at the ductal level. After 72 hours of extrauterine life, the ductus arteriosus is permanently closed. The foramen ovale is also functionally closed, and an adult-type circulatory pattern is established (Fig 1–11).

In prematurely born neonates and in neonates born at high altitude, constriction of the ductus after birth is less complete, and persistent patency of the ductus arteriosus is frequently seen. In premature newborns, the failure of com-

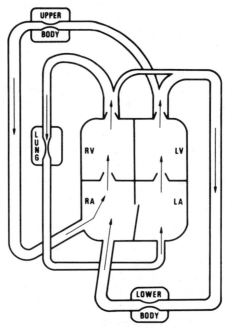

Fig 1–10.—The transitional circulation. There is an increase in left atrial pressure acting to close the foramen ovale, and the ductus arteriosus begins to close. The abbreviations are the same as in Figure 1–9.

plete constriction of the ductus is felt to be the result of less constrictor smooth muscle in the ductus walls. Persistent patency of the ductus after birth in premature infants has been implicated in the pathogenesis of bronchopulmonary dysplasia, a chronic pulmonary disease of premature newborns.

POSTNATAL DEVELOPMENT

The changes observed in postnatal pulmonary maturation are immense and must occur by various mechanisms. The saccular structure of the newborn lung must develop into the alveolar structures of the mature lung. The number of alveoli increases approximately tenfold, and the air-tissue interface increases to a magnitude 21 times that which exists in the newborn (Table 1–3). The interalveolar septa and alveolar walls undergo changes in morphology and relative size along with an increase in the lateral chest wall dimension. An integration of these processes results in the mature respiratory system. Pathologic derangement of any process may produce altered ventilatory or diffusion functions of the lung.

The respiratory system of the newborn infant, although developed sufficiently to support extrauterine respiration, soon would become inadequate if rapid postnatal growth and development did not occur. The lungs of an infant born prematurely after 28 weeks gestation who died of nonpulmonary causes

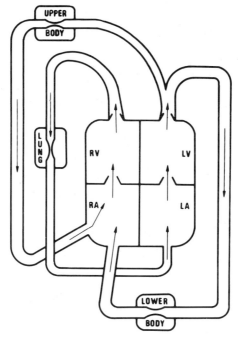

Fig 1–11.—The adult-type circulation.

after 6 days of life were noted to have the microscopic appearance of normal full-term newborn lungs. This observation suggests that the prematurely born infant who does not develop the respiratory distress syndrome may undergo accelerated pulmonary maturation.

At birth, the infant chest is cylindrical, with the anteroposterior diameter equal to or slightly greater than the transverse diameter. Following birth, there is more rapid growth of the transverse diameter. By about 3½ years of age,

TABLE 1–3.—EFFECT OF AGE ON LUNG SIZE*

	ALVEOLI ($\times 10^6$)	RESPIRATORY AIRWAYS ($\times 10^6$)	AIR-TISSUE INTERFACE (sq m)	BODY SURFACE AREA (sq m)
Birth	24	1.5	2.8	0.21
3 months	77	2.5	7.2	0.29
13 months	129	4.5	12.2	0.45
22 months	160	7.1	14.2	0.50
4 years	257	7.9	22.2	0.67
8 years	280	14.0	32.0	0.92
Adult	296	14.0	75.0	1.90
Approximate increase, birth to adult	10-fold	10-fold	27-fold	9-fold

*From Dunnill, M.S.: Postnatal growth of the lung, Thorax 17:329, 1962.

the adult chest wall configuration is attained, with the transverse greater than the anteroposterior diameter.

Chest wall growth reflects the underlying lung development. The conducting airways, while not adding new generations, grow by an increase in diameter and length. Tracheal and conducting airway diameters increase some threefold throughout the course of postnatal development into adulthood. Through the first 12 months of life, lung volume increases fourfold, and estimates have varied between 12-fold and 25-fold increases by 12 years. The greatest amount of change in volume and surface area during this time is accounted for by an increase in both size and number of the respiratory airways and alveolar structures (Table 1–3).

Postnatal development of the respiratory portion of the lung is evident in infants as early as the first 2 months of life. At birth, the respiratory portion of the infant lung consists of three generations of respiratory bronchioles and one order of alveolar ducts with alveolar sacs. Approximately 24 million rudimentary alveoli are present, but they are shallow and have an average diameter of only 50 μm. At 2 months, there are at least four orders of respiratory bronchioles and three orders of alveolar ducts. The alveolar sacs and alveoli range in diameter from 50 to 120 μm.

Opinion differs about the age at which the formation of new alveoli ceases. Increase in alveolar number has been felt by some to stop by the age of 8 years or even by 5 years. However, a study of the terminal respiratory units in fetal lungs and lungs of children up to the age of 12 years (see Table 1–1) showed some increase in alveolar numbers throughout this age span. Alveolar diameter has been found to increase most rapidly after the formation of new alveoli is almost complete. In older children, the range of alveolar diameter is 100 to 200 μm, while in the adult lung the range is 200 to 300 μm. The alveolar number in adults has been estimated to vary from 300 million to 600 million, depending on body size.

The histology of the respiratory portion of the adult lung differs in many ways from that of infants. Not only are alveolar architecture, alveolar walls, and respiratory airways different, but in the infant lung there is less provision for collateral alveolar ventilation through the pores of Kohn, since these pores apparently first appear in children after 1 to 2 years of age and subsequently increase in size and number. The bronchiolar–alveolar communications known as *canals of Lambert* have been observed in infants, but most of their development appears to come in children beyond 6 to 8 years of age.

Lung weight increases from approximately 60 gm at birth to 10 times this, or more. The lung differs from other organs in that its total volume increases more than its tissue mass, and thus it contains progressively more air per gram of tissue. The alterations in anatomy result in changes in pulmonary function.[2] For example, at birth and fully inflated, the lungs contain approximately 3 ml air per gram of tissue, whereas by 6 years of age they contain 8 ml air per gram of tissue.[17] The compliance of the lung also changes with lung growth. However, specific compliance, which is compliance per unit of lung volume,

TABLE 1–4.—More Common Congenital Anomalies of the Respiratory System*

ANOMALY	ORIGIN OF DEFECT	FIRST APPEARANCE	SEX CHIEFLY AFFECTED	RELATIVE FREQUENCY	REMARKS
Esophageal atresia, stenosis and tracheoesophageal fistula	Between 21 and 34 days	At birth	Equal	Common	
Posterolateral defects of the diaphragm (Bochdalek)	8th to 10th week	At birth or later	Equal	Common	Ipsilateral lung is hypoplastic
Congenital cysts of the respiratory tract:					
Bronchogenic cysts	6th to 7th week	Infancy, if at all	Equal	Uncommon	Compression of trachea may be fatal
Pulmonary cysts	24th week	Infancy and childhood	Male	Uncommon	Eventually fatal if untreated
Intralobar sequestration of the lung	8th weeks or later	At any period of life	Equal	Uncommon	Anomalous arterial supply usual
Extralobar sequestration of the lung (accessory lung)	6th week or later	At any period of life	Equal	Uncommon	Predominantly left-sided
Congenital tracheal stenosis	3d to 4th week	At birth	?	Rare	Usually fatal soon after birth
Tracheobronchomegaly	5th month (?)	Late childhood or later	?	Rare	
Atresia of the larynx	8th to 10th weeks	At birth	Equal	Uncommon	Fatal unless tracheostomy is performed at once
Laryngeal webs	10th week (?)	At birth, if large; asymptomatic, if small	Equal	Uncommon	
Tracheal atresia	3d to 4th week	At birth	Male	Very rare	Fatal at birth

*Adapted from Gray, S.W., and Skandalakis, J.E.: The Embryological Basis of Treatment of Congenital Defects (Philadelphia: W.B. Saunders Co., 1972).

is about 0.06 liter/cm H_2O/liter for all ages and lung sizes in normal individuals. The changes in pulmonary function with age are discussed in Chapter 9.

CONGENITAL ANOMALIES OF THE RESPIRATORY SYSTEM

Knowledge of the events of embryologic and postnatal development of the respiratory system provides an understanding of the etiology and clinical implications of congenital anomalies.[14] Infants with respiratory distress may have a congenital anomaly as the etiology of their symptoms. However, some anomalies may not be manifest until later in life. A clinical review of all congenital anomalies is available.[8] Table 1–4 presents the important features of these anomalies.

Tracheoesophageal anomalies present with the clinical features of excess salivation, respiratory distress, and the radiologic features of aspiration pneumonia. Atelectasis may be present, more commonly in the right upper lobe. Seventy-five percent of these anomalies are characterized by esophageal atresia with tracheoesophageal fistulas. Symptoms most commonly appear with the first feeding or during the first day of life. Immediate surgery is indicated, and the postoperative recovery period may be prolonged.

Diaphragmatic hernia may also present with symptoms during the first postnatal day. Because of its severe life-threatening nature when symptomatic, this anomaly must be corrected immediately. Most hernias occur into the left hemithorax through a posterior defect in the diaphragm (foramen of Bochdalek). The period following surgery is complicated by the fact that pulmonary development in the ipsilateral lung is retarded, with decreased numbers of bronchial and bronchiolar generations, decreased development of respiratory saccules, and concurrent delay in development of pulmonary arteriolar structure. The underdeveloped lung does mature following surgery, but pulmonary complications are encountered throughout early life. Congenital eventration of the diaphragm results from abnormal development of the diaphragm.

Pulmonary agenesis and tracheal stenosis result from maldevelopment of the lung buds in their early phases. Tracheal atresia and bilateral pulmonary agenesis are incompatible with life and cannot be corrected adequately.

Congenital pulmonary cyst are caused by the isolation of respiratory tissue from the rest of the lung at various stages of development. They may consist of purely alveolar or bronchial tissue or may contain a combination of tissues. Congenital lobar emphysema and congenital cystic adenomatoid malformation of the lung may stem from disordered embryonic development.

REFERENCES

1. Avery, M.E., Fletcher, B.D., and Williams, R.G.: *The Lung and Its Disorders in the Newborn Infant* (4th ed.; Philadelphia: W.B. Saunders Co., 1981).
2. Doershuk, C.F., Fisher, B.J., and Matthews, L.W.: Pulmonary physiology of the young child, in Scarpelli, E.M. (ed.): *Pulmonary Physiology of the Fetus, Infant and Child* (Philadelphia: Lea & Febiger, 1975).
3. Evans, H.E , Keeler, S., and Mandel, I.: Lung tissue elastin composition in new-

born infants with the respiratory distress syndrome and other diseases, J. Clin. Invest. 54:213, 1974.

4. Gluck, L., et al.: Diagnosis of the respiratory distress syndrome by amniocentesis, Am. J. Obstet. Gynecol. 109:440, 1971.
5. Hance, A.J., and Crystal, R.G.: The connective tissues of the lung—State of the art, Am. Rev. Respir. Dis. 112:657, 1975.
6. Inselman, L.S., and Mellins, R.B.: Growth and development of the lung, J. Pediatr. 98:1, 1981.
7. Kotas, R.V.: Estimate of pulmonary maturity, J. Pediatr. 81:378, 1972.
8. Landing, B.H.: Congenital malformations and genetic disorders of the respiratory tract. Am. Rev. Respir. Dis. 120:151, 1979.
9. Lauweryns, J.M., and Deuskens, J.C.: Neuroepithelial bodies in human infant bronchial and bronchiolar epithelium, Anat. Rec. 172:471, 1972.
10. Loosli, C.G., and Hung, K.S.: Development of pulmonary innervation, in Hodson, W.A. (ed.): *Development of the Lung, Volume 6: Lung Biology in Health and Disease* (New York: Marcel Dekker, Inc., 1977).
11. Milner, A.D., and Vyas, H.: Lung expansion at birth, J. Pediatr. 101:879, 1982.
12. Norman, I.C.S., et al.: Passage of macromolecules between alveolar and interstitial spaces in foetal and newly ventilated lungs of the lamb, J. Physiol. 210:151, 1970.
13. Polgar, G., and Weng, T.R.: The functional development of the respiratory system, Am. Rev. Respir. Dis., 120:625, 1979.
14. Reid, L.: The lung: Its growth and remodeling in health and disease, Am. J. Roentgenol. 129:777, 1977.
15. Reid, L.: Measurement of the bronchial mucous gland layer; a diagnostic yardstick in chronic bronchitis, Thorax 15:132, 1960.
16. Stahlman, M.T.: Structure and function in lung maturation, in Moore, Tom D. (ed.): *Lung Maturation and the Prevention of Hyaline Membrane Disease,* report of the seventieth Ross Conference on Pediatric Research, Columbus, Ohio 1976.
17. Thurlbeck, W.M.: Postnatal growth and development of the lung—State of the art, Am. Rev. Respir. Dis. 111:803, 1975.
18. Ville, C.A., Ville, D.B., and Zuckerman, J. (eds.): *Respiratory Distress Syndrome* (New York: Academic Press, 1973).

SUGGESTED READINGS

Farrell, P.M., and Avery, M.E.: State of the art—Hyaline membrane disease, Am. Rev. Respir. Dis. 111:657, 1975.

Hodson, W.A. (ed.): *Development of the Lung, Volume 6: Lung Biology in Health and Disease* (New York: Marcel Dekker, Inc., 1977).

Lung Maturation and the Prevention of Hyaline Membrane Disease, report of the seventieth Ross Conference on Pediatric Research, Ross Laboratories, Columbus, Ohio 1976.

Rudolph, A.M.: *Congenital Disease of the Heart* (Chicago: Year Book Medical Publishers, Inc., 1974).

Evaluation and Care of the Newborn Infant

WALDEMAR A. CARLO, M.D.
AVROY A. FANAROFF, M.B., F.R.C.P.E., D.C.H.
RICHARD J. MARTIN, M.B., F.R.C.P.(C)

2

Despite remarkable advances in neonatal care, respiratory diseases remain the most important cause of perinatal mortality. In recent years, chronic lung injury has evolved as a major cause of neonatal morbidity. The close interaction between the respiratory system and the various other organs necessitates that personnel administering respiratory care understand the many aspects of neonatal intensive care. This chapter reviews some of the present concepts of neonatal practice, especially as they relate to the respiratory system.

HIGH-RISK ANTICIPATION

Improved physiologic understanding and multiple technological advancements now provide the obstetrician with tools for objective evaluation of the in utero patient. In particular, specific information can now be sought and obtained relative to fetal growth (fetal ultrasound), well-being (estriols, fetal heart rate, fetal scalp pH), and functional maturity (lecithin:sphingomyelin ratio); these data are used to provide a rational approach to clinical management of the high-risk infant prior to birth. A substantial proportion of fetal malformations can now be specifically identified by antenatal ultrasound. Detailed reviews of the many new physical, hormonal, and biochemical approaches to prenatal and fetal assessment are available.

Many maternal, obstetric, or fetal factors alert the health care team to the birth of a high-risk infant (Table 2–1). In such a pregnancy, the fetus has a significantly increased chance of death, either before or after birth, or of later disability. Some fetuses may be damaged early, others late. Many infants will

28

TABLE 2–1.—ANTICIPATION OF HIGH-RISK INFANTS

Maternal Factors	Maternal age <16 yr or >40 yr
	Low socioeconomic status
	Poor nutrition
	Chronic disease
	hypertension
	diabetes mellitus
	cardiovascular
	pulmonary
	anemia
	renal
	Smoking, drug abuse, or alcoholism
	Underweight or overweight
	Hereditary anomalies
Obstetric Factors	Previous premature delivery or reproductive failures
	Previous or primary cesarean section
	Preeclampsia-eclampsia
	Gestational diabetes
	Pregnancy-induced hypertension
	Medications during pregnancy or labor
	Vaginal bleeding
	Premature onset of labor
	Prolonged rupture of membranes
	Prolonged gestation
	Prolonged or precipitous delivery
	Low urinary estriols
	Poly- or oligohydramnios
Fetal Factors	Prematurity
	Rh sensitization
	Congenital malformations
	Multiple pregnancy
	Abnormal pregnancy
	Abnormal presentation
	Intrauterine growth retardation
	Large for gestational age
	Congenital infection
	Cord accidents
	Immature L/S ratio
	Fetal heart rate abnormalities
	Fetal acidosis
	Birth trauma
	Meconium staining

be born prematurely or may be unusually small for their gestational age. A few will have grown too large or will have remained in utero too long. Each situation has its special hazards. Regardless of gestational age or birth weight, the extrauterine existence of the high-risk infant is compromised by a number of factors (prenatal, natal, or postnatal), and the baby is in need of special medical care.

It is most important to identify those infants at risk as soon as possible so that their problems may be anticipated and appropriate corrective measures taken. For example, in a pregnancy complicated by pre-eclamptic toxemia in which the mother develops hypertension, the fetus often grows poorly. It is less able to withstand the rigors of labor and hence more likely to be asphyxiated at birth. Therefore, preparations should be made in advance to resuscitate such infants promptly.

If due consideration is given to all of the factors mentioned in Table 2–1, it is possible to anticipate two thirds of the infants who will be distressed at delivery. Obviously, there are still a considerable number of infants who will be ill unexpectedly, and for this reason any hospital areas delivering infants should be maintained in a state of constant readiness.

ASPHYXIA AND RESUSCITATION

Only simple equipment is necessary for resuscitation. This should include a means for suctioning the infant, maintaining an airway, providing warmth and oxygen, and assisting the ventilation in a controlled manner, as well as being able to correct the attendant metabolic acidosis, if necessary.

Pathophysiology of Asphyxia

It should be noted that the fetus and newborn, compared to the adult, have a remarkable ability to withstand asphyxia or anoxia. This difference between the adult and the fetus or newborn depends on several physiologic factors. Our overall aim is survival without permanent impairment of any function, particularly that of the brain.

In order to establish a rational method of resuscitating an asphyxiated newborn, it is necessary to understand the pathophysiologic changes occurring with asphyxia. Since much of the information is obtained from animal experiments, caution must be exercised when applying these data to humans. Nevertheless, there appear to be close clinical analogies between the human infant and the rhesus monkey.

Initial experiments have revealed that the ability to withstand asphyxia decreases with increasing age from birth, and that animals asphyxiated by interruption of circulation survive for a shorter period of time than those merely deprived of oxygen. The early animal experiments also revealed that environmental temperature plays a significant role in the effects of asphyxia.

The physiologic effects of total asphyxia on the rhesus monkey fetus are considered in Figure 2–1. The effects on respiration, circulation, and blood gases were studied in monkeys following cesarean section delivery and immediate covering of the fetal head with a saline-filled rubber bag.

The initial effect of asphyxia is to produce a short period of rapid respiration followed by the onset of primary apnea that lasts about 1 minute and during which spontaneous respirations still can be induced by appropriate sensory

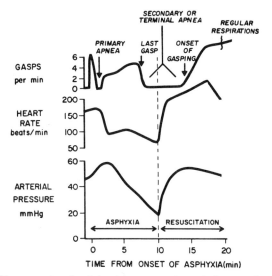

Fig 2–1.—Changes in physiologic parameters during asphyxia and resuscitation of the rhesus monkey fetus at birth. Rhesus monkeys were asphyxiated at birth by tying the umbilical cord while the head was in saline-filled rubber bag. Resuscitation was by positive-pressure ventilation. (From Fisher, D.E., and Paton, J.B.: Resuscitation of the newborn infant, in Klaus, M., and Fanaroff, A. [eds.]: *Care of the High-Risk Neonate* [2nd ed.; Philadelphia: W.B. Saunders Co., 1979].)

stimuli. During the period of primary apnea, the blood pressure is maintained or even slightly elevated, and the heart rate starts to fall but is often still faster than 100 beats per minute.

If the asphyxia is continued, the primary apnea is followed by a period of spontaneous, deep gasps occurring at a rate of 5 to 8 per minute, gradually becoming weaker over a period of 4 to 5 minutes, and terminating (the last gasp) after approximately 8 minutes of total anoxia. Secondary apnea then ensues, and if not reversed within minutes, death follows. During secondary apnea, the sensory stimuli mentioned above will not induce gasping or respiratory movements. Respiration can be initiated only by commencing some form of intermittent positive-pressure ventilation.

The recovery course from secondary apnea follows a definite sequence, with the onset of spontaneous gasping occurring before rhythmic respiration develops. The longer the delay in initiating adequate resuscitation measures (artificial ventilation) after the last gasp, the longer the time to the first gasp after resuscitation. For every 1-minute delay, the time to the first gasp is increased by about 2 minutes and the time to onset of rhythmic breathing delayed by an average of more than 4 minutes. The heart rate slows during the period of gasping; this is associated with a decrease in blood pressure and will cease during the period of secondary or terminal apnea. The skin becomes successively blue, blotchy, and then white in response to the circulatory failure that occurs with generalized peripheral vasoconstriction. It is thus apparent that the circulation also needs to be supported if the infant is in secondary apnea. Cardiac massage is often lifesaving.

During total asphyxia, pH progressively decreases, so that by the time secondary apnea has occurred, the pH is less than 7. Metabolic resuscitation with sodium bicarbonate is an important aspect of the resuscitation.

When confronted with an apneic newborn, it is difficult for the physician to determine quickly whether primary or secondary apnea is present. The latter must be assumed and resuscitative measures started at once. Retrospectively, on the basis of the infant's response, it may be possible to decide the degree of apnea at which resuscitation was started. If the color is restored before the onset of breathing, the infant is usually in secondary apnea. On the other hand, if gasping commences before or simultaneously with the onset of improvement in color, the infant has been in primary apnea. A number of infants in primary apnea will begin gasping while preparation is being made to start resuscitation with the initial handling, suctioning, or blowing of oxygen over the face. In primary apnea, the heart rate and blood pressure are maintained, and there is some muscle tone present. The vast majority of infants who require resuscitation will be in primary apnea.

Evaluation and Initial Resuscitation

The course of immediate management depends upon a critical evaluation of the severity of depression of the newborn infant. The Apgar score (Table 2–2) is most helpful in assessing the infant's condition. It is of paramount importance that the items comprising the Apgar score be checked in a systematic fashion at both 1 and 5 minutes, preferably by an independent observer rather than the person responsible for the resuscitation. If the Apgar score is between 7 and 10, very little resuscitation is required, unless the score drops suddenly several minutes after birth.

TABLE 2–2.—APGAR SCORING CHART

SIGN	0	1	2
Heart rate	Absent	Slow (below 100)	Over 100
Respiratory effort	Absent	Weak cry, hypoventilation	Good strong cry
Muscle tone	Limp	Some flexion of extremities	Well flexed
Reflex response Response to catheter in nostril or to other cutaneous stimulation	No response	Grimace	Cough, sneeze or cry
Color	Blue, pale	Body pink, extremities blue	Completely pink

An Apgar score between 4 and 6 indicates mild to moderate asphyxia. In this case, the airway should be suctioned gently, followed by the administration of oxygen. If there is not a prompt response, oxygen may be administered by positive pressure with mask and bag.

An Apgar score between 0 and 3 indicates prompt intervention as follows:

1. Clear the upper airway by a short period of gentle suction.
2. Establish adequate ventilation with oxygen by positive pressure, either with mask and bag or, preferably, with endotracheal tube. If there is no immediate response to mask and bag ventilation, an endotracheal tube should be passed and positive-pressure ventilation continued.
3. If bradycardia persists after ventilating the lungs a few times, closed chest cardiac massage should be commenced.
4. An umbilical venous catheter should be inserted and a 1 to 2 mEq/kg dose of sodium bicarbonate diluted with equal parts of sterile water administered over a 1-minute period (see below).
5. Heat loss should be minimized during resuscitation by keeping the infant warm and dry and the use of a radiant warmer. Try to maintain the skin temperature at around 36.5 C.

Every infant with meconium in the amniotic fluid or meconium staining requires the following:

1. Immediate suctioning of the nasopharynx by the obstetrician as soon as the head appears on the perineum.
2. Visualization of the cords by laryngoscopy immediately after delivery and direct suctioning of the trachea through an endotracheal tube. This is done prior to stimulation of the infant or positive-pressure ventilation.

During total asphyxia, dramatic changes in PCO_2 and HCO_3^- result in a combined respiratory and metabolic acidosis. Once adequate ventilation has been established, sodium bicarbonate may be required to treat the residual metabolic acidosis. Sodium bicarbonate should not be used in the treatment of a respiratory acidosis.

Infrequently, an infant may be depressed secondary to narcotic sedation of the mother, and improvement may occur after administration of a narcotic antagonist (naloxone hydrochloride 0.01 mg/kg given by umbilical or peripheral vein, intramuscularly, or subcutaneously). However, an airway should be established first and adequate ventilation initiated before this diagnosis is considered. Similarly, when hypovolemic shock is diagnosed, treatment with blood or a plasma expander may be required after clearing the airway and establishing good ventilation.

After successful resuscitation of the newborn infant, a feeding tube should be passed into the stomach and any secretions and/or air removed by gentle suction.

TABLE 2–3.—CHECKLIST OF MEDICATIONS AND EQUIPMENT
FOR NEONATAL RESUSCITATION

Radiant warmer
1 Laryngoscope handle with premature (Miller 0) and term infant (Miller 1) blades
Precut endotracheal tube, sizes, 2.5, 3.0, and 3.5
Adapters for endotracheal tubes
Bag and masks of various sizes
2 Infant airways
Syringes, sizes 1 cc, 3 cc, 5 cc, 10 cc
1 Umbilical vein catheterization set and extra catheters
1 Umbilical artery catheterization set and extra catheters
2 Nos. 5 and 8 French feeding tubes
2 30-ml ampules sterile distilled water
2 30-ml ampules sterile saline
Heparinized saline
2 10-cc vials diluted sodium bicarbonate (0.5 mEq/cc)
1 10-cc 10% glucose
1 10-cc 1:10,000 aqueous epinephrine
Naloxone
Atropine sulfate
Calcium gluconate
No. 23g scalp needles
No. 22g infusion catheters
Scissors
Scotch tape or equivalent
Blood pressure monitor
Cardiorespiratory monitor
Dextrostix
Three-way stopcocks, sterile
Stopcock plugs (needle caps)
Suction catheter
Tape measure
Disposable sterile gloves
Specimen tubes
Alcohol sponges
Preparation tray with Betadine
Thoracotomy tube set
Rubber bands
Lancets
2 Receiving blankets (warm)
Stethoscope
Oxygen hood
Thermometer
Hematocrit tubes
Intensive care record sheet
Transport information forms

Resuscitation Summary

1. Normal newborn infants may have a transient respiratory acidosis and hypoxia shortly after birth.
2. The asphyxiated newborn infant has more profound hypoxia and respiratory

acidosis. Additional metabolic acidosis may be found if asphyxia has been present for a short time. Such infants also may be hypothermic and require warming.

3. The resuscitation of the asphyxiated newborn must include both ventilatory and metabolic (bicarbonate) correction. Subsequently, arterial blood gases will determine further management.

4. Acidosis cannot be diagnosed clinically and must be assumed in any infant with a history of severe asphyxia.

5. Newborn infants may have cardiorespiratory problems because of asphyxia, maternal drugs (anesthesia, reserpine), intrathoracic disease (pneumothorax, diaphragmatic hernias, paralysis), anemia, hypotension, hypoglycemia, etc. The reason should be sought.

6. Stimulating drugs such as caffeine do not have a place in the treatment of asphyxia; however, antidotes should be considered (e.g., naloxone for narcotic depression).

A checklist of medications and equipment needed for resuscitation of newborn infants is provided in Table 2–3.

TRANSPORT

The development of neonatal intensive care units and the concept of regional centers for the care of sick infants have placed increased importance on methods of conveying the sick infant from the place of birth to specialized care centers. These intensive care units have been associated with a significant improvement in perinatal mortality.

Although the major emphasis has been on transportation from one hospital to another, it is equally important to have adequate facilities for transporting an infant within a hospital, from the delivery room either to the intensive care unit or to the operating room, x-ray department, or other areas of the hospital. At present, babies are being transported by specially equipped ambulances and vans that function as miniature intensive care units, and even by helicopter or airplane.

The transportation of a sick, small infant is a complex act requiring the coordinated efforts of a number of personnel and institutions. Though in most cases each act is simple, a single omission in the intricate chain may be detrimental to the infant's health. Communication and teamwork are the key to a successful transportation system. It is most important that the receiving unit be informed of the specific nature of the infant's problem in order that an appropriate plan of action may be formulated and any special preparations made.

The timing of the transport is particularly important for the premature infant. Approximately one third of all infant deaths occur within the first 24 hours following birth, and early treatment of many conditions appears to alter outcome favorably. Therefore, for whatever reason the physician considers referring an infant, be it an illness that cannot be handled properly at a particular hospital or inadequate equipment, we recommend early transportation.

We often have found it useful to have more than one individual on the transportation team—a physician and nurse or respiratory therapist. Before moving the infant, his condition should be stabilized so that the trip can be accomplished without catastrophe. In order for the transportation to be accomplished without damage to the infant, conditions such as pneumothorax, asphyxia, airway obstruction, abdominal distention, metabolic acidosis, hypoglycemia, and hypovolemia should be recognized and treated before transport.

Some type of assisted ventilation may have to be started before transportation. For apneic episodes and severe respiratory distress, a simple mask and bag are used for assisted ventilation. This support may be continued during transportation, which should be carried out in an optimally controlled environment. The baby should be kept warm and observed closely at all times.

Difficulties should be anticipated and provisions made for emergency treatment. The team must be in a position to promptly relieve airway obstruction, oxygenate, assist ventilation, correct acidosis, support circulation, control seizures, and maintain temperature during the trip. A bag containing medications and equipment necessary for resuscitation and other emergencies during transport should be replenished after each trip (Table 2–3). The major aim of the transport team is to improve the condition of the infant, and certainly the infant should arrive in no worse condition than he was in when he started. Notes made during the transport are essential for the physicians who will ultimately be caring for the infant.

A member of the transport team should have a brief discussion with the mother, if possible, and allow her to see the infant before leaving the referring hospital. Though it is obviously impossible to allay all of her fears, a short discussion about the transportation and the nature of the care the infant will receive in the intensive care unit is helpful. We have observed that most mothers believe that their baby probably will not survive when it is transferred, and they need reassurance to the contrary. In our unit, the mother can call directly into the intensive care unit 24 hours a day and may visit as soon as she is discharged. It is helpful to work closely with the father, who often accompanies the ambulance in his own car.

Problems of transportation often are related to the mechanical equipment. These may be minimized by careful maintenance (see chap. 5). It is often difficult to keep the baby warm during the trip. As this is so important, it is worth waiting until the baby has started to warm up before undertaking the journey. The transport incubator should be warmed on the way to the referring hospital. The battery should be spared by plugging it into the ambulance during all the trips. The oxygen concentrations required are obtained by use of plastic hoods and monitored with oxygen analyzers (chap. 5). Facilities for suctioning should be readily available in the transport vehicle.

Some ambulances are equipped with ventilators as well as cardiorespiratory and transcutaneous blood gas monitors. These might improve medical care during transport and assure that the infant is in optimal condition upon arrival at the receiving hospital.

TEMPERATURE

Environmental temperature has a measurable effect on morbidity and mortality. Preterm infants who are allowed to get cold have a significantly greater risk of dying than babies protected against heat loss during the early postnatal period. Therefore, heat control is one of the most important aspects of neonatal care.

A reduction in mortality is found when the infant is placed in a neutral thermal environment (that set of thermal conditions at which oxygen consumption is minimal, making less work for a deranged or immature cardiopulmonary system). This is usually accomplished by maintaining the infant's skin temperature at 36.5 C (98 F). The neutral thermal temperature results in the least amount of body metabolism, the lowest oxygen consumption, and optimal caloric requirements. Excessive cooling or overheating increases oxygen consumption. Cooling a newborn may produce or aggravate hypoxemia and a concurrent metabolic acidosis. Apneic spells sometimes occur during the warming of cold infants.

The infant loses heat according to physical laws governing evaporation, radiation, conduction, and convection. In the preterm infant, vulnerability to heat losses is increased due to the large surface area in proportion to body weight, thin epidermis, and decreased subcutaneous tissue. In addition, heat production is impaired due to decreased muscular activity (including lack of shivering) and dependence on the metabolic breakdown of triglyceride stored within brown fat.

A normal rectal temperature does not mean that the infant is in a neutral thermal environment. In fact, no single temperature measurement can determine the adequacy of thermal protection. The normal deep rectal temperature of a newborn ranges between 35.5 and 37.5 C. In young, low birth weight infants, if the incubator temperature is more than 2 to 3 C (3.6 to 5.4 F) cooler than the baby's skin temperature, it is likely that the infant is using up energy stores in trying to maintain a normal body temperature.

Delivery Room and Nursery

In the delivery room, resuscitative procedures should be performed with due attention to heat control. Evaporative loss is exaggerated in the delivery room (wet baby, wet towels, air conditioning). Evaporative losses may be reduced effectively by drying the infant immediately. Conductive losses can be eliminated by placing the infant on a warm towel or cloth. An overhead radiant warmer may provide a heat-gaining environment. Convective heat loss must be controlled by eliminating drafts in the room. Close maternal contact also offers a useful source of heat for the healthy infant. Use of the radiant warmer is ideal during resuscitation as the infant can be maintained nude and is readily accessible. Oxygen must be warmed and humidified.

While the use of radiant warmers is widespread in the delivery room or for the acutely ill neonate, they are used less widely for longer term care of sick infants. A substantial increase in insensible water loss occurs under radiant warmers, and this may be accompanied by an increase in metabolic rate. This is of particular concern in small preterm infants, in whom the ability to maintain caloric balance is already compromised.

Nursery temperature is usually maintained between 75 and 80 F. A healthy infant may be kept comfortable and normothermic if clothed in a shirt and diaper and loosely swaddled in soft blankets. The amount of swaddling and other protection needed may be determined only by routine monitoring of temperatures. Temperature of high-risk infants should be monitored very frequently.

Incubator

Small or sick infants require a controlled thermal environment such as an incubator. An attempt should be made to maintain abdominal skin temperature at 36.5 C. Table 2–4 provides the key for locating the neutral temperature if the walls of the incubator are warm and within 1 C of the incubator air temperature. If not, especially in a cool nursery, add 1 C to the temperature of the incubator setting for every 7 C that the incubator air temperature exceeds the room temperature. An alternative is to servo the incubator temperature to maintain abdominal skin temperature at 36.5 C. This also can be done by the nurse without automatic servo. Generally speaking, smaller infants in each weight group will require higher temperatures. Within each time range, the younger the infant, the higher the temperature required.

TABLE 2–4.—NEUTRAL THERMAL ENVIRONMENT TEMPERATURES*†

AGE AND WEIGHT	STARTING TEMPERATURE (CENTIGRADE)	RANGE OF TEMPERATURE (CENTIGRADE)
0–6 Hours		
Under 1,200 gm	35.0	34.0–35.4
1,200–1,500 gm	34.1	33.9–34.4
1,501–2,500 gm	33.4	32.8–33.8
Over 2,500 gm (and >36 weeks gestation)	32.9	32.0–33.8
6–12 Hours		
Under 1,200 gm	35.0	34.0–35.4
1,200–1,500 gm	34.0	33.5–34.4
1,501–2,500 gm	33.1	32.2–33.8
Over 2,500 gm (and >36 weeks gestation)	32.8	31.4–33.8
12–24 Hours		
Under 1,200 gm	34.0	34.0–34.5
1,200–1,500 gm	33.8	33.3–34.3
1,501–2,500 gm	32.8	31.8–33.8
Over 2,500 gm (and >36 weeks gestation)	32.4	31.0–33.7
24–36 Hours		
Under 1,200 gm	34.0	34.0–35.0
1,200–1,500 gm	33.6	33.1–34.2
1,501–2,500 gm	32.6	31.6–33.6
Over 2,500 gm (and >36 weeks gestation)	32.1	30.7–33.5

TABLE 2–4.—*Continued*

36–48 Hours

Under 1,200 gm	34.0	34.0–35.0
1,200–1,500 gm	33.5	33.0–34.1
1,501–2,500 gm	32.5	31.4–33.5
Over 2,500 gm (and >36 weeks gestation)	31.9	30.5–33.3

48–72 Hours

Under 1,200 gm	34.0	34.0–35.0
1,200–1,500 gm	33.5	33.0–34.0
1,501–2,500 gm	32.3	31.2–33.4
Over 2,500 gm (and >36 weeks gestation)	31.7	30.1–33.2

72–96 Hours

Under 1,200 gm	34.0	34.0–35.0
1,200–1,500 gm	33.5	33.0–34.0
1,501–2,500 gm	32.2	31.1–33.2
Over 2,500 gm (and >36 weeks gestation)	31.3	29.8–32.8

4–12 Days

Under 1,500 gm	33.5	33.0–34.0
1,501–2,500 gm	32.1	31.0–33.2
Over 2,500 gm (and >36 weeks gestation)		
4–5 Days	31.0	29.5–32.6
5–6 Days	30.9	29.4–32.3
6–8 Days	30.6	29.0–32.2
8–10 Days	30.3	29.0–31.8
10–12 Days	30.1	29.0–31.4

12–14 Days

Under 1,500 gm	33.5	32.6–34.0
1,501–2,500 gm	32.1	31.0–33.2
Over 2,500 gm (and >36 weeks gestation)	29.8	29.0–30.8

2–3 Weeks

Under 1,500 gm	33.1	32.2–34.0
1,501–2,500 gm	31.7	30.5–33.0

3–4 Weeks

Under 1,500 gm	32.6	31.6–33.6
1,501–2,500 gm	31.4	30.0–32.7

4–5 Weeks

Under 1,500 gm	32.0	31.2–33.0
1,501–2,500 gm	30.9	29.5–32.2

5–6 Weeks

Under 1,500 gm	31.4	30.6–32.3
1,501–2,500 gm	30.4	29.0–31.8

*For this table the authors had the walls of the incubator 1–2 C warmer than the ambient air temperatures.

†From Scopes, J., and Ahmed, I.: Range of critical temperatures in sick and premature newborn babies, Arch. Dis. Child. 41:417, 1966.

It is necessary to perform serial recordings of rectal, skin, and air temperatures during the care of babies, especially those in incubators. Usually, the skin temperature is the same as or slightly lower than the rectal temperature. If it is determined that the skin temperature is higher than the rectal temperature, it is likely that heat losses have been limited by environmental heating, and if the infant's body temperature increases, the fever is probably caused by overheating and not sepsis. On the other hand, if the skin is cooler than the rectal temperature, any fever would have to be explained on the basis of hypermetabolism, which may in turn reflect infection.

When infants are receiving oxygen in a hood, the hood temperature should be maintained within 1 C of incubator temperature in order to maintain a neutral thermal environment. Weaning involves a gradual lowering of incubator temperature in anticipation of transfer to an open crib. This can be done once the baby is sufficiently mature to maintain body temperature in the surrounding nursery environment of 75 F (24 C). At this time the infant should no longer require special observation or treatment.

UMBILICAL VESSEL CATHETERIZATION

A central catheter, inserted into the inferior vena cava via the umbilical vein or into the aorta via an umbilical artery, may be required in the management of the sick infant for intermittent or continuous monitoring of blood gas status and for parenteral infusion of fluids. Use of central catheters requires careful consideration of the risks involved and a decision that the need for the catheter outweighs the risk of the catheterization procedure and the subsequent presence of an indwelling catheter.

A major objective of umbilical arterial catheter placement is avoidance of the area of origin of the renal arteries around the level of the first lumbar vertebra (L1). A catheter tip placed at this level may occlude a renal artery or produce renal embolism or thrombosis. Due to the presence of other major arterial vessels at the thoracic and lumbar areas, desired vertebral positions for placement of the arterial catheter tip include T6 to T10 for high lines, and L3 to L4 for low lines. The length of insertion of the umbilical arterial catheter can be predetermined, using the graph in Figure 2–2.

An umbilical venous line should be advanced to the inferior vena cava, but if resistance is encountered it may be withdrawn until there is a good blood return. The position of either catheter should be verified radiologically. A lateral view will readily distinguish between an arterial and a venous line.

Infusion of a hypertonic solution of sodium bicarbonate or glucose has been responsible for liver necrosis and portal vein thrombosis if the umbilical venous catheter tip is in the portal vein. Other major complications of catheterization include thrombosis of the vessel around the catheter and subsequent release of microemboli on either the venous or the arterial side of the circulation.

In general, umbilical vein catheterization is technically easier. However, since monitoring the acid–base status and the adequacy of ventilation of the small, premature infant in cardiorespiratory distress is a major indication for catheterization, an umbilical artery catheter is required. Systemic blood pressure can be monitored continuously through this catheter.

The umbilical vein catheter should be removed as soon as possible and a peripheral venous catheter substituted, if required, for parenteral fluid therapy. In the undistressed newborn infant, under no circumstances should an umbilical

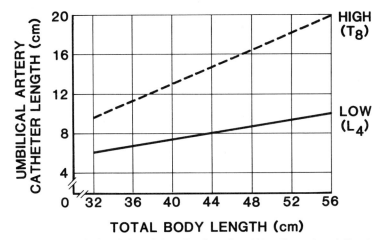

Fig 2–2.—Graph for determining the length of insertion of umbilical artery catheter for placement of its tip at high (8th thoracic) or low (4th lumbar) levels. The length of the umbilical stump should be added to the obtained value. (Adapted from Rosenfeld, W., et al.: J. Pediatr. 96:735, 1980; J. Pediatr. 98:627, 1981.)

vessel catheter be used for parenteral fluids when a peripheral intravenous catheter could be started via a scalp or peripheral vein.

A cord tie should be used before and after the catheter is inserted, and the catheter should be secured to the abdominal wall with skin tape. The risk of hemorrhage is minimized by tight connections and careful use of stopcocks. Careful observation for hemorrhage also is needed for some time following removal of the catheter.

OXYGEN THERAPY

Oxygen is the single most common therapeutic agent. Like many drugs given to infants in the neonatal period, it has many potential side effects. Therefore, it always should be used in a controlled fashion with careful monitoring by trained personnel.

Physiologic Considerations

Oxygen is carried by the blood in chemical combination with hemoglobin and, to a lesser extent, in physical solution. The oxygen taken up by both processes is dependent on the partial pressure of oxygen (Po_2). At ambient pressures, the amount of dissolved oxygen is only a small fraction of the total quantity carried in whole blood (0.3 ml O_2/100 ml plasma/100 mm Hg). Most of the oxygen in whole blood is bound to hemoglobin (1 gm hemoglobin combines with 1.34 ml oxygen at 38 C). The quantity of oxygen bound to hemoglobin is dependent upon the partial pressure as shown by the oxygen dissociation curve (Fig 2–3).

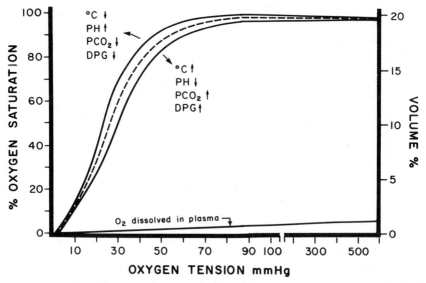

Fig 2–3.—Factors that shift the oxygen dissociation curve of hemoglobin. Fetal hemoglobin is shifted to the left as compared to the adult. (From Klaus, M., Fanaroff, A., and Martin, R.J.: Respiratory problems, in Klaus, M.H., and Fanaroff, A.A. [eds.]: *Care of the High Risk Neonate* [2nd ed.; Philadelphia: W.B. Saunders Co., 1979].)

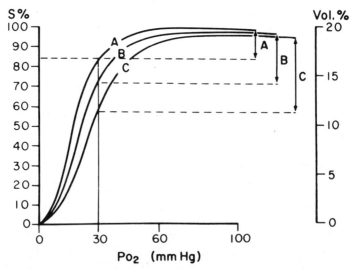

Fig 2–4.—The effect of three different oxygen dissociation curves of hemoglobin on the oxygen delivered at a tissue Po_2 of 30 mm Hg.

The blood is almost completely saturated* at an arterial oxygen tension (PaO_2) of 90 to 100 mm Hg. The dissociation curve of fetal blood is shifted to the left, and at any PaO_2 less than 100 mm Hg, fetal blood binds more oxygen. The shift is the result of the lower content of diphosphoglycerate. (The pH, PCO_2, temperature and 2,3-diphosphoglycerate influence the position of the dissociation curve.)

Figure 2–4 illustrates that at an alveolar PO_2 of 100 mm Hg, the three different blood samples have very similar saturations and O_2 content. However, if we assume a tissue PO_2 of 30 mm Hg, each sample will unload different amounts of oxygen per 100 ml plasma (A–3 ml, B–5 ml, C–7.0 ml) to the tissues. The clinical significance of this is that the sick neonate's blood will take up more oxygen at an alveolar PO_2 of 40 mm Hg, but the tissue PO_2 will drop to a very low level in order to unload adequate amounts of oxygen. The shift makes clinical recognition of hypoxia more difficult since cyanosis will be observed at a lower oxygen tension. Cyanosis is first observed at saturations of 75 to 85%, which relates to oxygen tensions of 32 to 42 mm Hg on the fetal dissociation curve. Cyanosis in the adult is observed at higher tensions. The flattening of the upper portion of the S-shaped dissociation curve makes it almost impossible to estimate oxygen tensions accurately above 60 to 80 mm Hg from arterial oxygen saturation data.

Figure 2–5 illustrates the pH, $PaCO_2$, HCO_3^-, and PaO_2 in normal infants breathing room air. Note the presence of respiratory acidosis in the first minutes of life.

The partial pressure of oxygen in arterial blood not only depends on the ability of the lung to transfer oxygen, but is modified by shunting of venous blood into the systemic circulation through the heart or lungs. Breathing 100% oxygen for a prolonged time will correct desaturation secondary to both diffusion abnormalities and inadequate ventilation. Measurements of arterial PaO_2 while the patient is breathing 100% oxygen are therefore useful diagnostically in determining whether arterial desaturation is caused by a right-to-left shunt, diffusion abnormalities, or inadequate ventilation. If no right-to-left shunt is present, the arterial PO_2 after breathing 100% oxygen is equal to the atmospheric pressure minus the partial pressures of alveolar carbon dioxide and water vapor.

Placing a baby in 100% oxygen therefore may help to differentiate cyanosis of cardiac causation from that of pulmonary causation. It is rare in a baby with cyanotic congenital heart disease, and hence a fixed anatomical shunt from right to left, for the PaO_2 to be raised above a level of 80 to 100 mm Hg while he is breathing 100% oxygen. The differentiation between cyanotic congenital heart disease and persistent fetal circulation may be difficult. While both conditions are characterized by severe hypoxemia in 100% FiO_2, infants with per-

---

*The arterial oxygen saturation is the actual oxygen bound to hemoglobin, divided by the capacity of hemoglobin for binding oxygen.

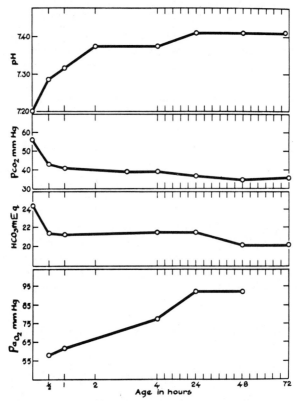

Fig 2–5.—The arterial pH, Pco_2, HCO_3 and PaO_2 during the first hours and days of life. (From Klaus, M.: Respiratory function and pulmonary disease in the newborn, in Barnett, H. [ed.]: *Pediatrics* [15th ed.; New York: Appleton-Century-Crofts, 1972].)

sistent fetal circulation may demonstrate a markedly improved oxygenation during hyperventilation, which would not be expected with primary heart disease.

During the first days of life, 20% of the cardiac output normally is shunted from right to left. It is not known whether this shunt is primarily at the foramen ovale, ductus arterious, or within the lungs. In contrast, in the adult, the shunt from right to left is only 5% of the cardiac output.

Clinical evidence of hypoxia in the newborn may include pallor, tachycardia, abdominal distention, tachypnea and cyanosis, increased activity, and decreased rectal temperature. If hypoxia persists, acidosis increases, pH drops, and heart rate and blood pressure will then fall.

Clinical Uses of Oxygen

Clinical conditions for which oxygen therapy may be necessary in the newborn include asphyxia neonatorum; common respiratory problems such as the respiratory distress syndrome, meconium aspiration, bacterial pneumonia, and pneumothorax; shock; apneic spells; congenital heart disease with right-to-left circulatory shunt; persistent fetal circulation; and many other respiratory problems.

Cyanosis is related to a variety of factors such as oxygen saturation of the blood, hemoglobin concentration, character of the hemoglobin, and perfusion of the skin. In some infants, cyanosis is not evident until very low arterial oxygen tension occurs, while on the other hand, peripheral cyanosis due to local circulatory inadequacy may occur despite normal arterial oxygen tension. It is always important to differentiate between central cyanosis, which implies desaturation of the blood, and peripheral cyanosis (or *acrocyanosis,* as it is commonly called), which is usually normal in the first 2 to 3 days of life, but may be associated with polycythemia or poor peripheral circulation. Evaluation of the oral mucosa provides the best clinical assessment of oxygenation.

When an infant requires supplemental oxygen, careful control of environmental concentration and measurement of arterial tension are essential. In low birth weight infants in particular, there is a fine dividing line between the therapeutic benefits of oxygen and its toxic effects on the eyes and lungs. The desired levels of arterial oxygen tension will be considered in the detailed discussion of the respiratory distress syndrome.

Though oxygen often is needed in the treatment of a severe apneic episode and for a few minutes thereafter, its continued use is contraindicated if there is no ongoing hypoxia. If there is persistent hypoxemia between apneic episodes, the number of apneic periods can be reduced markedly if the oxygen concentration is increased slightly, but careful monitoring is required to prevent hyperoxia.

Oxygen Monitoring

Although arterial oxygen tension has traditionally been monitored by intermittent sampling from indwelling arterial catheters placed in the aorta or radial artery, methods have recently been developed for continually monitoring oxygen tension both intra-arterially and transcutaneously. The principle of transcutaneous oxygen monitoring is that warming the skin to approximately 44 C allows arterialization of the capillary bed and diffusion of oxygen through the skin surface underlying the electrode. Devices that measure oxygen saturation noninvasively have been recently developed. The obvious advantages to continuous monitoring of oxygen tension include instant detection of changes in the infant's condition, easier adjustment of ventilator settings, and observation of the deleterious effects of the many interventions on sick infants. These include such minor manipulations as taking vital signs, altering the position of the infant, and feeding the infant. Continuous oxygen monitoring is an adjunct and not a substitute for intermittent blood sampling in the very sick neonate. There is an excellent correlation between transcutaneous and arterial PO_2 in the neonate (Fig 2–6A) although the results of transcutaneous monitoring may not be as accurate in infants with severe hypotension, those with poor tissue diffusion, and when PaO_2 exceeds 100 mm Hg. The electrode site should be changed every 4 hours to prevent skin burns.

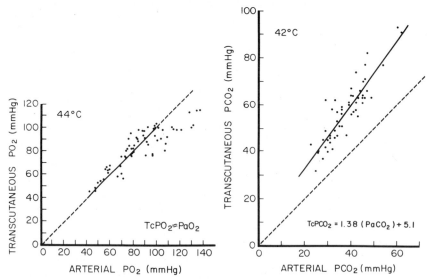

Fig 2–6.—A, Correlation between transcutaneous and arterial Po_2 in preterm infants with RDS, **B,** Correlation between transcutaneous and arterial Pco_2 in preterm and term infants with cardiopulmonary diseases. (From Martin, R.J., Robertson, S.S., and Hopple, M.M.: Crit. Care Med. 10:679, 1982; and Martin, R.J., Fanaroff, A.A., and Skalina, M.E.L.: The respiratory system; The respiratory distress syndrome and its management, in Fanaroff, A.A., and Martin, R.J. [eds.]: *Behrman's Neonatal-Perinatal Medicine* [3rd ed.; St. Louis: C.V. Mosby Co., 1983]).

Transcutaneous measurements of Pco_2 also correlate with $PaCO_2$ (Fig 2–6B), although hypoperfusion may cause elevated transcutaneous Pco_2 measurements. The longer response time of the transcutaneous CO_2 measurements has somewhat limited its clinical usefulness.

RESPIRATORY PROBLEMS

Respiratory problems are responsible for most morbidity and mortality in infants. However, considering the complexity of the pulmonary and hemodynamic changes occurring after delivery, it is surprising that most infants make the transition from intra- to extrauterine life so smoothly and uneventfully.

The treatment required by the sick preterm or full-term infant can be administered only by pooling the resources of many present-day delivery units. The application of the principles discussed in this section requires not only some special equipment but, more important, skilled nurses, respiratory therapists, a laboratory equipped for 24-hour blood gases, and a physician who is readily available to the unit 24 hours a day.

Once the respiratory diagnosis has been made, it is necessary to determine whether the neonatal unit has all the facilities that might be needed during the course of the illness.

Respiratory Distress

Respiratory problems in the early neonatal period present with a combination of symptoms, including cyanosis, grunting, tachypnea, nasal flaring, and retractions. The onset of these symptoms necessitates early and vigorous intervention to establish the etiology and initiate early therapy.

As indicated earlier, cyanosis is observed only with a very low PaO_2 in newborn infants. A grunting sound made during expiration and produced by expiring against a partially closed glottis is considered abnormal if it persists beyond the first 30 minutes of life. Respiratory rates up to 60 per minute are normal in the first hours of life. Rates above this require careful attention. The persistence of retractions, flaring, the use of accessory respiratory muscles, and powerful diaphragmatic action during respiration are indicative of increased respiratory effort and warrant investigation.

Even while administering emergency therapy, the initial objective is to establish an etiology for the respiratory symptoms. A major error in care can easily be made if other organ systems are not considered initially. Not every cyanotic, rapidly breathing infant has hyaline membrane disease. Low blood volume, hypoglycemia, hypothermia, congenital heart disease, cerebral hemorrhage, or even the effect of drugs may all mimic primary respiratory disorders. Appropriate care depends on the diagnosis.

A working classification of some of these disorders is presented in Table 2–5. Whenever faced with these respiratory symptoms, the physician's next steps (following a history-taking and physical examination including blood pressure and temperature) should be to obtain a chest x-ray film, a central hematocrit (peripheral hematocrits are usually higher than intravascular hematocrits), a blood sugar, and an arterial blood gas.

TABLE 2–5.—DIFFERENTIAL DIAGNOSIS OF NEONATAL RESPIRATORY DISTRESS

RESPIRATORY DISORDERS		
COMMON	LESS COMMON	MECHANICAL
Respiratory distress syndrome	Pulmonary hemorrhage	Upper airway obstruction
Transient tachypnea	Pulmonary hypoplasia/agenesis	Tracheal lesions
Meconium aspiration	Congenital lung cysts, tumors	Rib cage anomalies
Pneumonia	Congenital lobar emphysema	Extrinsic masses
Pneumothorax/air leaks	Tracheoesophageal fistula	Diaphragmatic hernia
		Abdominal distension
		Pleural effusion/chylothorax

EXTRAPULMONARY DISORDERS		
CARDIAC/VASCULAR	METABOLIC	NEUROLOGIC/MUSCULAR
Hypovolemia	Acidosis	Cerebral edema
Anemia	Hypoglycemia	Cerebral hemorrhage
Polycythemia	Hypothermia	Drugs
Persistent fetal circulation	Hyperthermia	Muscle disorders
Cyanotic heart disease		Spinal cord problems
Congestive heart failure		Phrenic nerve damage

In many cases, arterial catheterization will be required. The decision to catheterize the umbilical artery depends on the infant's condition. We catheterize the umbilical artery and/or vein during the first 15 minutes of life if metabolic resuscitation is required or if the infant remains severely distressed, as defined by continued hypoxemia with or without hypotonia and severe respiratory efforts. On the other hand, if the infant has tachypnea and grunting with retractions but is active and pink, we place an arterial catheter only if oxygen requirement persists above an FiO_2 of 40%.

Respiratory Distress Syndrome

Respiratory distress syndrome (RDS) should be anticipated in immature infants especially if there is a history of maternal bleeding, maternal diabetes, perinatal asphyxia, or erythroblastosis. Expiratory grunting or whining is observed when the infant is not crying. This important sign sometimes may be the only indication of disease, while a decrease in grunting may be the first sign of improvement. Intercostal and subcostal retractions are secondary to a combination of decreased lung compliance and increased chest wall compliance. Nasal flaring, cyanosis in room air, rapid respiration, diminished air entry, and edematous extremities occur early in the disease. The chest x-ray film reveals a reticulogranular, ground-glass appearance with air bronchogram.

Physiologic abnormalities include reduced compliance (Fig 2–7), large areas of underperfused lung (up to 50 to 60%), a large right-to-left shunt, reduced

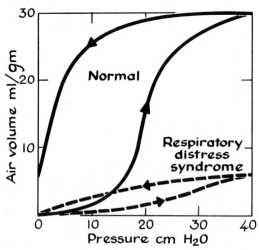

Fig 2–7.—Air pressure-volume curves of a normal and abnormal lung. Volume is expressed as milliliters of air per gram of lung. The lung from an infant with the respiratory distress syndrome accepts a smaller volume of air at all pressures. Note also that the deflation pressure-volume curve closely follows the inflation curve. (From Klaus, M.: Respiratory Function and Pulmonary Disease in the Newborn, in Barnett, H. [ed.]: *Pediatrics* [15th ed.; New York: Appleton-Century-Crofts, 1972].)

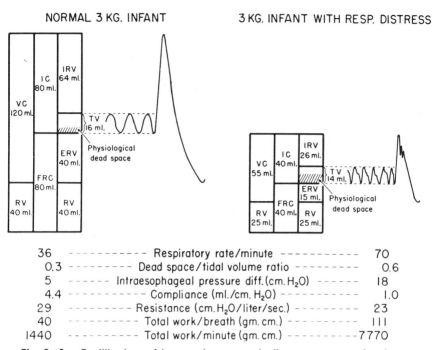

NORMAL 3 KG. INFANT   3 KG. INFANT WITH RESP. DISTRESS

36	- - - - - - - - - -	Respiratory rate/minute	- - - - - - - - - -	70
0.3	- - - - - - - - -	Dead space/tidal volume ratio	- - - - - - - - -	0.6
5	- - - - - -	Intraesophageal pressure diff. (cm. H_2O)	- - - - - -	18
4.4	- - - - - - - - - -	Compliance (ml./cm. H_2O)	- - - - - - - - - -	1.0
29	- - - - - - - - -	Resistance (cm. H_2O/liter/sec.)	- - - - - - - - -	23
40	- - - - - - - - -	Total work/breath (gm. cm.)	- - - - - - - - -	111
1440	- - - - - - - - -	Total work/minute (gm. cm.)	- - - - - - - - -	7770

Fig 2–8.—Partitioning of lung volumes and other measures of pulmonary function in a normal infant and in one with RDS. (From Avery, M., Fletcher, B., and Williams, R.: *The Lung and its Disorders in the Newborn Infant.* [4th ed.; Philadelphia, W.B. Saunders Co., 1981].)

lung volume, decreased pulmonary capillary blood flow, and decreased alveolar ventilation despite an increased minute ventilation and increased work of breathing (Fig 2–8). These changes result in hypoxemia, metabolic acidosis, and often an increased $PaCO_2$.

Gross pathologic findings include collapsed, firm, and dark red lung. Microscopic examination shows alveolar collapse, overdistention of alveolar ducts, and pink-staining membrane on alveolar ducts (the hyaline membrane). The muscular portion of pulmonary arteriolar walls is thickened, and the lumen is small. Lymphatic vessels are distended. In addition, pulmonary surfactants are altered, deficient, or absent. Perfusion studies of the vascular tree reveal a severely reduced arterial bed with blockage near the pulmonary arterioles. Biochemical analysis reveals that the lung contains decreased phospholipid and surface-active lipoprotein fractions.

ETIOLOGY.—In the past 25 years, numerous theories explaining the respiratory distress syndrome (RDS) or hyaline membrane disease (HMD) have been proposed and rejected. The most attractive proposal at present is that the disease is the result of a primary absence, deficiency, or alteration of the highly surface-active alveolar lining layer, the pulmonary surfactant. Surfactant, a lipoprotein, binds to the internal surface of the alveolus and markedly weakens surface tension at the air–water interface, thereby reducing the pressure and tending to collapse the alveolus. By equalizing the forces of surface tension in units of varying size, it is a potent factor against atelectasis and is essential for normal respiration. Alteration or absence of the pulmonary surfactant would lead to the sequence of events shown in Figure 2–9, resulting in decreased lung compliance (stiff lung) and thus an increase in the work of breathing. The additional work would soon tire the infant, leading to a sequence of reduced alveolar ventilation, atelectasis, and alveolar hypoperfusion. Asphyxia would induce pulmonary vasoconstriction, and blood would bypass the lung through fetal pathways (patent ductus, foramen ovale), lowering pulmonary blood flow, and a vicious cycle would be promoted. The resultant ischemia would reduce lung metabolism and surfactant production further. The degrees of pulmonary hypoperfusion and surfactant deficiency vary with each infant.

PREVENTION.—Major efforts at treating this disease focus on its prevention. Numerous studies have noted the inexcusably high incidence of this disorder following elective cesarean sections done without previous adequate documentation of pulmonary maturity from amniotic fluid testing. The prolongation of pregnancy with bed rest and/or drugs that inhibit premature labor (e.g., tocolytic agents such as ritodrine) will reduce the incidence of this disease.

After the observation that glucocorticoid-induced acceleration of lung maturation in preterm lambs, Liggins and Howie first showed in a double-blind prospective study that maternal treatment with betamethasone prevented the development of RDS in the offspring. The precise mechanisms involved in lung maturation are unclear, but decreased endogenous steroids have been observed in cord blood of infants who subsequently developed RDS. Since the observations of Liggins and Howie in 1972, several prospective studies including a large collaborative multicenter trial have confirmed these observations, although limitations in the effectiveness of this treatment have been found. The reduced incidence of RDS was mainly due to an effect in singleton female

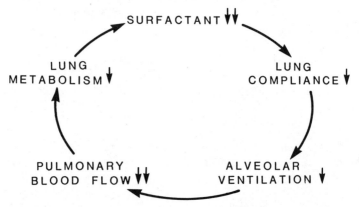

Fig 2–9.—Alveolar function in the respiratory distress syndrome.

infants, and no benefit was observed in male infants. Similarly, steroid treatment was more effective in Hispanics and North American Indians. Other studies have shown reduced morbidity and mortality associated with RDS. Complications of therapy have usually been limited to an increase in maternal postpartum infection, and long-term follow-up of the children at up to 6 years has shown no differences between treated and control groups. It seems, therefore, that steroids are indicated in selected preterm deliveries for the prevention of RDS.

The clinical course of RDS can be divided into acute and recovery phases. The acute phase lasts until it is reasonably certain that the infant will survive. During the acute phase, every maneuver is directed at increasing the chance of recovery. The infant is placed in a neutral thermal environment (see the earlier section on temperature) to reduce oxygen requirements and CO_2 production. For an infant with severe pulmonary involvement this step alone may be life-saving. To meet fluid and partial caloric requirements, the infant is initially given 65 ml/kg/24 hours of 10% glucose intravenously, gradually increasing up to 120 to 150 ml/kg/day by day 7. To meet the immediate and changing oxygen, metabolic, and ventilatory requirements of the infant, we closely monitor color, activity, heart rate, skin or rectal temperature, and pH, $PaCO_2$, PaO_2, and HCO_3^- at a minimum of every 4 hours. Respiration is monitored continuously to prevent a long apneic period.

Most important in the prescription are skilled nursing, respiratory therapy, and physician management. Vital signs and observations must be made so as not to disturb the infant continually; yet the patient always must be observed. The real skills of a unit can be tested by noting closely the care given an infant with RDS. Is the environmental oxygen at the correct percentage, temperature, and flow rate? Is the arterial oxygen permitted to go too high or too low for a prolonged period? Is the unit anticipating the future needs of the infant or always treating complications?

Our general plan is to maintain the PaO_2 in the abdominal aorta between 50 and 80 mm Hg and the pH above 7.25 (with alkali if metabolic acidosis is present). The production of lecithin, the principal component of pulmonary surfactant, is maximal at a pH of 7.4. To prevent the toxic effects of hyperosmolar solutions, we are cautious about using $NaHCO_3$ and limit the total amount of alkali administered to 8 mEq/kg/24 hours, if possible.

Between 3 and 4 days, most infants will start the recovery phase. This phase is usually preceded by a period of diuresis in which urine output exceeds fluid intake with a simultaneous improvement in lung compliance. Respiratory rate and retractions will decrease, and PaO_2 will rise. During this phase, expertise in oxygen management is required. The PaO_2 should be kept below 80 mm Hg, but if environmental oxygen is decreased too rapidly, PaO_2 may drop farther than expected.

During the recovery phase, the umbilical arterial catheter is removed when the PaO_2 has been adequate for several hours at an ambient oxygen concentration of less than 40%. It should be emphasized that any increase in environmental oxygen concentration can result in arterial oxygen tensions that are toxic to the retina if maintained for a prolonged period. We continue to lower ambient oxygen in small decrements, closely monitoring the infant's clinical state (i.e., respiratory rate, heart rate, color, abdominal distention). As the infant recovers, apneic periods can occur but they do not have the ominous significance that they have in the acute phase. (For further details see Table 2–6.)

OXYGEN ADMINISTRATION.—The use of a small hood (see chap. 5) over the infant's head will prevent fluctuation of the oxygen concentration when the incubator is opened. The temperature of the oxygen must be warmed to that of the incubator and checked hourly. The flow into the hood must be at least 7 liters per minute to prevent CO_2 accumulation. Improper oxygen administration can be disastrous for the small infant and result in brain, lung, or eye damage or death.

The following points should be observed during the administration of high-concentration oxygen.

1. Peripheral cyanosis may be present in a neonate with a normal or high arterial oxygen tension.
2. The environmental oxygen should be monitored at least hourly in all infants receiving supplementary oxygen or assisted ventilation.
3. Management of oxygen therapy without arterial oxygen tension determinations is dangerous. We measure PaO_2 continuously or at least every 4 hours (night and day) if the infant is receiving supplemental oxygen. This may be modified for infants with chronic lung disease (see below).
4. Attempt to maintain arterial oxygen tension between 50 and 80 mm Hg during the acute phase of respiratory distress.
5. Some infants recovering from respiratory disease (severe RDS, bronchopulmonary dysplasia) may require slightly increased oxygen concentrations (25 to 30%) for prolonged periods. These infants should have a transcutaneous or arterial Po_2 determination at least every day. Caution should be exercised when transcutaneous assessment of blood gases is used to estimate absolute arterial values in infants with BPD. Although there is a good correlation between transcutaneous and arterial Po_2, the latter is underestimated by transcutaneous measurements in these patients. Furthermore, transcutaneous Pco_2 overestimates arterial Pco_2. The mechanisms underlying these discordances still need to be elucidated. When the environmental oxygen is to be lowered, observe these infants closely for pallor, tachycardia, tachypnea, abdominal distention, and a decrease in body temperature.
6. Small infants with respiratory problems cannot usually maintain adequate tissue oxygenation for a prolonged period if PaO_2 falls between 30 and 40 mm Hg, and they require some supplemental oxygen.
7. Long periods of time in any supplemental oxygen can result in retrolental fibroplasia in preterm infants.
8. Every preterm infant receiving additional oxygen should be examined at least once shortly before discharge by an experienced ophthalmologist.

TABLE 2–6.—Essentials of Care for Infants with Respiratory Distress

TREATMENT	LOGIC
1. a. Trained nurses (ratio of at least 1:1 or 1:2) and monitoring equipment. b. Available physician.	1. Early management of complications and notification of change in course (i.e., apnea, bleeding from catheter).
2. a. Precise temperature control to maintain infant in neutral temperature (includes oxygen hood).	2. Maintain minimal oxygen consumption and carbon dioxide production.
3. a. pH, PaO$_2$, PaCO$_2$, and HCO$_3^-$ measurement every 4 hours (at least); maintain PaO$_2$ at 50–80 mm Hg. b. Measure blood pressure. c. Attempt to keep pH >7.25. If PaCO$_2$ > 55, consider changing treatment. d. Lower environmental oxygen slowly when RDS infant is still acutely ill. Continuous monitoring of oxygen is ideal. e. Limit NaHCO$_3$ to 8 mEq/kg/day	3. a,c. To determine requirements for oxygen and additional HCO$_3^-$. Permits continual assessment of infant's condition and limits toxic effects of oxygen. b. Rule out hypovolemia and/or hypotension. d. Prevents greater than expected drop in PaO$_2$ when environmental oxygen is reduced. e. Prevents hypernatremia and may reduce risk of intraventricular hemorrhage.
4. IV glucose 65 ml/kg first day, gradually increasing up to 120–150 cc/kg/day by day 7. Determination of body weight, urine output, and serum electrolytes help determine fluid requirements.	4. Meets a portion of the large caloric requirements. Excessive fluid administration may increase the incidence of patent ductus arteriosus.
5. Controlled oxygen administration warmed and humidified, using a hood.	5. Prevents large swings in environmental oxygen and decreases water requirements.
6. Continually monitor respiration, heart rate, and temperature.	6. Prevents hypoxemia and acidemia with apneic episodes.
7. Frequent determinations of blood sugar and hematocrit (Na, K, and Cl every 24–48 hours).	7. Necessary for calculating general metabolic requirements.
8. Transfuse if initial central hematocrit < 40 or if hematocrit < 40 during acute phase of illness.	8. For adequate oxygen-carrying capacity.
9. Record all observations (laboratory, nurse notes, etc.) on single form.	9. Permits immediate correlations of many variables.
10. Urinary pH, output, osmolality.	10. Evaluation of blood flow to the kidney; an increase in output occurs as the infant starts to improve.
11. Obtain blood culture; treat with a penicillin and aminoglycoside until cultures available.	11. Cannot radiographically separate RDS from Group B streptococcal and other bacterial pneumonias.
12. Minimize routine procedures such as suctioning, handling, ausculation, etc.	12. Prevents iatrogenic drops in PaO$_2$.

Oxygen Toxicity

High concentrations of oxygen at atmospheric pressures can affect the stability of the red cell membrane and possibly alter the neonatal brain. Serious toxicity has been a major clinical problem in the retina and lung.

THE RETINA.—The effect of oxygen on the retinal vessels depends upon (1) the stage of development of the retinal vessels, (2) the length of exposure to oxygen, and (3) the partial pressure of oxygen in the arterial blood. If only the eyes of susceptible young animals are exposed to oxygen by cupping the eye, no toxic effects are observed. The first stage of retinal vessel disease is vasoconstriction. The vasoconstricting effects of very short periods of oxygen exposure are reversible. Pronounced vasoconstriction is not observed when the retina is fully vascularized. In the full-term human neonate, the temporal portion of the retina is still sensitive at birth, but no lasting damage has been observed.

The second stage is the proliferative phase, in which new vessels grow from the capillaries and sprout through the retina into the vitreous. These vessels are usually permeable, and hemorrhages and edema sometimes follow. Organization of the hemorrhages that enter the vitreous can produce traction on the retina and may result in detachment and blindness. Depending on the severity of the retinal detachment, the changes are classified as stages III, IV, or V.

To prevent retinal damage, the arterial oxygen tension must be kept below the level that stimulates vasoconstriction. The exact concentration that is toxic is unknown. For the sick infant the general practice is to maintain the PaO_2 between 50 and 80 mm Hg. For the well, small premature infant, 40 to 60 mm Hg may be adequate. Vitamin E prophylaxis may reduce the incidence or severity of RLF, although further studies are needed to determine its full clinical usefulness.

THE LUNG.—Since Northway's description of chronic pulmonary disease following prolonged ventilatory assistance and high inspired oxygen concentration in infants with RDS, bronchopulmonary dysplasia (BPD) has been recognized with increasing frequency. Although the precise etiology is controversial, BPD is probably caused in part by use of high airway pressures and oxygen concentration in association with endotracheal intubation. While high pressures are destructive to the alveolar and bronchial linings, oxygen metabolism produces hydroxyl and superoxide radicals that alter the structural integrity of the lung cells and may decrease ciliary activity. In addition, infection and uninhibited proteolytic enzymes together with immaturity and malnutrition may be contributing factors in the development of BPD. Initial radiographic and pathologic findings are indistinguishable from severe RDS, but subsequent progressive changes are characteristic (see Table 2–7).

Cautious weaning from assisted ventilation using intermittent mandatory ventilation is preferable, allowing the infant to gradually develop a compensated respiratory acidosis. FiO_2 may be weaned with the use of arterial blood gases,

TABLE 2–7.—Classification of Bronchopulmonary Dysplasia

STAGE	POSTNATAL AGE	CHEST X-RAY	LUNG PATHOLOGY
Stage I	2–3 days	Granular pattern with air bronchogram	Hyaline membranes, atelectasis metaplasia and necrosis of bronchiolar mucosa Loss of ciliated cells Lymphatic dilatation
Stage II	4–10 days	Increased lung density	Thickening of basement membrane Necrosis and repair of alveolar epithelium Onset of emphysematous changes
Stage III	10–20 days	Small radiolucent areas	Alveolar coalescence → emphysematous changes Bronchial mucosal metaplasia and hyperplasia with increased mucus
Stage IV	>1 month	Enlargement of hyperlucent areas with strands of intervening density	Group of emphysematous alveoli Increased collagen and elastin

transcutaneous monitoring, echocardiographic assessment of relative pulmonary artery pressure, as well as general clinical condition. Tracheostomy may be indicated for the infant requiring prolonged periods of assisted ventilation, but patients can usually be managed with endotracheal intubation for as long as 2 months or more without developing major tracheal complications. If there is clinical suspicion that bronchospasm is a major contributing factor, a trial with bronchodilators may be indicated. Fluid restriction has been used when cor pulmonale and right-sided heart failure supervene. Most recently, the acute use of furosemide has been shown to improve pulmonary function in these patients, although its chronic use can result in increased incidence of patent ductus arteriosus. Home oxygen therapy is an alternative when the recovery period is prolonged.

Several studies have attempted to prevent the development of BPD by giving vitamin E, but the most recent results are discouraging. Several long-term follow-up studies indicate that the incidence of neurologic handicaps in infants with BPD is comparable to that of infants with severe RDS requiring assisted ventilation who did not develop BPD. Some evidence of pulmonary dysfunction has been reported to persist for up to 8 years in BPD survivors. Nonetheless, further data on the long-term outcome of BPD needs to be collected.

ASSISTED VENTILATION

Although mechanical ventilation in infants was reported sporadically during the 1940s, it was not until the late 1960s that its use in neonates became more widespread. Over the last 15 years, it has become apparent that mechanical ventilation of sick neonates has contributed substantially to a reduction in perinatal mortality.

Continuous Positive Airway Pressure by Endotracheal Tube, Negative Chamber, and Nasal Tubes

The application of continuous positive airway pressure (CPAP) throughout the respiratory cycle constituted a major breakthrough in the treatment of severe RDS. Gregory's studies demonstrated that gas exchange in RDS can be improved significantly by applying a constant positive pressure to the airway. CPAP is probably the first method that should be used to support ventilation of the infant severely ill with RDS.

Because of surfactant deficiency in the infant with RDS, alveoli tend to collapse easily. The resulting atelectatic areas of lung are the sites of shunting from right to left. When alveoli are prevented from closing by a continuous positive transpulmonary pressure being maintained throughout the respiratory cycle, functional residual capacity increases, and there is improved ventilation of perfused areas of lung, resulting in a marked decrease in intrapulmonary shunt. We administer CPAP whenever more than 70% oxygen is needed to maintain a PaO_2 greater than 50 to 60 mm Hg. Continuous positive transpulmonary pressure may be achieved by applying either CPAP or continuous negative pressure (CNP) to the body wall. CPAP is most useful in infants with decreased lung compliance even though an increase in dynamic lung compliance has not been observed when infants with RDS receive CPAP. In infants with normal lung compliance, high CPAP is more likely to result in complications such as air leaks, air trapping, and impairment of venous return.

ENDOTRACHEAL TUBE CPAP.—The technique for applying CPAP was developed primarily by Gregory and his colleagues, and a modification is shown in Figure 2–10. A suitable air/O_2 mixture (total flow not exceeding 5 liters per minute) passes through a humidifier. Gas passes to the elbow, which is attached to an endotracheal tube. The screw clamp on the reservoir bag is used to control the flow of gas and maintain a constant positive pressure within the system, as indicated on the pressure manometer. The side-arm ends under a 15-cm column of water. This acts as a safety valve. Applying CPAP with an endotracheal tube was most successful initially, but alternative methods that have been developed avoid the risks of intubation.

A continuous airway pressure of 8 cm H_2O is used to initiate the therapy. If this fails to produce an improvement in 20 minutes, 10 and 12 cm of H_2O are tried. These positive pressures at the airway are not transmitted completely to the pleural space because of the severely reduced pulmonary compliance. Hence, venous return and cardiac output are usually not compromised.

An improvement in arterial O_2 tension usually occurs on applying CPAP. Priority then should be given to reducing environmental oxygen until 40% is reached. Then the level of CPAP may be reduced slowly 1 cm H_2O at a time. Total weaning from CPAP may take several days.

NASAL TUBES CPAP.—CPAP or CNP has been applied successfully via endotracheal tube (Gregory), sealed head chamber (Gregory), pressurized plastic bag enclosing the head of the infant (Barrie), and nasal mask (Harris), modified

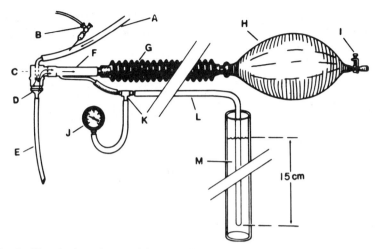

Fig 2–10.—System for applying continuous positive airway pressure (CPAP) through an endotracheal tube during spontaneous breathing. **A,** gas flow; **B,** oxygen sampling port; **C,** normal elbow (modified T-piece); **D,** endotracheal tube connector; **E,** endotracheal tube; **F,** Sommers T-piece; **G,** corrugated anesthesia hose; **H,** reservoir bag (500 ml) with open tail piece; **I,** screw clamp; **J,** aneroid pressure manometer; **K,** plastic T-connector; **L,** plastic tubing (1 cm internal diameter); **M,** underwater "pop-off." Arrows indicate direction of gas flow. (Adapted from Gregory, G., et al.: Treatment of the idiopathic respiratory distress syndrome with continuous positive airway pressure, N. Engl. J. Med. 284:1333, 1971.)

negative-pressure respirator (Vidyasagar), and plastic body chamber (Fanaroff). However, all of these methods are associated with potentially undesirable complications. The endotracheal tube is irritating to the airway, interferes with the normal ciliary clearing of the trachea, and may easily become occluded or dislodged. The positive-pressure hood, plastic head bag, and CNP body chamber all tend to isolate the infant and prevent accessibility without temporary interruption of therapy. Potentially harmful effects of positive pressure to the eyes, cooling of the face, high sound levels, and fluctuations of oxygen concentration are problems presented by several of the systems. Use of nasal tubes for the application of CPAP has been shown to be successful, with fewer complications.

We have designed an apparatus that cannulates both nares for the administration of CPAP. Our nasal piece (Fig 2–11)* is molded from Silastic† and strapped to the infant's head in the same manner as oxygen prongs are used in older children. During nasal CPAP the infant is easily accessible without interruption of therapy, and some of the complications mentioned above are avoided. With the exception of substitution of the CPAP nasal cannula for the

---

*Sherwood Medical, St. Louis, Missouri.
†Dow Corning Company, Midland, Michigan 48640.

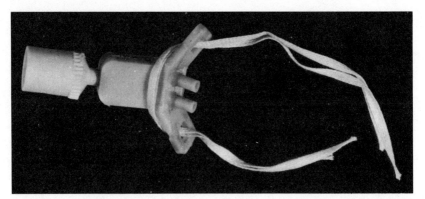

Fig 2–11.—Silastic device for administration of nasal CPAP. (From Kattwinkel, J., et al.: A device for administration of continuous positive airway pressure by the nasal route, Pediatrics 52:131, 1973.)

endotracheal tube and insertion of an orogastric tube, the rest of the apparatus is essentially identical with that described by Gregory et al.

CPAP significantly improves arterial oxygenation in infants with RDS, shortens the exposure time to high concentrations of oxygen, and arrests the downhill progression of the disease, thus lessening the need for mechanical-assisted ventilation. Application of CPAP by the nasal technique appears to be effective, simple, inexpensive, safe, and readily available to any intensive care nursery.

Despite its widespread acceptance, the use of CPAP nasal cannula may result in an added resistance to the airway, thus increasing the work of breathing. The incidence of pneumothoraces and other air leaks does not appear to be increased as a result of the appropriate use of CPAP. If CPAP fails to maintain the arterial gases adequately, intermittent bagging using the CPAP setup may prove useful to prevent endotracheal intubation in some infants. Continuous distending pressure when administered in association with assisted mechanical ventilation is known as positive end-expiratory pressure (PEEP). The indications and complications of PEEP are comparable to those of CPAP.

MECHANICAL VENTILATION

If CPAP fails to maintain adequate ventilation or if apnea occurs, mechanical ventilation is required. Mechanical ventilation is part of the supportive management of newborn infants with respiratory failure. The primary objective of mechanical ventilation is to undertake gas exchange for the infant until there is recovery from the potentially reversible pathologic process that has caused respiratory failure. Hence, it follows that prior to instituting therapy the following facilities must be available:

1. Continuous expert nursing and medical care.
2. A suitable mechanical ventilator and respiratory therapy support.
3. Arterial blood gas determinations to monitor therapy.

Indications

Some of the conditions noted in Table 2–6 can be associated with respiratory failure in the newborn infant. If respiratory failure ensues, these conditions may be managed with mechanical ventilation. Infants with RDS constitute the largest number of patients receiving mechanical ventilation.

Respiratory failure is present when the $PaCO_2$ is increased, and this is usually associated with hypoxemia and acidosis. We usually start assisted ventilation when one or more of the following criteria are met during the acute stage of RDS:

$$PaCO_2 > 55$$
$$pH \quad < 7.20$$
$$PaO_2 \quad < 50 \text{ in a } 100\% \text{ } FiO_2$$

These blood gas parameters must be considered in conjunction with the clinical condition of the infant. If the infant is clinically stable, a repeat blood gas is recommended. On the other hand, signs of clinical deterioration such as apnea, bradycardia, and hypotension would necessitate immediate action.

Special Considerations

Regardless of the type of ventilator used, warming and humidification of the inspired gases are essential to prevent tracheal damage, excessive thermal loss or impaction of secretions during prolonged mechanical ventilation.

Meticulous attention to detail is mandatory while maintaining infants on ventilators. All ventilators and ventilator equipment must be sterilized carefully and monitored for bacterial contamination before use. Bacterial colonization of the humidifier and tubing may be minimized by changing the humidifier and ventilator tubing at least every 24 hours.

When endotracheal intubation and intermittent positive-pressure ventilation are used, the intubation should be accomplished as aseptically as possible and under a radiant warmer. A tube of appropriate external diameter should be selected to fit loosely in the trachea in order to prevent complications from circular compression of the mucosa, which may cause ischemia and necrosis with subsequent strictures. For suggested guidelines of various sizes of endotracheal tubes, see Table 6–2.

The laryngoscope should have a Miller 0 or 1 blade. The visualization of the glottis may be facilitated by slight extension of the neck and pressure on the glottis. The following guideline for length of orotracheal insertion approximated from Figure 2–12 facilitates emergency intubation:

INFANT WEIGHT	ENDOTRACHEAL TUBE LENGTH
1000 gm	7 cm
2000 gm	8 cm
3000 gm	9 cm

At these lengths, the distal end of the endotracheal tube should be at the mid-

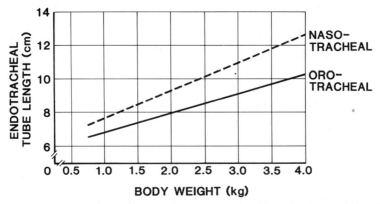

Fig 2–12.—Graph for determination of length of insertion of endotracheal tubes. The tip of the endotracheal tubes is aimed at the midtrachea. (Adapted from Tochen, M.L.: J. Pediatr. 95:1050, 1979, and Coldiron, J.S.: Pediatrics 41:823, 1968.)

trachea, but radiographic confirmation is essential. The tube should be secured so that movement of the head and neck will not dislodge it. Use of lightweight plastic connectors will prevent kinking. If repeated attempts at intubation are required, the infant should be allowed to recover with manual ventilation and oxygenation between attempts. Greater air entry in the right than left hemithorax suggests that the tube has passed into the right main stem bronchus and it must be slowly withdrawn until bilateral air entry returns. Radiographic confirmation of tip position is still mandatory.

For nasotracheal intubation, the lubricated tube is passed through the nares, visualized in the oropharynx, and guided into the glottis. McGill forceps may be needed, but a stylet should not be used. A program of pulmonary physiotherapy should be initiated to facilitate mobilization of pulmonary secretions. This usually is carried out by both nursing and respiratory therapy staffs, with position changes of the infant made every 2 to 4 hours and percussion and vibration of the chest done before suctioning of the airways. In the acutely ill infant with minimal mucus production, physiotherapy and tube suctioning should be performed less frequently.

Suctioning is potentially dangerous because it may introduce infection, result in a hypoxic episode from the discontinuing of ventilation, and produce traumatic lesions in the trachea at the site of the suction catheter tip. The infant should be suctioned briefly, using a strict sterile technique with disposable gloves and suction tubes, and must be allowed to recover between episodes of suctioning. Routine instillation of saline facilitates removal of secretions; however, if adequate humidification is used, this usually is not necessary. Changing of an endotracheal tube is indicated if the tube becomes dislodged or blocked. Routine tube changes probably are not indicated.

Since tracheostomy for prolonged mechanical ventilation of the newborn is fraught with the hazards of tube displacement, infection, and inability to extubate because of the development of stenosis, it has been superseded in most centers by prolonged periods of endotracheal intubation.

Muscle relaxants such as pancuronium bromide (Pavulon) have been employed in the care of selected severely ill neonates to produce muscle paralysis during assisted ventilation. A recent controlled trial was unable to show improved gas exchange or ability to reduce ventilator settings in infants treated with pancuronium bromide, although the paralyzed infants had less hypoxia or hyperoxia than control subjects. In another controlled study, infants given pancuronium bromide required oxygen supplementation for a shorter duration. Nonetheless, there is much controversy on the benefits and side effects (intraventricular hemorrhage) of muscle relaxants.

We prefer to restrict the use of muscle relaxants to patients that "fight" the ventilator and, despite ventilatory support with high peak inspiratory pressures (>30 mm Hg), have poor oxygenation. In preterm infants who are at risk for intraventricular hemorrhage, we try to limit muscle paralysis. An initial dose of 0.05 to 0.1 mg/kg IV may be followed by 0.03 to 0.1 mg/kg IV with the reappearance of movements that might interfere with ventilation. Continuous monitoring of the infant is necessary because of the potential risk of inadvertent extubation. Once it is estimated that muscle paralysis is not required, the infant may be allowed to spontaneously recover muscle activity. Rarely, it may be necessary to reverse muscle paralysis with administration of atropine 0.01 mg/kg IV and neostigmine 0.08 mg/kg IV. Several other sedative medications have also been used, but controlled studies have been performed only with phenobarbital. A 71% reduction in intraventricular hemorrhage that was found in an initial study has not been confirmed by subsequent data.

Use of Ventilators

The principles and mechanics of the different types of ventilators used are discussed in Chapter 6. Only respirators appropriate for ventilating newborn infants should be used. To obtain the best results, each intensive care unit should become very familiar with the type of equipment available. We strongly urge that not more than two different types of ventilators be used in any single neonatal intensive care nursery. This will permit the physicians, nurses and therapists to understand their use completely.

When mechanical ventilation is initiated, complete responsibility for the infant's gas exchange is undertaken. Hence, monitoring of the patient is vital and requires, ideally, one nurse per patient for continuous observation and frequent blood gas determinations. If continuous blood gas monitoring is not available, we determine arterial blood gases within 10 to 15 minutes of any change in ventilator settings, immediately if the infant's condition changes markedly, or at a minimum of every 4 hours. Our goal is to maintain the PaO_2 between 50 and 80 mm Hg, the $PaCO_2$ between 35 and 45 mm Hg, and the pH above 7.25 during the acute stage of RDS.

Respiratory frequency and peak inspiratory pressure (PIP) or tidal volume (in volume ventilators) determine minute ventilation and consequently CO_2 elimination. Reynolds and Boros have observed that mean airway pressure correlates with oxygenation in infants with RDS. Ventilator changes that augment this pressure include increase in PEEP and PIP or prolongation of inspiratory phase. The concentration of oxygen used should initially correspond to that necessary to maintain an adequate PaO_2 during spontaneous ventilation. Effective mechanical ventilation sometimes may result in striking increases in oxygen tension; therefore, it is important to follow and monitor these infants closely after beginning mechanical ventilation to prevent the development of retrolental fibroplasia and pulmonary oxygen toxicity.

When the clinical condition of the infant suddenly worsens, or if the blood gases demonstrate a fall in the PaO_2 and a rise in the $PaCO_2$, one or more clinical complications may have occurred:

1. Plugging of the endotracheal tube.
2. Malfunction of the respirator, disconnection of tubing, etc.
3. Displacement of the tube into a main-stem bronchus or into the pharynx.
4. Pneumothorax.
5. Sepsis, cerebral hemorrhage, patent ductus arteriosus or other complications.

The first step is to disconnect the respirator, suction the endotracheal tube, and institute bag breathing. If the condition improves, a mucous plug was probably removed; however, the ventilator and its connections should be checked carefully. If the bagging did not result in improvement, the endotracheal tube may need to be repositioned or replaced. Transillumination of the thorax is performed to diagnose a pneumothorax, which may need to be treated prior to radiographic confirmation.

Mechanical assistance of the infant is not the only component of the therapy that needs careful attention. Fluid therapy, temperature control, maintenance of the neutral thermal environment, correction of acidosis, and provision of calories are all of paramount importance in order to insure not only survival but also intact survival.

Complications of Assisted Ventilation

Some of the most common complications of mechanical ventilation include pneumothorax, pneumomediastinum, or interstitial emphysema. Trauma from the tube can cause tracheal lesions that can result in stenosis. Some of the complications of mechanical ventilation are listed in Table 2–8.

Precautions should be taken to prevent these complications. Careful attention to aseptic techniques will reduce the incidence of infection; monitoring of the oxygen and reducing its concentration as early as possible will limit the incidence of retrolental fibroplasia and bronchopulmonary disease.

Weaning from the Respirator

We usually begin to wean the infant from the respirator when the concentration of inspired oxygen is 60% or lower. Once ventilator settings have been de-

TABLE 2–8.—Complications of Assisted Ventilation

Pulmonary air leaks	Pneumothorax, pneumomediastinum, pulmonary interstitial emphysema, etc.
Endotracheal tube accidents	Displacement, dislodgement, occlusion, postextubation atelectasis, esophageal perforation
Tracheal lesions	Erosion, granuloma, subglottic stenosis
Infection	Pneumonia, septicemia, meningitis
Chronic lung disease	Bronchopulmonary dysplasia
Miscellaneous	Intracranial hemorrhage, patent ductus arteriosus, retrolental fibroplasia

creased via intermittent mandatory ventilation (see chap. 6), the infant may be given an opportunity to breathe spontaneously through the endotracheal tube.

An endotracheal CPAP or PEEP of at least 2 cm H_2O should be maintained to compensate for the absence of "physiologic" CPAP provided by the upper airway during normal breathing. Postextubation atelectasis is common in preterm infants recovering from RDS and may occur in over 50% of those weighing less than 1000 grams. In a prospective study, postextubation atelectasis occurred more frequently after nasotracheal than orotracheal intubation in infants weighing less than 1500 gm, while no difference was observed in larger infants. Use of nasal CPAP after extubation in infants with resolving RDS has resulted in improved oxygenation and CO_2 elimination, as well as a lower incidence of atelectasis.

High-Frequency Ventilation

While the etiology of major complications of mechanical ventilation (bronchopulmonary dysplasia, air leaks) is unclear, high ventilatory pressures and the resultant barotrauma are thought to be major contributory factors. Newer modes of assisted ventilation such as high-frequency positive-pressure ventilation, high-frequency oscillation (HFO), and high-frequency jet ventilation (HFJV) deliver small volumes of gas at fast frequencies in order to limit the development of high peak inspiratory pressures.

We have used HFJV at rates of 250/min in 12 preterm infants with severe RDS for short periods and observed adequate gas exchange at peak inspiratory and mean airway pressures lower than those required during conventional ventilation. A typical example of the marked reduction in airway pressures possible during HFJV is shown in Figure 2–13. Pokora used a similar system to ventilate 10 neonates with respiratory failure and intractable air leaks and observed a reduction in alveolar arterial Po_2 gradient and $PaCO_2$ when compared to a period on conventional ventilation. In adult cats with meconium aspiration, Mammel has shown that conventional ventilation was superior to HFJV. In this study there was increased pulmonary artery pressure and resistance, and lower oxygenation during HFJV.

Both Marchak and Frantz employed HFO at rates of 480 to 1800/min (8 to 30 Hz) to adequately ventilate a total of 24 infants with RDS. Five of the

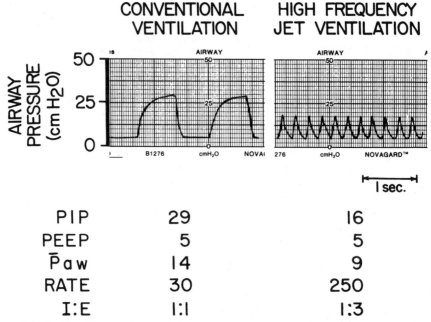

	CONVENTIONAL VENTILATION	HIGH FREQUENCY JET VENTILATION
PIP	29	16
PEEP	5	5
P̄aw	14	9
RATE	30	250
I:E	1:1	1:3

Fig 2–13.—Comparison of the positive-pressure actual recording of the pressure waveform during both conventional positive-pressure ventilation and high-frequency jet ventilation in one infant. The values for the various airway pressures, rate (frequency), and I.E. ratio are presented for comparison.

infants treated by Frantz had interstitial emphysema and showed a marked improvement in blood gases and subsequent resolution of their pulmonary air leaks. Although these preliminary data are encouraging, larger controlled trials are required to determine whether high-frequency ventilation is superior to conventional ventilation and whether complications from barotrauma are reduced by this therapy.

Surfactant

Soon after the observations that RDS was associated with deficiency or inactivation of lung surfactant, efforts were made to treat neonates with surfactant replacement. Initial studies were unsuccessful probably because only one component of lung surfactant, dipalmitoyl phosphatidylcholine (DPPC), was being administered. Although recent studies have shown that lung surfactant is a mixture of various phospholipids including DPPC and phosphatidylglycerol (PG), the components of lung surfactant that have the appropriate surface active, absorptive, and spreadable properties have not yet been determined. This lack of understanding has delayed the development of effective surfactant replacement preparations. In addition, the optimal mode of delivery of surfactant (aerosol vs. direct tracheal instillation), as well as the time of treatment (before the first breath vs. during the course of worsening RDS), are unknown at this moment.

Various kinds of surfactant preparations including natural, artificial, or a combination, are presently being evaluated. Fujiwara reported in 1980 that the tracheal instillation of a lyophilized surfactant (including components of animal surfactant) improved ventilatory status in a small group of preterm infants with RDS within 3 hours of treatment. However, the development of a patent ductus arteriosus in most subjects, the lack of a control group, and use of animal products raised further questions. A year later, Morley reported that treatment of 22 preterm infants using a powdered artificial surfactant that contained DPPC and PG reduced the need for assisted ventilation during the first day of life and subsequently decreased mortality. Although a control group was studied, randomization was not performed, and patients in each group may have received different medical attention. In addition, treatment was given before a definitive diagnosis of RDS was proved. Furthermore, there was no difference in the requirement of ventilatory assistance 24 hours after surfactant treatment. Recently, Hallman isolated human surfactant from pooled amniotic fluid and treated five preterm infants with severe RDS. They observed a marked reduction in $AaDO_2$ and ventilatory pressure needed that paralleled radiographic improvement. These three human studies suggest the feasibility of treating neonates with RDS with surfactant replacement in the near future.

Meconium Aspiration/Persistent Fetal Circulation

Meconium-stained amniotic fluid is present in about 9% of all pregnancies, but occurs uncommonly in the preterm delivery, almost never before 34 weeks. It may be a sign of fetal distress, especially when accompanied by late fetal heart rate deceleration or fetal acidosis. Therefore, if meconium is noticed during labor, arrangements must be made in case resuscitation is required at birth. Nasopharyngeal and oropharyngeal suctioning using a DeLee catheter, before delivery of the thorax is important to reduce the risk of postnatal aspiration. Immediately after the infant is born, direct laryngoscopy with endotracheal intubation should be performed and meconium aspirated from the trachea. This procedure should be rapidly and skillfully repeated until the trachea has been cleared and further resuscitation can commence. The presence of meconium in the trachea does not imply subsequent respiratory problems. Gregory reported that while meconium was aspirated from the trachea of 56% of all infants who were born covered with meconium, only half of these had radiographic changes, and one-third became sick. None of the infants without meconium in the trachea became sick, although some did have radiographic changes. In another study of meconium-stained infants, a significant decrease in neonatal mortality was observed in the group that received endotracheal suctioning at birth. Although carefully controlled randomized studies have not been performed to substantiate the practice of endotracheal suctioning of meconium-stained infants, we recommend this approach until further data are available.

Two overlapping clinical presentations have been observed in symptomatic infants who passed meconium before birth. One group, in whom pneumonitis (secondary to aspirated meconium) predominates, develop respiratory distress with tachypnea, patchy infiltrates on x-ray examination, and an oxygen requirement that may be mild to severe. Pulmonary air leaks are a common complication in infants with meconium aspiration syndrome and may be due to a ball-valve mechanism and the irregular distribution of ventilation caused by the meconium itself. There is no place for systemic glucocorticoids in the management of the pneumonitis that accompanies this disorder. In contrast, another group of infants manifests primarily severe hypoxemia. The term *persistent fetal circulation* (PFC) has been coined for this clinical presentation, but this entity may also be seen associated with metabolic disturbances such as hypoglycemia, hypocalcemia, or polycythemia, pulmonary diseases such as pneumonia or hypoplastic lungs, sepsis, and birth asphyxia. The common underlying pathophysiologic process involves an abnormal persistent elevation of pulmonary vascular resistance with consequent extrapulmonary right-to-left shunt through the foramen ovale and the ductus arteriosus. Recently, increased muscularization of the pulmonary vessels has been observed in infants with PFC who died very early in the neonatal period, implying that the process started prenatally.

The diagnosis of PFC may be supported by noninvasive heart ultrasonography with the observation of an increased ratio of systolic pre-ejection period to ejection time of the pulmonary valve, and the finding of right-to-left shunt at the foramen ovale. A heart ultrasound is also useful to exclude structural heart disease. Nonetheless, similar ultrasound findings may be observed in other neonatal respiratory disorders such as RDS. A gradient between preductal and postductal Po_2 may be observed if the right-to-left shunt is occurring at the ductus arteriosus and verified by transcutaneous monitoring. Marked fluctuations of PaO_2 even in the absence of this preductal to postductal gradient suggest a variable shunt and exclude a fixed anatomic lesion of the heart.

Infants with PFC occasionally improve with oxygen delivered by hood, but usually require assisted ventilation, although CPAP may be sufficient to improve oxygenation in some cases. Alkalosis and/or hypocapnia decrease pulmonary vascular resistance, and in the infant with a poor response to conventional assisted ventilation, hyperventilation may be beneficial. Hyperventilation to the point of decreasing the $Paco_2$ to 20 to 25 mm Hg and increasing the pH to 7.55 to 7.6 may be required, but the potential risk of decreased cerebral perfusion must be considered. Developmental examinations at 1 to 3 years of age were normal in a group of eight infants who were treated with hyperventilation during the neonatal period. Nonetheless, longterm outlook in these patients probably depends to a large extent on the severity of the initial asphyxial insult.

Attempts to decrease pulmonary vascular resistance with the use of vasodilators such as tolazoline has been effective in some intractable cases. Tolazoline may be used as a bolus dose of 1 to 2 mg/kg followed by a maintenance dose of 1 to 2 mg/kg/hr. Continuous Po_2 monitoring must be employed. Improved oxygenation is sometimes seen immediately after tolazoline is given, but about two-thirds of the infants develop hypotension and hemorrhagic manifestations while impaired renal function is also common. Selective pulmonary vasodilators such as prostaglandin D_2 are presently under evaluation to determine their usefulness in PFC. Recently, the use of inotropic agents has been proposed to increase systemic vascular resistance and to reduce the right-to-left shunting, although these too require further evaluation. High-frequency jet ventilation has been found to be of no benefit in an animal model of meconium aspiration. In uncontrolled studies, term infants with intractable respiratory failure, some secondary to eliminate MAS/PFC, have been successfully treated with extracorporeal membrane oxygenation (ECMO). This highly experimental technique may have numerous advantages, but should only be used by highly specialized teams in selected patients and under carefully designed study protocols.

Pneumonia

Pneumonia is one of the most common causes of respiratory distress in the neonate. Pneumonia may be acquired prenatally, during labor and delivery, or postpartum, and apart from aspiration pneumonia, is most frequently caused by bacteria, viruses, or fungi. Frequently, signs of respiratory distress, especially grunting, are accompanied by temperature instability, apnea, hypotension, and other signs of sepsis, together with laboratory evidence of infection (high or low WBC count, increased immature neutrophils, marked metabolic acidosis, and infiltrates on x-ray examination). Group B streptococcal pneumonia, the most frequent bacterial pneumonia, may present early after birth with radiographic evidence of patchy infiltrates or a diffuse granular process indistinguishable from RDS. This has prompted administration of antibiotics to many neonates with respiratory distress until a bacterial etiology may be ruled out. *Listeria* pneumonia may have the same clinical presentation as streptococcal pneumonia. Gram-negative bacilli, especially *Escherichia coli* and *Klebsiella,* also are occasionally acquired prenatally or intrapartum, presenting during the first 3 days of life, but may present later if the hospital course is prolonged. Pseudomonal, staphylococcal, and fungal pneumonias typically present after the first few days of life. *Pseudomonas* is likely to be the pathogen when prolonged respiratory therapy has been required. Fungal pneumonia, especially by *Candida,* is frequently seen in very low birth weight infants with prolonged hospitalization and multiple antibiotic courses. Viral pneumonias may present early or late in the neonatal period. Although chlamydial infection occurs in the perinatal period, pneumonitis usually presents after the third week of life.

Bacterial pneumonia in the initial neonatal period may be appropriately treated with a penicillin (penicillin or ampicillin) and an aminoglycoside (gentamycin or kanamycin) until pathogenic identification is obtained. Later in the neonatal period, the possibility of other pathogens may necessitate modification of this antibiotic therapy.

Apnea

Preterm neonates frequently experience pauses in their breathing of variable duration. Short respiratory pauses are usually benign. Short pauses recurring repetitively in a regular pattern are called periodic breathing. This breathing, normal in neonates, is not accompanied by signs of clinical deterioration and requires no treatment. Periods of absent respiration of more than 10 to 15 seconds are generally defined as apneas and may be accompanied by bradycardia or cyanosis. Recent observations in neonates indicate that nasal airflow may be absent despite the presence of respiratory efforts. Apneas have subsequently been classified as follows: obstructive apnea—respiratory efforts occur during the absence of airflow; central apnea—a complete absence of respiratory effort and airflow; and mixed apnea—a combination of both patterns. Airway obstruction at the oropharynx is thought to occur in obstructive or mixed apneas.

It has commonly been accepted that apneic episodes in preterm infants are rare during the first day of life. While in infants with mild to moderate RDS respiratory pauses and apneas are rare during the acute illness, these events are as common in healthy infants throughout the first week of life (Fig 2–14). These findings are consistent with previous observations of Daily, who found that the incidence of long apneas (>30 secs) was unchanged throughout the first 10 days of life. In contrast, in adequately oxygenated infants with RDS, apneas usually do not appear until the lung disease resolves.

By far the most common apnea in neonates is idiopathic apnea of prematurity. Diagnosis is based upon the exclusion of a variety of apnea-related conditions (Fig 2–15) that must be considered and ruled out because they require

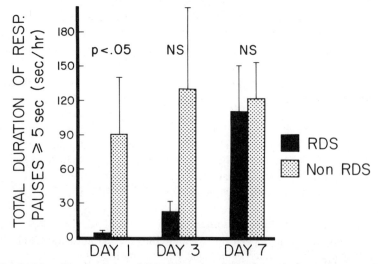

Fig 2–14.—Comparison of the total duration of respiratory pauses greater than 5 seconds in two groups of preterm infants with or without RDS, during the first week of life. (From Carlo, et al.: Am. Rev. Respir. Dis. 126:103, 1982.)

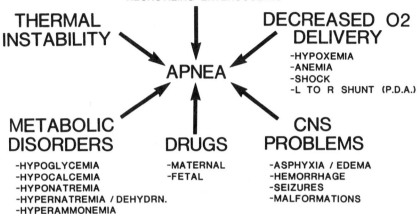

Fig 2–15.—Specific causes of apnea to be considered in the differential diagnosis of apnea of prematurity.

specific therapy. Treatment for idiopathic apnea of prematurity depends on the severity of the clinical presentation. While tactile stimulation or water beds may be adequate for mildly sick infants, low CPAP (3 to 5 cm H_2O), or theophylline (or caffeine) may be required for sicker ones. CPAP has been shown to preferentially resolve obstructive apnea, while theophylline is beneficial for all types. Severely apneic infants may require endotracheal intubation and assisted ventilation.

Transient Tachypnea of the Newborn

This syndrome, not always transient, usually follows an uneventful term pregnancy and is first detected in the transitional care nursery if the infant has a persistently high respiratory rate. This entity occurs more frequently in infants delivered by cesarean section. Cyanosis is not a prominent feature, although a few infants may require 35 to 40% oxygen to remain pink. Air exchange is good with no rales, rhonchi, or intercostal retractions, and expiratory grunt may be present but arterial pH and $PaCO_2$ measurements should be within normal limits. The chest x-ray film reveals central perihilar streaking and usually can be distinguished from meconium aspiration or RDS.

In most cases, respirations decrease gradually during the first 3 days of life, and the infant is usually able to go home when the mother is discharged from the hospital. The pathogenesis has not been clarified; however, it has been suggested that this syndrome may be secondary to slow absorption of lung fluid. Fluid remaining in the periarterial tissue would explain the x-ray findings, and lung compliance would be decreased because of the additional fluid. The infant's increased respiratory rate then would minimize respiratory work. The syndrome appears to be self-limited, and there have been no reported complications.

Pneumothorax and Other Air Leak Syndromes

An asymptomatic pneumothorax is found in about 1% of all routine newborn chest radiographic examinations. Considering the very high intrathoracic pressures recorded during the first minutes of life, it is surprising that pneumothorax is not a more frequent occurrence. Pneumothorax and other air leak syndromes are common complications in infants with RDS occurring in as many as one third of those requiring assisted ventilation. In infants with meconium aspiration syndrome, the incidence of air leaks may be even higher.

Macklin described the path of the air after rupture: air from the ruptured alveolus dissects up the vascular sheath into the mediastinum and from there may continue into the pleural or pericardial cavities. In some series, as many as half of the symptomatic patients had aspirated meconium or blood. This suggests that obstruction with a ball-valve action may be the basis for the rupture.

Pneumothorax should be suspected in any newborn with respiratory distress, or in a baby on a respirator whose condition suddenly worsens. Cyanosis, tachypnea, grunting, and flaring of the nares are often observed. Percussion is sometimes helpful, but a shift of the apical impulse is usually more easily noted. Auscultation may be misleading because of the wide referral of breath sounds. The sudden onset of a tense, distended abdomen is often a useful clinical feature signifying a pneumothorax. Hypotension or hypertension may be present.

If the pneumothorax is asymptomatic and the infant is free of underlying respiratory disease, no specific therapy is necessary, but color, heart rate, respiratory rate, and blood pressure should be closely observed. If respiratory distress is noted, a thoracostomy tube should be placed in the midaxillary or anterior axillary line. The effectiveness in evacuating a pneumothorax depends on achieving anterior placement of the tip of the thoracostomy tube. Lung perforation, a major complication of thoracostomy, may occur in as many as 25% of treated infants and can be prevented in part, by careful insertion technique, especially by eliminating the use of a trocar. Partial obstruction of the thoracic aorta may be observed when a posterior chest tube pushes on mediastinal structures.

Pulmonary interstitial emphysema and pneumomediastinum do not require evacuation, but should alert the clinician to the possibility of other subsequent air leaks, and efforts should be aimed at reducing barotrauma. Rarely, selective bronchial intubation of the nonemphysematous side has been performed in the treatment of interstitial emphysema. Pneumopericardium, on the other hand, has specific clinical manifestations including hypotension, muffled heart sounds, and decreased pulse pressure. Evacuation is usually required. Massive air embolism usually presents with rapid cardiopulmonary deterioration, and air bubbles may be observed in blood obtained from indwelling arterial catheters in patients ventilated at extremely high pressures. There is no specific treatment, and prognosis is poor.

A high-intensity transilluminating light using a fiberoptic probe is especially helpful in quickly diagnosing a pneumothorax. If the infant's clinical condition is relatively stable, it is wise to check the diagnosis radiographically prior to treatment.

SUGGESTED READINGS

General References

Avery, M.E., Fletcher, B.D., and Williams R.G.: *The Lung and Its Disorders in the Newborn Infant* (4th ed.; Philadelphia: W.B. Saunders Co., 1979).
Fanaroff, A.A., and Martin, R.J. (eds.): *Behrman's Neonatal-Perinatal Medicine* (3rd ed., St. Louis: C.V. Mosby Co., 1983).
Klaus, M., and Fanaroff, A. (eds.): *Care of the High-Risk Neonate* (2nd ed., Philadelphia: W.B. Saunders Co., 1979).

Asphyxia and Resuscitation

Adamsons, K., Jr., et al.: The treatment of acidosis with alkali and glucose during asphyxia in foetal rhesus monkey, J. Physiol. 169:679, 1963.
Beard, R.W., and Nathaniels, P.W. (eds.): *Fetal Physiology and Medicine - The Basis of Perinatology* (London: W.B. Saunders Co., 1976).
Carson, B.S., et al.: Combined obstetric and pediatric approach to prevent meconium aspiration syndrome, Am. J. Obstet. Gynecol. 126:712, 1976.
Dawes, G.: *Foetal and Neonatal Physiology* (Chicago: Year Book Medical Publishers, Inc., 1968).
Dawes, G., Hibbard, E., and Windle, W.: The effect of alkali and glucose infusion on permanent brain damage in rhesus monkeys asphyxiated at birth, J. Pediatr. 65:801, 1964.

Transportation

American Academy of Pediatrics' Committee on Fetus and Newborn: *Guidelines for Perinatal Care* (Evanston, Ill.: American Academy of Pediatrics, 1983), p. 185.
Segal, S. (ed.): *Manual for the Transport of High-Risk Newborn Infants: Principles, Policies, Equipment, Techniques* (Vancouver: Canadian Pediatric Society, 1972).

Temperature Control

Adamsons, K., Jr.: The role of thermal factors in fetal and neonatal life, Pediatr. Clin. North Am. 13:599, 1966.
Hey, E.: The relation between environmental temperature and oxygen consumption in the newborn baby, J. Physiol. 200:589, 1969.

Umbilical Vessel Catheterization

Rosenfeld, W., et al.: A new graph for insertion of umbilical artery catheters below the diaphragm, J. Pediatr. 96:735, 1980.

Rosenfeld, W., et al.: Evaluation of graphs for insertion of umbilical artery catheters below the diaphragm, J. Pediatr. 98:627, 1981.

Oxygen Therapy

Duc, G.: Assessment of hypoxia in the newborn: Suggestions for a practical approach, Pediatrics 48:469, 1971.

Ehrenkranz, R.A., et al.: Amelioration of bronchopulmonary dysplasia after vitamin E administration, N. Engl. J. Med. 299:564, 1978.

Emery, J.R., and Peabody, J.L.: Are we misusing transcutaneous PO_2 and PCo_2 measurements in infants with bronchopulmonary dysplasia?(abstract), Pediatr. Res. 17:374A, 1983.

Kao, L.C., et al.: Furosemide acutely decreases airway resistance in chronic bronchopulmonary dysplasia, J. Pediatr. 103:624, 1983.

Kinsey, V., Jacobus, J., and Hemphill, F.: Retrolental fibroplasia: Cooperative study of retrolental fibroplasia in the use of oxygen, Arch. Ophthalmol. 56:481, 1956.

Northway, W., Rosan, R., and Porter, D.: Pulmonary disease following respiratory therapy, N. Engl. J. Med. 276:357, 1967.

Rome, E.S., et al.: Limitations of transcutaneous PO_2 and PCO_2 monitoring in infants with bronchopulmonary dysplasia, Pediatrics 74:217, 1984.

Saldanah, R.L., Cepeda, E.E., and Poland, R.L.: The effect of vitamin E prophylaxis on the incidence and severity of bronchopulmonary dysplasia, J. Pediatr. 101:89, 1982.

Smyth, J.A., et al.: Pulmonary function and bronchial hyperreactivity in long-term survivors of bronchopulmonary dysplasia, Pediatrics 68:336, 1981.

Wedig, K.E., et al.: Bronchopulmonary dysplasia, in Nussbaum E., and Galant, S. (eds.): Clinical Approaches In Pediatric Respiratory Disorders. (San Diego, CA, Academic Press, Inc. 1983).

Respiratory Distress Syndrome

Avery, M.E., Fletcher, B.D., and Williams, R.G.: *The Lung and Its Disorders in the Newborn Infant* (4th ed.; Philadelphia: W.B., Saunders Co., 1979).

Ballard, P.L., et al.: Fetal sex and prenatal betamethasone therapy, J. Pediatr. 97:451, 1980.

Bancalari, E., et al.: Muscle relaxation during IPPV in prematures with RDS(abstract), Pediatr. Res. 14:590, 1980.

Berman, L.S., et al.: Optimum levels of CPAP for tracheal extubation of newborn infants, J. Pediatr. 89:109, 1976.

Clyman, R.I., et al.: Increased shunt through the patent ductus arteriosus after surfactant replacement therapy, J. Pediatr. 100:101, 1982.

Collaborative Group on Antenatal Steroid Therapy: Effect of Antenatal dexamethasone administration on the prevention of respiratory distress syndrome, Am. J. Obstet. Gynecol. 141:276, 1981.

Crone, R.K., and Favorito, J.: The effects of pancuronium bromide on infants with hyaline membrane disease, J. Pediatr. 7:991, 1980.

Donn, S.M., et al.: Prevention of intraventricular haemorrhage in preterm infants by phenobarbitone. A controlled study, Lancet 2:215, 1981.

Engelke, S.C., Roloff, D.W., and Kuhns, L.R.: Postextubation nasal continuous positive airway pressure, Am. J. Dis. Child 136:359, 1982.

Farrell, P.M., and Avery, M.E.: Hyaline membrane disease, Am. Rev. Respir. Dis. 111:657, 1975.

Finer, N.N., and Tomney, P.M.: Controlled evaluation of muscle relaxation in the ventilated neonate. Pediatrics 67:641, 1981.

Fujiwara, T., et al.: Artificial surfactant therapy in hyaline membrane disease, Lancet 1:55, 1980.

Green, T.P., et al.: Furosemide promotes patent ductus arteriosus in premature infants with respiratory-distress syndrome, N. Engl. J. Med. 308:743, 1983.

Hack, M., et al.: Neonatal respiratory distress following elective delivery: A preventable disease? Am. J. Obstet. Gynecol. 126:43, 1976.

Hallman, M., et al.: Isolation of human surfactant from amniotic fluid and a pilot study of its efficacy in respiratory distress syndrome, Pediatrics 71:473, 1983.

Heaf, D.P., et al.: Changes in pulmonary function during the diuretic phase of respiratory distress syndrome, J. Pediatr. 101:103, 1982.

Liggins, G.C., and Howie, M.B.: A controlled trial of antepartum glucocorticoid treatment for prevention of the respiratory distress syndrome in premature infants, Pediatrics 50:515, 1972.

MacArthur, B.A., et al.: School progress and cognitive development of 6-year-old children whose mothers were treated antenatally with betamethasone, Pediatrics 70:99, 1982.

Morgan, M.E.I., et al.: Does phenobarbitone prevent periventricular hemorrhage in very low birth weight babies?: A controlled trial, Pediatrics 70:186, 1982.

Morley, C.J., et al.: Dry artificial lung surfactant and its effect on very premature babies, Lancet 1:64, 1981.

Murphy, B.E.P.: Cortisol and cortisone levels in the cord blood at delivery of infants with and without the respiratory distress syndrome, Am. J. Obstet. Gynecol. 119:1112, 1974.

Najak, Z.D., et al.: Pulmonary effects of furosemide in preterm infants with lung disease, J. Pediatr. 102:758, 1983.

Notter, R.H., and Shapiro, D.L.: Lung surfactant in an era of replacement therapy, Pediatrics 68:781, 1981.

Papageorgiou, A.N., et al.: The antenatal use of betamethasone in the prevention of respiratory distress syndrome: A controlled double-blind study, Pediatrics 63:73, 1979.

Perelman, R.H., and Farrell, P.M.: Analysis of causes of neonatal death in the United States with specific emphasis on fatal hyaline membrane disease, Pediatrics 70:570, 1982.

Pollitzer, M.J., et al.: Pancuronium during mechanical ventilation speeds recovery of lungs of infants with hyaline membrane disease, Lancet 1:346, 1981.

Spitzer, A.R., and Fox, W.W.: Postextubation atelectasis-role of oral versus nasal endotracheal tubes, J. Pediatr. 100:806, 1982.

Stark, A.R., Bascom, R., and Frantz, I.D., III,: Muscle relaxation in mechanically ventilated infants, J. Pediatr. 94:439, 1979.

Taeusch H.W. Jr., et al.: Risk of respiratory distress syndrome after prenatal dexamethasone treatment, Pediatrics 63:64, 1979.

Tochen, M.L.: Orotracheal intubation in the newborn infant: A method for determining depth of tube insertion, J. Pediatr. 95:1050, 1979.

Whitfield, J.M., and Jones, M.D. Jr.: Atelectasis associated with mechanical ventilation for hyaline membrane disease, Crit. Care Med. 8:729, 1980.

Assisted Ventilation

Bland, R.D., et al.: High frequency mechanical ventilation in severe hyaline membrane disease: An alternative treatment? Crit. Care Med. 8:275, 1980.

Carlo, W.A., et al.: Decrease in airway pressure during high-frequency jet ventilation in infants with respiratory distress syndrome, J. Pediatr. 104:101, 1984.

Chatburn, R.L., and McClelland, L.D.: A heat and humidification system for high frequency jet ventilation. Respir. Care 27:1386, 1982.

Fanaroff, A., et al.: Controlled trial of continuous negative external pressure in the treatment of severe respiratory distress syndrome, J. Pediatr. 82:921, 1973.

Frantz, I.D., III, Werthammer, J., and Stark, A.R.: High-frequency ventilation in premature infants with lung disease: Adequate gas exchange at low tracheal pressure, Pediatrics 71:483, 1983.

Gregory, G., et al.: Treatment of the idiopathic respiratory distress syndrome with continuous positive airway pressure, N. Engl. J. Med. 283:1333, 1971.

Kattwinkel, J., et al.: A device for administration of continuous positive airway pressure by the nasal route, Pediatrics 52:131, 1973.

Mammel, M.C., et al.: Comparison of high-frequency jet ventilation and conventional mechanical ventilation in a meconium aspiration model, J. Pediatr. 103:630, 1983.

Marchak, B.E., et al.: Treatment of RDS by high-frequency oscillatory ventilation: A preliminary report, J. Pediatr. 99:287, 1981.

Pokora, T., et al.: Neonatal high-frequency jet ventilation, Pediatrics 72:27, 1983.

Reynolds, E.: Effect of alterations in mechanical ventilator settings on pulmonary gas exchange in hyaline membrane disease, Arch. Dis. Child. 46:246, 1971.

Special Conference Report. High frequency ventilation for immature infants. Report of a conference, March 2–4, 1982. Pediatrics 71:280, 1983.

Meconium Aspiration/Persistent Fetal Circulation

Brett, C., et al.: Developmental follow-up of hyperventilated neonates: Preliminary observations, Pediatrics 68:588, 1981.

Carson, B.S., et al.: Combined obstetric and pediatric approach to prevent meconium aspiration syndrome, Am. J. Obstet. Gynecol. 126:712, 1976.

Drummond, W.H., et al.: The independent effects of hyperventilation, tolazoline, and dopamine on infants with persistent pulmonary hypertension, J. Pediatr. 98:603, 1981.

Fox, W.W., et al.: The therapeutic application of end-expiratory pressure in the meconium aspiration syndrome, Pediatrics 56:214, 1976.

Goetzman, B.W., et al.: Neonatal hypoxia and pulmonary vasospasm: Response to tolazoline, J. Pediatr. 89:617, 1976.

Gregory, G.A., et al.: Meconium aspiration in infants—A prospective study, J. Pediatr. 85:848, 1974.

Kirkpatrick, B.V., et al.: Use of extracorporeal membrane oxygenation for respiratory failure in term infants, Pediatrics 72:872, 1983.

Murphy, J.D., et al.: The structural basis of persistent pulmonary hypertension of the newborn infant, J. Pediatr. 98:962, 1981.

Riggs, T., et al.: Persistence of fetal circulation syndrome: An echocardiographic study, J. Pediatr. 91:626, 1977.

Soifer, S.J., Morin F.C., III, and Heymann, M.A.: Prostaglandin D_2 reverses induced pulmonary hypertension in the newborn lamb, J. Pediatr. 100:458, 1982.

Starks, G.C.: Correlation of meconium-stained amniotic fluid, early intrapartum fetal pH, and Apgar scores as predictors of perinatal outcome, Obstet. Gynecol. 56:604, 1980.

Ting, P., and Brady, J.P.: Tracheal suction in meconium aspiration, Am. J. Obstet. Gynecol. 122:767, 1975.

Truog, W.E., et al.: Effects of PEEP and tolazoline infusion on respiratory and inert gas exchange in experimental meconium aspiration, J. Pediatr. 100:284, 1982.

Yeh, T.F., et al.: Roentgenographic findings in infants with meconium aspiration syndrome, JAMA 242:60, 1979.

Pneumothorax and Air Leaks Syndromes

Brans, Y.W., Pitts, M., and Cassady, G.: Neonatal pneumopericardium, Am. J. Dis. Child. 130:393, 1976.

Brooks, J.G., et al.: Selective bronchial intubation for the treatment of severe localized pulmonary interstitial emphysema in newborn infants, J. Pediatr. 91:652, 1977.

Fletcher, B.D.: Medial herniation of the parietal pleura: A useful sign of pneumothorax in supine neonates, Am. J. Roentgenol. 130:469, 1978.

Goldberg, R.N.: Sustained arterial blood pressure elevation associated with pneumothoraces: Early detection via continuous monitoring, Pediatrics 68:775, 1981.

Gooding, C.A., et al.: Medially deployed thoracostomy tubes: Cause of aortic obstruction in newborns, ARJ 136:511, 1981.

Henderson-Smart, D.J.: Massive air embolism in a neonate with respiratory distress, Med. J. Aust. 2:641, 1975.

Kuhns, L.R., et al.: Diagnosis of pneumothorax or pneumomediastinum in the neonate by transillumination, Pediatrics 56:355, 1975.

Lipscomb, A.P., et al.: Pneumothorax and cerebral haemorrhage in preterm infants, Lancet I:414, 1981.

Madansky, D.L., et al.: Pneumothorax and other forms of pulmonary air leak in newborns, Am. Rev. Respir. Dis. 120:729, 1979.

Moessinger, A.C., Driscoll, J.M., Jr., and Wigger, H.J.: High incidence of lung perforation by chest tube in neonatal pneumothorax, J. Pediatr. 92:635, 1978.

Ng, K.P.K., and Easa, D.: Management of interstitital emphysema by high-frequency low positive-pressure hand ventilation in the neonate, J. Pediatr. 95:117, 1979.

Pneumonia

Baker, C.S.,: Group B streptococcal infections in neonates, Pediatr. Rev. 1:5, 1979.

Leonidas, J.C., et al.: Radiographic findings of early onset neonatal group B streptococcal septicemia, Pediatrics 59:1006, 1977.

Phillip, A.G., and Hewitt, J.R.: Early diagnosis of neonatal sepsis, Pediatrics 65:1036, 1980.

Transient Tachypnea of the Newborn

Avery, M.E., Gatewood, O.B., and Brumley, G.: Transient tachypnoea of newborn. Possible delayed resorption of fluid at birth, Am. J. Dis. Child. 111:380, 1966.

Apnea

Carlo, W.A., et al.: The effect of respiratory distress syndrome on chest wall movements and respiratory pauses in preterm infants, Am. Rev. Respir. Dis. 126:103, 1982.

Daily, W.J.R., Klaus, M., and Meyer, H.P.B.: Apnea in premature infants: Monitoring, incidence, heart rate changes, and an effect of environmental temperature, Pediatrics 45:510, 1969.

Henderson-Smart, D.J.: The effect of gestational age on the incidence and duration of recurrent apnea in newborn babies, Aust. Paediatr. J. 17:273, 1981.

Korner, A.F., et al.: Effects of waterbed flotation on premature infants: A pilot study, Pediatrics 56:361, 1975.

Miller, M.J., Carlo, W.A., and Martin, R.J.: Continuous positive airway pressure selectively reduces obstructive apnea in preterm infants. J. Pediatr. 106:91, 1985.

Myers, T.F., et al.: Low dose theophylline therapy in idiopathic apnea of prematurity, J. Pediatr. 96:99, 1980.

Perlstein, P.H., Edwards, N.K., and Sutherland, J.M.: Apnea in premature infants and incubator-air-temperature changes, N. Engl. J. Med. 282:461, 1970.

Roberts, J.L., Mathew, O.P., and Thach, B.T.: The efficacy of theophylline in premature infants with mixed and obstructive apnea and apnea associated with pulmonary and neurologic disease, J. Pediatr. 100:968, 1982.

Shannon, D.C., et al.: Prevention of apnea and bradycardia in low birthweight infants, Pediatrics 55:589, 1975.

Thach, B.T., and Stark, A.R.: Spontaneous neck flexion and airway obstruction during apneic spells in preterm infants, J. Pediatr. 92:275, 1979.

Uauy, R., et al.: Treatment of severe apnea in prematures with orally administered theophylline, Pediatrics 55:595, 1975.

Respiratory Diseases and Treatment

CAROLYN M. KERCSMAR, M.D.
ROBERT C. STERN, M.D.

3

THE CONDITIONS discussed in this chapter account for virtually all admissions of infants for pediatric pulmonary disease after the newborn period. Enough information about the pathophysiology of each disease is included to explain the role of the respiratory therapist in the treatment. The chapter begins with a consideration of the rationale for oxygen and mist therapy. Details concerning the techniques of supplying this therapy are found in Chapter 5. Sections covering atelectasis, pneumothorax, and respiratory failure are followed by discussion of the individual disease entities.[5]

OXYGEN THERAPY

Hypoxemia occurs very early in both acute and chronic pulmonary diseases. Although there is a mechanism to minimize the effect of localized pulmonary disease by decreasing perfusion to the more severely affected areas, some intrapulmonary shunting of blood inevitably occurs. Metabolic alterations to reduce the effect of hypoxemia (such as a rise in the level of red blood cell 2,3-diphosphoglycerate, rise in hematocrit value, and the renal compensation for respiratory acidosis) help, but hypoxemia still can be a substantial stress to the patient. Increasing the environmental oxygen concentration results in elevations of arterial P_{O_2} in such patients and therefore eliminates or decreases the stress of hypoxemia.

Oxygen therapy has three primary drawbacks:

1. In patients with chronic hypercapnia, hypoxemia is the most important stimulus to continued respiration. A sudden increase in the arterial P_{O_2} of such patients may increase the degree of hypoventilation by decreasing the frequency and depth of breathing. Fortunately, chronic hypercapnia is ex-

tremely unusual in patients with pediatric pulmonary disease (except in those with cystic fibrosis).

2. Oxygen is very drying and has other direct toxicity effects on the respiratory epithelium. Humidification of oxygen or use of an oxygen tent with mist is helpful in minimizing this problem.

3. Patients with chronic illness occasionally become rapidly dependent on oxygen therapy. This may delay their discharge from the hospital or necessitate oxygen therapy at home.

Supplemental oxygen is, therefore, theoretically useful in treating virtually all acute pediatric pulmonary diseases (including pneumonia, bronchiolitis and asthma). The decision to use it will depend primarily on the degree of illness and the patient's acceptance of the mask or tent (see chap. 5). Oxygen therapy in the treatment of chronic pulmonary disease is a more complicated problem and will depend, in addition to the above factors, on the response of the arterial P_{CO_2} to the use of oxygen and on the rapidity with which the individual patient can be weaned to room air.

MIST THERAPY

According to its advocates, mist tent therapy for lung disease has two major aims. The first is to prevent insensible water loss and thereby help ensure adequate hydration. Although overhydration has not been shown clearly to be therapeutically useful in thinning respiratory secretions, dehydration does dry secretions and make them viscous and hard to clear. A mist tent may also be helpful in administering supplemental oxygen by ameliorating its drying effect and by eliminating the need for nasal cannulas or masks.

The second major objective of mist therapy is to supply water down to and including the relatively small airways to maintain full humidification or to aid in thinning secretions (see chap. 5). There is considerable controversy at present concerning the usefulness of mist for this purpose. It is agreed that during nasal breathing most large mist particles (greater than 5–6 μm) do not penetrate beyond the nose. Newer mist generators are capable of producing water particles that are in the theoretically optimal range to reach the small airways (1–5 μm). These particles are achieved by using distilled water with either 5% propylene glycol or dilute saline with ultrasonic nebulizers.

There are several possible drawbacks to mist tent therapy. With inadequate sterilization procedures the tent can become the vehicle for spreading pathogens. This problem is related to poor technique and is not an inevitable hazard. Patients with voluminous secretions may become acutely more dyspneic if mist therapy mobilizes secretions more quickly than they can be cleared. If this occurs, mist therapy should be discontinued temporarily and respiratory physical therapy (postural drainage with clapping and vibration) instituted. The same patient may benefit later from mist therapy. A rare patient may develop bronchospasm with mist, as a reaction to either the water or the propylene glycol. It may not be possible to use mist therapy if this occurs; however, the same patient may tolerate mist at a later time. Another potential hazard of mist therapy is that the patient may be obscured by the mist, thus making intermittent nursing observation more difficult. This is particularly true of croup patients who are treated in "steam rooms."

Large-particle mist therapy is also a time-honored and well-accepted treatment for croup (see chap. 5).

ATELECTASIS

Complete obstruction of an airway (from extrinsic compression, inflammatory obstruction, mucus plug or foreign body) results in slow resorption of air distal to the point of obstruction and subsequent collapse of that portion of lung. Microscopic areas of collapse commonly occur in patients with cystic fibrosis secondary to the retention of viscous mucus that blocks small bronchioles. Obstruction of larger bronchi (as with a foreign body) results in segmental or lobar atelectasis. The blood flowing through an atelectatic area is not oxygenated, and a degree of systemic hypoxemia results. Normal areas of lung are able to compensate for the collapsed area by increasing their elimination of carbon dioxide, preventing systemic hypercapnia.

Atelectasis compromises the mucociliary apparatus and eliminates the effect of cough for the area involved, thus making it more susceptible to infection. Chronic infection in an atelectatic area leads to irreversible bronchiectasis or abscess formation that may then endanger other portions of the lung.

TREATMENT.—Atelectasis is a symptom of another underlying disease, and diagnostic efforts will be in progress simultaneously with the initiation of therapy. Bronchoscopy usually is done early to help rule out the possibility of a foreign body, to suction the airway involved for removal of any mucus plug and to obtain material for culture. Intermittent positive-pressure treatments, occasionally with a decongestant (e.g., phenylephrine) or a bronchodilator (e.g., isoproterenol), may be useful in helping to reexpand the involved lung (see chap. 5). Incentive spirometry is commonly used in the treatment and prevention of atelectasis in postoperative patients and may also be useful in other types of atelectasis as well (see chap. 5). Systemic antibiotics and oral bronchodilators also may be needed.

Continuing collapse, particularly when associated with infection, may necessitate lobectomy to protect the remaining lung.

PLEURAL EFFUSION

The normally expanded lung is immediately adjacent to but not physically joined with the chest wall. The lungs and the internal thoracic wall are each covered by a pleura; a potential space exists between them. Accumulation of fluid within this space results from many intrathoracic diseases as well as some systemic disorders. As the amount of fluid increases, respiration becomes compromised.

The amount of fluid within the pleural cavity is determined by several factors. High pleural capillary hydrostatic pressure and interstitial hydrostatic pressure favor fluid transudation into the pleural space. Reabsorption of pleural fluid occurs largely secondary to high plasma oncotic pressure. Normally the balance between these forces is such that only a very small amount of intrapleural fluid is present.

PATHOPHYSIOLOGY.—Pleural fluid accumulates when the rate of formation exceeds the rate of reabsorption. Inflammatory processes increase capillary permeability, allowing accumulation of pleural fluid. Even normal reabsorptive mechanisms may then be inadequate. Elevated systemic hydrostatic pressures also may result in increased pleural fluid. When lymphatic drainage is obstructed, pleural fluid accumulates due to impaired reabsorption. As capillary osmotic pressure falls, as in hypoproteinemic states, fluid transudation occurs. Major clinical conditions that produce pleural effusions include parenchymal lung infection, malignancy, congestive heart failure, collagen vascular disease, hypoproteinemia, and uremia.[1]

CLINICAL PRESENTATION.—Small pleural effusions may be asymptomatic. Large amounts of accumulated pleural fluid restrict lung expansion, and respiratory distress ensues. Depending on the size of the effusion, the degree of respiratory embarassment may be mild or severe. When effusions result from inflammatory processs, chest pain is often prominent. Symptoms produced by an underlying disease process may also be the predominant features.

DIAGNOSIS.—Physical examination of the patient with pleural effusion reveals dullness to percussion over the affected hemithorax. Breath sounds are typically decreased or absent; however, infants may exhibit normal or tubular breath sounds. Fremitus is decreased, and a pleural friction rub may be heard.

X-ray films usually reveal loss of the costovertebral angles and cardiophrenic angles, and a density obscuring the underlying lung parenchyma, but approximately 300 to 400 ml of fluid must have accumulated before these radiologic findings will occur. Ultrasound of the thorax can usually identify much smaller amounts of fluid.

Thoracentesis can be performed for both diagnostic and therapeutic purposes. The aspirated fluid can be identified as exudate, transudate, empyema (infected fluid), blood, or chyle. Exudates and transudates can be differentiated on the basis of serum and pleural fluid proteins and lactic acid dehydrogenase (LDH). A pleural-fluid serum protein ratio above 0.5 and/or a pleural-fluid serum LDH ratio above 0.6 and/or an absolute pleural fluid LDH greater than 200 IU describe an exudate. Bacteriologic cultures of pleural fluid are almost always obtained. Specimens of pleural fluid should be sent for cytologic examination if a malignancy is possible.

THERAPY.—Treatment includes measures directed at the underlying disease process. When respiratory compromise is significant, removal of pleural fluid may be beneficial. Therapeutic thoracentesis is often not needed in patients with pneumococcal pneumonia, congestive heart failure, or marked hypoproteinemia because effusions accompanying these disorders usually resolve with appropriate medical therapy. Clinical judgment must be exercised in all cases, however. When pleural effusion is likely to recur, an indwelling chest tube may be placed for continuous drainage. In the case of malignant effusion, a sclerosing agent such as talc can be instilled through the chest tube into the thoracic cavity. This procedure may prevent reaccumulation of the fluid.

PNEUMOTHORAX

The left and right pleural cavities in humans are separated completely by the mediastinum. Free air in one of the pleural cavities (pneumothorax) interferes with expansion of the lung. Pneumothorax can result from entry of air through the chest wall (as in penetrating trauma) or leakage from the lung itself (as from a ruptured cyst). If the leak allows free passage of air, the lung on that side collapses in proportion to the amount of free air that enters the thorax before equilibrium is reached. If the leak is a "ball valve" type in which air enters the pleural space with inspiration but cannot escape during expiration, a tension pneumothorax is said to be present. In this circumstance, the pressure of free air on the involved side of the chest may be sufficient to cause the mediastinum to shift toward the normal lung and restrict its expansion as well.

Pneumothorax may occur spontaneously in apparently healthy individuals, particularly in young men. However, in children, it usually results from chronic obstructive pulmonary disease with the rupture of a bleb.

The severity of the symptoms arising from sudden pneumothorax varies with both the amount of lung collapse and the degree of antecedent lung disease. A pneumothorax in an individual with normal or near-normal lungs generally causes sudden, severe dyspnea and chest pain. When pneumothorax is secondary to long-standing pulmonary disease, it tends to occur on the side with more extensive involvement. Since the patient already has made physiologic adjustments to shunt pulmonary blood flow away from the more diseased lung, the increase in symptoms is often surprisingly small, and the pain may be minimal. Occasionally, pneumothorax may be discovered in such patients by routine follow-up chest x-ray films at a time when no new symptoms are present.

TREATMENT.—Small pneumothoraces, especially if asymptomatic, frequently are left untreated. If the defect that caused the leakage of air already has healed, the free air gradually will be resorbed, and the lung will expand completely again. Administration of 100% oxygen may hasten resolution by increasing the nitrogen gradient between the pleural space and the blood. With more complete collapse, especially if there is evidence of a ball valve effect, insertion of a chest tube with continuous suction is indicated to evacuate the air. The tube can be removed after the leak has stopped, and, frequently, other specific treatment is not required. Recurrent pneumothorax requires more drastic surgical treatment (through as small an incision as possible) consisting of removal of blebs and pleural abrasions or instillation of an irritant such as silver nitrate, Atabrine, or tetracycline into the pleural space to stimulate scarring and adhesion of the lung to the chest wall. Frequently, both excision of abnormal lung and a scarifying procedure are done. All patients with bilateral pneumothorax should be treated with chest tubes because of the possibility of additional leakage with progression to life-threatening restriction of the expansion of both lungs.

Treatment of underlying chronic pulmonary disease with antibiotics, physical therapy, or aerosols is continued, although the presence of chest tubes and pleural pain will limit the amount of physical therapy the patient can tolerate. Supplemental oxygen may be required. In general, if surgical treatment is indicated, it is wise to proceed before continued chest pain and suboptimal treatment of the underlying disease further weaken the patient. With good supportive care, the necessary surgical procedures and anesthesia can be carried out safely in chronic pulmonary patients.

Most patients with pneumothorax require oxygen therapy either until the chest tube is inserted or, if no surgical treatment is started, until the free air is partially resorbed. Routine aerosol treatment should continue. Positive-pressure treatments may be used, but the possibility that they may keep a leak from sealing or produce another pneumothorax (even on the opposite side) must be considered.

RESPIRATORY FAILURE

In patients with any progressive pulmonary disease involving either obstruction of the airways or destruction of pulmonary tissue, hypoxemia occurs relatively early. All blood passing through the alveoli normally is completely oxygenated. Thus, if there is localized disease and oxygenation is incomplete, the remainder of the lung cannot compensate fully by increasing the oxygen supply to the blood. Although perfusion of diseased areas of the lungs generally is reduced, enough blood does go to these areas to result in systemic hypoxemia. Hypoxemia tends to become more severe with progression of the underlying disease.

In the normal lung the elimination of carbon dioxide is not being carried out at a maximal rate. In fact, the ability to increase the elimination of CO_2 during times of metabolic acidosis constitutes one of the primary mechanisms of defense against changes in blood pH. Thus, the normal person can decrease his Pa_{CO2} voluntarily by hyperventilation. With steadily increasing pulmonary disease, localized areas of lung that are severely involved gradually may become unable to do their share of CO_2 elimination. At first, this deficiency can be compensated for by hyperventilation of the portions of more normal lung. In this way, the Pa_{CO2} can be maintained at normal levels until late in the course of progressive pulmonary disease. However, when the arterial P_{CO_2} begins to rise, the clinician knows that vast areas of lung are working very poorly and that the remaining, more normal lung cannot compensate adequately even with maximal effort. This is alveolar hypoventilation. Clearly, a rise in arterial P_{CO_2} is ominous. Any patient with an elevated arterial P_{CO_2} is said to be in respiratory failure.

An elevated or rising $PaCO_2$ not only has grave import as a guide to the adequacy of ventilation, but in itself constitutes a risk to the patient. First, the inability to maintain or to lower arterial PcO_2 deprives the body of its primary defense against metabolic acidosis. A simultaneous disease process resulting in acidosis will, therefore, put the patient in great danger. Second, at very high levels, carbon dioxide acts as an anesthetic on the central nervous system and as a respiratory depressant.

An intensive attack on the underlying pulmonary disease is required and may include antibiotics, postural drainage, bronchodilators, and/or corticosteroids.[4] Respiratory therapy measures will assist both in the treatment of the underlying disease and in the management of the respiratory failure itself.

PEDIATRIC DISEASE ENTITIES

Acute Upper Airway Obstruction

Rapidly increasing upper airway obstruction results in a characteristic progression of symptoms and physical findings (Table 3–1). At first, there is only a hoarse voice and a barking cough. Inspiration then becomes increasingly difficult and is associated with a rasping sound called *stridor*. Further obstruction results in severe dyspnea and the associated hypoxia is reflected clinically by restlessness and air hunger (usually with pallor) and then florid cyanosis. As shown in Table 3–1, the patient rapidly tires and hypercapnia occurs, which together with severe hypoxia can quickly lead to coma and death. This progression can be extremely rapid; the sequence from initial barking cough, or stridor, to death may occur in as little as ½ to 2 hours.

The symptom complex frequently referred to as *croup* has an initial clinical presentation that often includes inspiratory difficulties, a barking cough, and stridor. A wide range of underlying conditions can cause acute airway obstruction. Proper treatment of croup requires correct diagnosis of the underlying cause as well as immediate measures to relieve or circumvent the obstruction if necessary. Most acute airway obstruction results from infection. Infection of the epiglottis and surrounding tissues (epiglottitis or, more correctly, supraglottitis) is always life-threatening (see below).

Most cases of croup are caused by viral infection of the subglottic area,

TABLE 3–1.—SEQUENCE OF EVENTS IN PROGRESSIVE UPPER
AIRWAY OBSTRUCTION

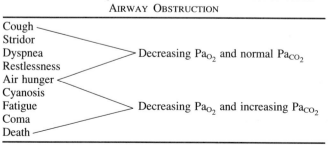

although the disease can also result from neck trauma with bleeding into the tissues of the airway, an allergic reaction with edema, or a foreign body. In patients with diphtheria, a membrane can form in the upper airway and cause obstruction. Diphtherial croup, which caused the death of many infants and children until an effective immunization method was developed, has become a very rare disease in this country. However, the recent increase in the number of inadequately immunized children in the United States may result in new outbreaks of the disease.

EPIGLOTTITIS

Epiglottitis (supraglottitis) results from bacterial infection and subsequent inflammatory edema of the supraglottic laryngeal structures, primarily the epiglottis and hypopharynx. While the aryepiglottic folds and arytenoids may also exhibit marked swelling, the vocal cords, subglottic tissues, and trachea are usually not involved; simultaneous pneumonia is uncommon. Complete airway obstruction can occur precipitously. Epiglottitis, therefore, constitutes a true pediatric emergency; all providers of health care for children must be able to diagnose and treat this life-threatening disease rapidly.

ETIOLOGY.—Epiglottitis is almost always caused by *Hemophilus influenzae* type b. Although several other common respiratory tract pathogens, such as beta-hemolytic streptococcus, pneumococcus, and *Staphylococcus aureus* have been implicated in epiglottitis, they are, at most, rare causes of the disease. Viruses have not been demonstrated as etiologic agents in eipglottitis. *H. influenzae* is commonly found in the nasopharynx of asymptomatic children. Although carriage does not appear to predispose to infection, it does contribute to spread of disease.

EPIDEMIOLOGY.—Epiglottitis probably accounts for approximately 10 to 15% of all systemic *H. influenzae* infections. Most illness occurs in the early winter and spring. Children under 2 years of age rarely contract epiglottitis, and the peak age of incidence is between 3 and 6 years. Epiglottitis is not uncommon, however, in those aged 6 to 8 years. There is no appreciable male/female predominance in the incidence of epiglottitis.

CLINICAL MANIFESTATIONS.—Typically, children with epiglottitis develop acute febrile illness without a significant prodrome. Fever is usually significant (>39 C) and is accompanied by a variable degree of respiratory distress. The child is initially hoarse, or even aphonic, and complains of a sore throat. Drooling is often a prominent feature. Inspiratory stridor may be marked unless obstruction has already limited airflow.

Physical examination characteristically reveals a febrile, toxic-appearing child in moderate or marked respiratory distress. Inspection shows moderate to severe retractions. If the degree of respiratory obstruction is severe, the patient may also show altered (depressed) mental status. However, the hypoxemia and discomfort may produce marked agitation. As swelling progresses, the child assumes a position of sitting up, leaning forward with the chin thrust outward in an attempt to maintain the airway. Cough is not a prominent feature. Complete airway obstruction can occur abruptly and may be precipitated by numerous (often unnecessary) manipulations of the patient.

Management of children with epiglottitis involves appropriate confirmation of the diagnosis, establishment of an adequate airway, and antibiotics. Strict attention to the clinical history should arouse suspicion early in cases of epiglottitis. Once the diagnosis is entertained, the child should be made as comfortable and relaxed as possible while preparations for further procedures are rapidly made. Physical examination must be performed briefly and include no unnecessary anxiety-provoking procedures. Notably, the child should be seated on a parent's lap, and no attempt should be made to examine the pharynx directly. Pharyngeal examination can precipitate laryngospasm. Oxygen may be offered by mask, but care must be taken that the child does not become frightened and that signs of respiratory failure and hypercarbia are not masked. X-ray films of the lateral neck reveal a swollen protuberant epiglottis, but such studies are rarely needed. Patients with suspected epiglottitis should never be sent to the radiology department alone; radiographic studies should be performed rapidly and in the presence of a physician who is prepared to establish an artificial airway. The diagnosis of epiglottitis is confirmed by direct visualization of a swollen, inflamed epiglottis. This procedure is carried out only in the operating room with experienced anesthesiologists and surgeons in attendance. An airway is established via naso- or orotracheal intubation; tracheostomy is performed only if intubation is not possible. Nasotracheal tubes are usually better tolerated and certainly incur less morbidity than does tracheostomy. The patient is then further cared for in an intensive care unit. Mechanical ventilation is rarely necessary in uncomplicated cases, and humidified air or oxygen is all that is required. Careful observation is necessary to aid in keeping the airway free of inspissated secretions and to prevent accidental extubation. The duration of intubation varies between 12 hours and 5 days, but most patients are ready for extubation in 36 to 48 hours. In an intensive care setting with appropriate personnel immediately available for reintubation, the endotracheal tube may be safely removed. There is no conclusive evidence that administration of corticosteroids facilitates extubation.

The majority of patients will have *H. influenzae* recovered from blood cultures. Swabs of the epiglottis may also be positive. Intravenous antibiotic therapy with ampicillin and/or chloramphenicol should be instituted promptly pending culture and sensitivity reports. Intravenous therapy is usually necessary for only several days, and oral antibiotics then substituted.

Deaths from epiglottitis are preventable if the disease is recognized rapidly and treated aggressively. In the absence of placement of an artificial airway, mortality ranges from 6 to 25%, while those managed with either endotracheal intubation or tracheostomy have less than 1% mortality.

LARYNGOTRACHEOBRONCHITIS (CROUP)

Acute laryngotracheobronchitis (LTB, croup) is characterized primarily by laryngeal and subglottic inflammation leading to some degree of upper airway obstruction. The degree of lower respiratory tract involvement varies, but frank pneumonia occasionally develops. Most croup results from viral infection of the upper and/or lower respiratory tract; allergic mechanisms have been postulated to play a role in spasmodic croup. Children whose subglottic airways are congenitally narrow or have been compromised by disease or previous intubation are sometimes very susceptible to viral croup and may develop life-threatening obstruction.

ETIOLOGY.—Most croup is caused by parainfluenza viruses; adenoviruses, respiratory syncytial viruses, and influenza are less frequent etiologic agents. Parainfluenza is a ubiquitous virus. However, among the serotypes some seasonal variation does exist. Type 1 predominates in the autumn, and large outbreaks occur in even-numbered years. Epidemics of Type 2 parainfluenza peak in the fall months of odd-numbered years, but the outbreaks are much less predictable. Type 3 virus is endemic.

EPIDEMIOLOGY.—Type 1 and Type 2 parainfluenza are the major causes of croup in children aged 8 to 30 months. Primary infection with Type 3 has a peak occurrence in infancy. More young boys develop serious croup secondary to Types 1 and 2 parainfluenza than do girls. Parainfluenza Type 3 produces identical infection rates in both sexes. Repeated episodes of croup are not uncommon.

CLINICAL MANIFESTATIONS.—Children with croup have laryngeal and subglottic narrowing secondary to inflammatory edema. They present with a mildly febrile illness whose major features are barking cough and stridor. Children with viral croup often have had other symptoms of respiratory illness (e.g., coryza, cough, etc.) for several days before the stridor develops. The symptoms usually worsen gradually and may increase at night or when the child attempts to sleep. Physical examination typically reveals a febrile child in mild to moderate respiratory distress. Slight coryza may be evident, but examination of the pharynx is usually normal. Chest wall and suprasternal retractions may be prominent as the airway obstruction progresses. Unless pneumonia or profound upper airway obstruction is present, auscultation of the thorax is unremarkable. A lateral neck x-ray film usually is normal, although subglottic edema can occasionally be seen. The epiglottis is normal. The anteroposterior (AP) chest or neck film often demonstrates the subglottic narrowing. While the white blood cell count may be slightly elevated, there are no other characteristic features of the complete blood count. When involvement of the lower airways accompanies croup, edema and secretions lead to significant ventilation-perfusion abnormalities. A marked degree of hypoxia may therefore be reflected in the arterial blood gas. Other signs of hypoxemia such as anxiety, tachypnea, and trachycardia can also occur and usually precede cyanosis.

Spasmodic croup typically occurs in boys between 2 and 4 years of age. The onset of upper airway obstruction is acute and usually has no obvious infectious prodrome. Symptoms characteristically first appear at night, with the child awakening from sleep with stridor and a barking cough. No fever is present. The physical appearance is otherwise not unlike that seen in infectious croup. The symptoms, however, often remit dramatically with exposure to cool humidified air. The observation that some patients improve after vomiting has led to the fairly widespread practice of inducing vomiting (e.g., with syrup of ipecac). If such treatment is ineffective, however, the patient will still have respiratory symptoms, but then will also be vomiting.

TREATMENT.—The vast majority of children with croup can be successfully managed at home. Fewer than 10% of children with croup require hospital admission. The mainstay of therapy is cool, humidified air, (i.e., large-particle mist). At home, this may involve sitting with the child in the bathroom with a hot shower going to steam up the room. Cold-mist vaporizers may also be used. These are safer than hot-air nebulizers, as there is no risk of accidental burning or overwarming of the child. It is unclear whether there is any other advantage of cool air over warm air.

Children with croup who present to the emergency room with moderate-to-marked stridor while at rest usually require hospitalization. The in-hospital treatment of croup generally includes large particle mist and close observation, and may include oxygen and intravenous hydration. Although it is important to minimize anxiety-provoking procedures such as blood drawing, careful attention to the child's respiratory status must be maintained constantly.

Laboratory procedures and nonpertinent physical examinations should be postponed. Parents are encouraged to stay with and comfort the child. Frequent monitoring of vital signs is mandatory, as rising respiratory and pulse rates often herald hypoxemia. Hypercarbia is often a late finding and is preceded by fatigue, increased chest wall retractions, and change in vital signs. Arterial blood gases should be examined only when there is difficulty in assessing the child clinically. Sedation is not recommended as it may lead to further respiratory depression.

Humidity is usually supplied either via a "fog room" or a "croup tent." The fog room allows the patient substantial freedom as well as direct contact with a parent. While oxygen can be readily mixed into the croup tent, children are often frightened when confined. Moreover, it is sometimes difficult to view patients adequately in a misty oxygen tent. Although many children with croup demonstrate hypoxemia, oxygen administration is often not necessary. However, severe hypoxemia must be avoided. Some children are frightened by a face mask thus making oxygen delivery difficult; a parent may be recruited to both comfort the child and hold the oxygen mask. Patients receiving oxygen must be carefully monitored, as relief from hypoxemia may temporarily mask progression of airway obstruction.

It is important to maintain adequate hydration during the acute illness. Water losses from the respiratory tree are minimized while the child is in a humidified enviroment. With the aid of a parent or skilled nurse, most children with croup may be fed orally. Intravenous fluids for hydration may be necessary when patients are unable to tolerate oral feedings.

The role of corticosteroids in the treatment of croup remains controversial. Reported studies do not clearly show that they are useful, but many patients receive corticosteroids early in the disease in order to reduce or prevent inflammatory obstruction. In the dosage schedules administered, there is little likelihood of toxicity. Their actual role in treatment of croup awaits future definitive studies.

Aerosolized racemic epinephrine given with or without positive pressure is a useful adjunct in the treatment of patients with acute laryngotracheobronchitis. Racemic epinephrine is composed of equal parts of D and L isomers of epinephrine. The L isomer is 15 to 20 times more active than the D form. The drug's presumed action is to reduce the inflammatory edema in the subglottis by virtue of its vasoconstrictive properties. A 1:8 dilution can be given as often as every 30 minutes. Intermittent positive pressure administration is probably unnecessary, and simple nebulization with oxygen will suffice. Because rebound edema can occur up to several hours following an aerosol, racemic epinephrine should not be administered to outpatients.

Croup is infrequently severe enough to warrant an artificial airway; under 5% of all children admitted to the hospital with croup require tracheostomy or endotracheal intubation. Nevertheless, hospital areas used for croup treatment must be equipped with a laryngoscope and various sizes of oro- and nasotracheal tubes.

OTHER CAUSES OF ACUTE UPPER AIRWAY OBSTRUCTION

Less common causes of croup can usually be ruled out by historical data or simple laboratory determinations. It is important that they be kept in mind, however, since the treatment required may be substantially different from that described above for viral laryngotracheobronchitis.

Foreign-body aspiration can often be diagnosed by history; a sudden inexplicable choking spell while a child is eating or playing with a small toy may be followed by croup symptoms. Some foreign bodies are visible on x-ray films, but usually they are lucent and not visualized. Emergency laryngoscopy/ bronchoscopy is indicated if there is a reasonable chance of foreign-body aspiration.

Allergic croup is fairly uncommon. Usually a history of exposure to a new allergen (e.g., a cat) is easily obtained. These patients may respond to subcutaneous administration of epinephrine. Upper airway obstruction as part of a generalized severe allergic reaction (anaphylaxis) caused by insect sting, ingestion of an allergen (e.g., nuts), or exposure to a potent inhalant allergen is easily diagnosed by history and physical findings (e.g., urticaria or recent bee sting).

Other less common causes of croup include injury to the neck with bleeding into the soft tissues and hypocalcemia with tetany of the laryngeal muscles.

Foreign-Body Aspiration

Although young children frequently put small objects into their mouths, aspiration is uncommon. Occasionally, however, an object too large to be eliminated by the mucociliary clearance system gains access to the tracheobronchial tree and is not expelled immediately by coughing. When this occurs, respiratory symptoms inevitably result, although there may be a delay of hours to days.

If the aspirated object is large enough to occlude the upper airway completely, death from asphyxia occurs quickly. In adults, this may be a more common problem than is generally appreciated. The so-called cafe coronary (a previously well adult dies suddenly while eating in a restaurant) is more likely to be food aspiration than heart disease and if recognized can be treated using the Heimlich maneuver (see below). There are also well-established reports of complete upper airway occlusion by a foreign body in children, but this appears to be exceedingly rare. Immediate treatment at the scene of the event determines the outcome. In older children and adults the diagnosis is made by the extremely sudden onset of aphonia with respiratory distress. An attempt to remove the foreign body by grasping it from above with two fingers or an improvised forceps is occasionally successful but has the risk of impacting the object more firmly into the larynx, converting a partial or nearly complete obstruction into a complete obstruction. Similarly, when a person is thought to have ingested a large foreign body, the common practice of turning him or her upside down and pounding on the back has the disadvantage of potentially impacting the foreign body into the larynx from below.

For older children, the method of treatment introduced by Heimlich[3] is safer and quite effective. In this technique, the "rescuer" either (1) pushes his fist sharply into the epigastrium toward the chest while standing in front of the patient or kneeling at his side or (2) pulls his clasped hands up into the epigastrium while positioned behind the patient. Success with this technique has been reported in all age groups, including infants. Some authorities warn that abdominal thrust may result in serious trauma to the abdominal viscera, notably liver laceration, when the Heimlich maneuver is performed on young children. The current recommendations of the American Academy of Pediatrics for the first aid of the choking, breathless child who cannot cough are to deliver four back blows using the heel of the hand to the area just below and between the child's shoulder blades. The child should first be placed in the head down and prone position. If breathing does not resume, the child is turned over and placed in a supine position on the rescuer's arm. With the opposite hand, the rescuer gives the child four chest thrusts, as is done in external cardiac compression. The mouth should then be inspected for a foreign body. Failure to resuscitate breathing necessitates mouth-to-mouth ventilation. The sequence of maneuvers is repeated if ventilation is not established.

Smaller objects usually impact in one of the mainstem or lobar bronchi and cause more chronic symptoms. The right lung is more often involved than the left. Most likely, an immediate choking episode, possibly with cyanosis, accompanies every aspiration. Although it may be relatively brief and thus go unnoticed by the parents or baby-sitter, it is worth asking about. A surprisingly long asymptomatic interval ranging from hours to weeks may then pass before the patient becomes symptomatic with recurrent lobar pneumonia or intractable wheezing, which is often incorrectly diagnosed as asthma. The wheezing is usually, but not always, unilateral and unresponsive to bronchodilator therapy. Hemoptysis is a rare presenting symptom of foreign-body aspiration.

Diagnosis is made on the basis of history, suggestive symptoms, and radiologic evaluation.. Chest x-ray films including inspiration and expiration films or fluoroscopy of the chest during breathing are necessary and reveal a shift of the mediastinum away from the side of the foreign body during expiration. The foreign body acts as a valve that allows the ipsilateral lung to fill during inspiration but prevents it from emptying completely during expiration until an overinflated equilibrium is established. The normal lung will continue to expand and lose volume as expected during the breathing cycle.

The present treatment of choice is removal of the foreign body by endoscopy under anesthesia. Occasionally, the object cannot be adequately grasped through the rigid bronchoscope, and a thoracotomy is necessary either to "milk the foreign body toward the mouth or, rarely, to enter the lung to remove it. If the nature of the foreign body is known, it may be wise for the endoscopist to practice with a duplicate object to ensure that the equipment is theoretically able to grasp it.

The administration of aerosols with isoproterenol followed by postural drainage with clapping has recently been introduced as an alternative to endoscopy for removal of foreign bodies. Although this technique has undoubtedly been successful, it does not appear to have substantial advantages over the endoscopic approach. In any case, it should not be used for longer than overnight or 24 hours before endoscopy is done.

Asthma

Asthma is a syndrome characterized by intermittent, reversible airway obstruction occurring secondary to bronchial hyperreactivity. The resulting episodes of wheezing and shortness of breath are usually of sudden onset. Some patients exhibit elements of obstructive lung disease between acute attacks.

PATHOPHYSIOLOGY.—Several pathophysiologic pathways may lead to bronchial obstruction. Vigorous contraction of the smooth muscle surrounding the bronchial lumen narrows the airway and decreases ventilation. The presence and reactivity of bronchial smooth muscle exists in all individuals and is not unique to asthmatics. Normally, contraction and relaxation of bronchial musculature helps maintain the correct balance between ventilation and hemodynamic perfusion. For instance, in areas of lung receiving substantial blow flow, bronchial wall relaxes normally to increase alveolar air supply. Similarly, poor perfusion stimulates bronchial constriction to "shunt" air to better-perfused segments. The arterial oxygen concentration is thus maintained at optimal levels. Furthermore, bronchial constriction in response to inhalation of toxic gases (e.g., sulfur dioxide) or particulates (e.g., smoke) can serve as a protective mechanism until escape from the noxious agent is achieved. In asthma, the bronchial smooth muscle is hyperactive and contracts in response to numerous, often nontoxic, stimuli. Common triggers include extrinsic allergens, such as dust, molds, pollen; exercise accompanied by inhalation of cold air; changes in ambient temperature and/or barometric pressure; nonspecific irritants such as pollutants and chemical sprays; viral respiratory infections. Moreover, the sensitivity to any one irritant varies among asthmatics and varies with time. Emotional upset may aggravate bronchospasm.

Associated with bronchospasm are mucosal edema and an increase in tracheobronchial mucus secretion. Vasoactive substances such as histamine and leukotrienes probably mediate, at least in part, both the bronchial muscle constriction and the increased mucus secretion and are released in response to the same stimuli that cause bronchoconstriction. Such agents also facilitate the production of edema fluid within the bronchial epithelium. Moreover, the mucus glands within the same epithelium are also stimulated and release excess secretions into the bronchial lumina. If infection is involved in the asthmatic attack, an inflammatory cellular infiltrate may be present as well. Because the resultant bronchial obstruction is not associated with an appropriate adjustment in blood supply, a ventilation-perfusion mismatch occurs. Hypoxemia develops, and the patient hyperventilates in an attempt to compensate. Hyperinflation and air-trapping ensue. Although the increased respiratory rate initially leads to hypocapnea, hypercapnea may develop if the attack progresses and the patient fatigues. Arterial blood gases then reveal hypoxemia and respiratory acidosis.

EPIDEMIOLOGY.—Asthma may have its onset at any age. In some series, nearly 30% of asthmatic children had the onset of their disease within the first 6 months of life. It is, however, sometimes difficult to distinguish between the infant who wheezes secondary to the inflammatory obstruction of a viral respiratory infection (see bronchiolitis) and the one who indeed has asthma. Labelling infants as having asthma, wheezy bronchitis, asthmatic bronchitis, or recurrent bronchitis without appropriate diagnostic and therapeutic maneuvers as well as a prolonged period of obstruction is unwarranted. Few new cases of asthma are diagnosed during adolescence. The incidence increases in young adulthood. While some studies indicate that there is no difference in the incidence of asthma between the sexes, others suggest that males are affected slightly more often, particularly in the group with severe disease.

The natural history of childhood asthma remains somewhat confusing. It appears that up to 80% of asthmatic children have the presentation of their illness prior to age 5 years. Most experience a remission of symptoms within 6 to 10 years of onset. In some studies, patients with onset of disease before age 6 months appeared more likely to develop more severe and persistent disease. However, other studies indicate that the age of onset of illness is not correlated with subsequent severity or outcome. Factors that fairly consistently herald a worse prognosis are severe illness at onset and family history of atopic disease.

DIFFERENTIAL DIAGNOSIS.—Although asthma is the leading cause of wheezing in childhood, numerous other clinical entities are characterized by respiratory distress and wheezing (Table 3–2). Since some nonasthmatics may respond at least in part to bronchodilators, the correct diagnosis can be elusive. A complete history and physical examination of all children presenting with wheezing is mandatory.

CLINICAL PRESENTATION.—Physical findings in children with asthma vary with the severity of their disease. Patients with mild asthma usually have a normal physical examination and normal pulmonary function tests between acute attacks. Those with more severe disease may exhibit chest wall deformity (pectus carnatum) as well as some degree of wheezing even when otherwise symptom-free. Chronic cough without episodic wheezing may be a manifestation of asthma. Pulmonary function testing reveals some obstructive lung disease, which usually improves following a bronchodilator aerosol. Chronic severe asthma may involve growth failure.

TABLE 3–2.—DIFFERENTIAL DIAGNOSIS OF WHEEZING

DIAGNOSIS	EXAMPLES OF HELPFUL IMFORMATION
Allergic asthma	Family history, seasonal occurrence
Bronchiolitis	Age group, preceding upper respiratory infection symptoms
Cystic fibrosis	History of abnormal stools, salty sweat, failure to thrive, chronic cough
Reaction to infection (e.g., pneumonia and bronchitis)	Chest x-ray appearance, cough, fever
Reaction to nonspecified irritants	History of exposure, presence of chemicals in home, chemical odor of breath
Heart failure	Known congenital heart disease, murmur
Foreign body	History of aspiration, unequal breath sounds, radiologic appearance
Vascular ring	Progressive symptoms, esophogram appearance
Neuroblastoma	Mass in chest on x-ray, anemia
Hyperventilation	Dyspnea out of proportion to amount of wheezing and aeration, history of emotional problems
Reaction to cold	History of exposure
Organic phosphorus poisoning	Pinpoint pupils, diarrhea, history of insecticide use
Tumor of the airway	Marked difference in finding over each lung

Patients experiencing an acute asthmatic attack generally demonstrate tachypnea and tachycardia, the degree depending in part on the severity of the attack. Unless pronounced hypoxemia and hypercarbia are present, the sensorium is usually clear. Most children demonstrate some anxiety due to dyspnea, hypoxia, and fear. Further observation may reveal use of accessory respiratory muscles; nasal flaring and intercostal retractions are common findings even with mild respiratory distress. Marked sternal and suprasternal retractions herald more profound respiratory embarrassment; however, fatigue may result in markedly decreased respiratory effort and obscure these findings. Cyanosis is absent unless hypoxemia is marked. The thorax may show an increased anteroposterior diameter as well as hyperresonance to percussion; hyperinflation and air trapping account for these findings. Auscultation typically reveals wheezing over all lung fields. Although primarily an expiratory noise, wheezing may also occur during inspiration as the degree of bronchoconstriction increases. Absence of wheezing in a patient who exhibits other signs of marked respiratory distress is an ominous finding; such a phenomenon occurs when bronchospasm is so profound that air exchange is insufficient to produce audible wheezes. Scattered rales and rhonchi are not uncommon and may not indicate infection. Unequal breath sounds commonly reflect patchy areas of bronchoconstriction but may also indicate atelectasis, infiltrate, or even pneumothorax.

LABORATORY FINDINGS.—Hypoxemia occurs early in acute asthmatic attacks and may be marked by the time the patient presents for treatment. Arterial blood gases in moderately ill patients reveal $PaCO_2$ of 20 to 30 mm Hg and PaO_2 in the 50 to 60 mm Hg range. As the attack worsens and the patient fatigues, hypercarbia ensues and the PaO_2 drops. Combined respiratory and metabolic acidosis then develops. Chest x-ray films display hyperinflation; atelectasis secondary to mucus plugging may also occur. Pneumomediastinum and/or subcutaneous emphysema are more uncommon findings. Pneumonic infiltrates may be present if lower respiratory tract infection has occurred.

Status asthmaticus is defined in various ways but most commonly refers to failure to control an acute asthmatic attack following the administration of two or three subcutaneous epinephrine injections. Patients require hospital admission for more rigorous treatment. Patients in status asthmaticus exhibit various degrees of illness, ranging from mild distress to respiratory failure. If left untreated, these patients often fatigue and deteriorate. Deaths occur in status asthmaticus patients who have inordinately delayed medical care, receive inappropriate/inadequate therapy, or have other serious illnesses.

TREATMENT.—Patients with chronic asthma are usually maintained on oral bronchodilators, such as theophylline and/or beta-adrenergic agonists. The outpatient management of chronic asthma is not relevant to this discussion and will not be pursued. For infrequent acute attacks or for individuals with exercise-induced asthma, a pressurized, metered-dose inhaler of isoetharine, metaproterenal, or salbutamol may be useful. Inappropriate use of such inhalers (e.g., too frequent, too high dose) has been associated with paradoxical bronchospasm, cardiac arrhythmias, and sudden death.

The patient who presents to the emergency room with an acute asthmatic attack receives several therapies. Since many moderately ill asthmatics exhibit a significant degree of hypoxia, oxygen, preferably humidified, is suggested for all acutely ill asthmatics presenting to the hospital and/or emergency room. Since childhood asthmatics do not have chronic hypercarbia, the risk of oxygen-induced hypoventilation and apnea is negligible. Therefore, the concentration of administered O_2 is not critical and should be high enough (30–50%, FiO_2) to relieve the patient's hypoxia rapidly. Although some young children may be frightened, a parent can hold the face mask and calm the child. Moreover, relief of hypoxia often eases anxiety. Positive pressure O_2 may provide fatigued patients with some rest but is often not tolerated well by children. Furthermore, positive pressure increases the risk of pneumothorax and/or pneumomediastinum.

Nebulized sympathomimetic drugs such as isoetharine, isoproterenol, or terbutaline are frequently necessary. These drugs are administered in normal saline and should be propelled by O_2, not compressed air. Because of drug-induced pulmonary vasodilation, the $\dot{V}/\dot{Q}$ mismatch, which typically accompanies acute asthma, can be worsened. Increasing the FiO_2 helps alleviate this problem. In children old enough to cooperate (>3 years) the aerosol should be delivered via a mouthpiece instead of a face mask to facilitate better distribution in the tracheobronchial tree.

When respiratory failure is imminent or has occurred, the patient should be managed in an intensive care unit. When appropriate intravenous bronchodilators, corticosteroids, and frequent aerosol treatments fail to relieve the bronchoconstriction, other therapies are instituted. Intravenous isoproterenol is a potent bronchodilator and may obviate the need for mechanical ventilation. It is not a benign drug, however, and patients must be carefully monitored for hypoxemia, tachyarrythmias, and/or myocardial necrosis. Despite intravenous isoproterenol, some patients will require intubation and mechanical ventilation. Most patients will require high pressures to deliver an adequate tidal volume. Volume ventilators are, therefore, preferred. Frequent arterial blood gas sampling is required for optimal management of such severely ill patients. Most patients can be successfully weaned from the ventilator within 2 to 3 days.

Bronchiolitis

During the first two years of life bronchiolitis is the most common lower respiratory tract infection. Many infants younger than 6 months of age fall victim to the disease. Since bronchiolitis may closely resemble asthma, the two entities are often confused. Correct diagnosis is made only by consideration of the epidemiology and clinical and laboratory findings associated with the disease.

ETIOLOGY.—Bronchiolitis most often results from respiratory syncytial virus (RSV) infection. RSV is an enveloped RNA virus, a member of the paramyxovirus group. The virus is shed in nasopharyngeal secretions and may be identified by the cytopathic effect it produces on certain cultured cell lines. It takes approximately 4 days for the virus to product its pathologic effect on cell cultures; immunofluorescence techniques applied to contaminated nasopharyngeal secretions may yield far more rapid, although somewhat less sensitive and less specific results.

While RSV infection accounts for the vast majority of bronchiolitis, several other viruses can also cause the syndrome. Certain types of adenovirus, parainfluenza virus Type 3, and, more rarely, influenza virus have all been associated with bronchiolitis. *Mycoplasma pneumoniae* may cause bronchiolitis infrequently, but no true bacteria are known etiologic agents for the syndrome.

CLINICAL MANIFESTATIONS.—Bronchiolitis symptoms include fever, cough, tachypnea, and dyspnea. The illness usually begins as a simple "cold" with nasal congestion and some cough. The symptoms worsen over a few days, with cough and wheeze becoming prominent. Respiratory distress may be severe enough to interfere with feeding. Young infants (<3 months) may have apnea. Physical examination usually reveals a mildly febrile infant in some degree of respiratory distress. Auscultation of the chest reveals occasional fine rales and wheezing. Chest x-ray film is typically clear except for hyperinflation. While the illness is usually self-limited and resolves in several days, severe pneumonia can develop. When pneumonia does develop, the chest x-ray film shows a diffuse interstitial infiltrate and/or segmental involvement including atelectasis.

Hypoxemia is present in nearly all infants hospitalized with bronchiolitis. The degree of arterial desaturation is variable but may be as low as 85%. The hypoxemia may be protracted and persist for days. Hypercarbia is much less common.

EPIDEMIOLOGY.—Epidemics of RSV infections usually start in midwinter and persist through early spring. The outbreaks last 1 to 5 months. The interepidemic intervals are alternately long (13 to 16 months) and short (7 to 12 months). RSV is virtually never present in the community during August and September. Parainfluenza Type 3 is essentially endemic and frequently occurs even during epidemics of other viral agents. Adenovirus is also present year-round, but incidence peaks in November through July.

AGE.—RSV infects all age groups, including adults. Asymptomatic illness is rare. The majority of infections occur in individuals aged 3 weeks to 24 months, with infants younger than 1 year incurring the highest infection rate. Reinfections are common, and immunity is incomplete. RSV can readily occur in neonates, although relatively infrequently. The presentation may be atypical, and a significant percentage of patients have only nonspecific findings, such as lethargy, poor feeding, irritability, and apnea. Parainfluenza also infects all age groups, but infants most frequently. Adenovirus bronchiolitis/pneumonia is most prevalent between 3 and 18 months of age.

SEX.—When only minor illness is considered, there is no difference in incidence between the sexes. Severe bronchiolitis and other lower tract disease (i.e., disease severe enough to require medical attention) does, however, exhibit a 2:1 male/female predominance.

MORBIDITY AND MORTALITY.—Approximately 1% of infants younger than 2 years of age with uncomplicated bronchiolitis will require hospitalization. Mortality for hospitalized infants under 1 year of age is 1 to 3%. Neonatal mortality may reach 20%.

If bronchiolitis and pneumonia are caused by adenovirus, the syndrome of bronchiolitis obliterans may ensue. Bronchiolitis obliterans is characterized by a necrotizing lesion of the bronchioles and alveoli, leading to obstruction of the small airways. This complication is characterized by episodes of wheezing, pneumonia, and atelectasis for a period of weeks to months. While recovery may be complete, more than half of the patients have some degree of permanent lung damage and abnormal pulmonary function.

TREATMENT.—Bronchiolitis is largely self-limited, requiring only supportive care. Antibiotics and corticosteroids have no proven efficacy; if a superimposed bacterial infection is suspected or documented, appropriate antibiotic therapy is indicated. The majority of infants, however, do well at home without specific medical intervention. Since affected infants are uniformly tachypneic, slow, frequent feedings are advised to maintain adequate nutrition and hydration. The chance of aspiration is reduced by avoiding the prone position. Although a cool mist vaporizer is often recommended, its actual efficacy is unproven. Such treatment probably serves as a hydration source for the tachypneic infant. Moreover, some feel that humidified inspired air aids in hydration of respiratory secretions thereby rendering them more easily cleared from the respiratory tract. Cool mist is favored because hot air may be a safety hazard.

More severely affected infants require hospitalization and more vigorous respiratory care. Since hypoxemia is a universal finding in such patients, oxygen therapy is indicated. The best way to administer humidified oxygen to infants is with a tent. Some older infants become inconsolable in mist tents and may tolerate face mask oxygen better. Although the pathophysiology of asthma and bronchiolitis are quite different, the symptoms, particularly dyspnea and wheezing, are similar.

Bronchodilator drugs, effective in asthma, are frequently administered to infants in whom the diagnosis of bronchiolitis and/or asthma is suspected. Infants presenting with a first episode of wheezing are often given isoproterenol or isoetharine aerosols or subcutaneous epinephrine as a therapeutic trial. If improvement is noted, the infant is usually then given an oral or intravenous bronchodilator such as aminophylline. Great care must be taken in administering such drugs, as they have no proven efficacy in viral bronchiolitis. Improvement that may occur following bronchodilators is often subjectively assessed and is minimal at best. Aminophylline kinetics are markedly altered in infants under 6 months old, such that the serum half-life is significantly prolonged compared to that of older children and adults. If the drug is given in a routine fashion, serious overdosing can occur; aminophylline toxicity can cause nausea, vomiting, fever, irritability, cardiac arrhythmias, seizures, and even death. Treatment of aminophylline overdosage is difficult as the drug is not dialyzable, and other means of rapid elimination are not readily available.

A small percentage of young infants (younger than 3 months old) admitted to the hospital with bronchiolitis will develop severe disease and respiratory failure. Such children require intensive care, which may include endotracheal intubation, and mechanical ventilation is often necessary to relieve profound hypoxemia and hypercarbia. The need for intensive treatment of this magnitude is variable but rarely may be necessary for several weeks. While the viral infection and secondary inflammation may subside within days, damage secondary to oxygen toxicity, barotrauma, and mechanical ventilation may ensue. Infants developing these problems are at high risk for chronic pulmonary disease.

Bronchitis

Inflammation of the major airways (bronchitis) can result from a variety of infectious agents and from chemical irritants. Usually, bronchitis is a self-limited disease that resolves even without specific treatment. Acute bronchitis is encountered frequently in children. Under certain conditions bronchitis may become a chronic problem requiring more intensive attention. The response of the major airways to inflammation is similar to that of the rest of the respiratory tract: mucus production is increased, and there is hypertrophy and proliferation of the mucus-producing structures, which can occur at the expense of the ciliated epithelium. A cycle is then set up in which ongoing inflammation leads to increased secretions and decreased mucociliary clearance. Infection eventually may spread to the smaller airways, resulting ultimately in bronchiectasis and bronchiolectasis. Therapy aimed at interrupting this cycle is most effective before irreversible damage occurs but is useful in treating even advanced disease (Fig 3–1).

Acute bronchitis usually requires little if any treatment beyond short courses of antibiotics and expectorants. In general, suppression of cough should be avoided unless the cough interferes significantly with sleep or is painful enough (either throat or muscular pain) to cause involuntary or voluntary inhibition of its forcefulness.

In adults, a productive cough for 3 months of the year for 2 or more successive years is arbitrarily defined as chronic bronchitis. Diagnosis is more difficult in young children for whom definitive clinical criteria have not been established. Chronic bronchitis usually requires more intensive treatment measures: longer antibiotic courses, decongestant aerosols, physical therapy to aid in clearing of secretions, expectorants, and possibly a mist tent or cold mist vaporizers. This treatment must be carried out long enough to allow the hypersecretory state to resolve completely. Coexisting sinusitis, allergy, or other underlying respiratory problems will require specific therapy as well.

Respiratory therapy generally will not be needed in treating the usual patient with acute bronchitis. In patients with established chronic bronchitis, aerosol treatment (see chap. 5) with bronchodilators (e.g., isoproterenol) may be used either alone or in combination with physical therapy (see chap. 7). Oxygen and positive-pressure treatment should not be necessary for uncomplicated chronic bronchitis.

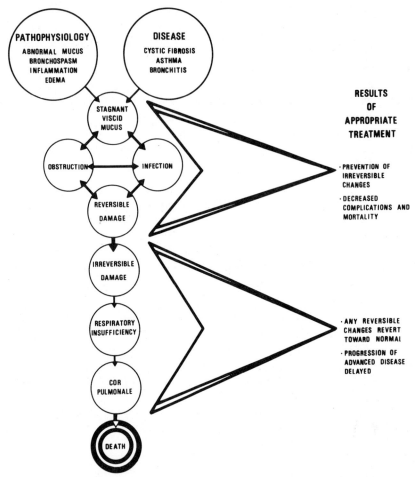

Fig 3–1.—Pathophysiology of progressive bronchitis in children. Early treatment of chronic bronchitis *(upper arrow)* can reverse pathologic changes toward normal and prevent progression in areas that are still normal. Treatment after irreversible histologic changes have occurred *(longer arrow)* is less effective in that it can retard but not prevent the inevitable progression of bronchiectasis.

Dyskinetic Cilia Syndrome

The cilium is a cellular organelle that exists as a projection on certain epithelial cells. Normal cilia are anchored to the cellular cytoplasm by a basal body, and each contains two central and nine peripheral microtubules that course its entire length. The microtubules are loosely bound to one another by radial spokes; an adenosine triphosphatase (ATPase) within the cilia generates the energy whereby the microtubules slide along adjacent microtubules. This sliding action provides for ciliary motion. Cilia beat in a coordinated fashion, typically at

1000 cycle/min. Such wavelike motion is necessary to effectively clear secretions from the tracheobronchial tree.

Ciliated cells cover the mucosa of the nasal cavity, the sinuses, the middle ear, and the airways of the lung. Ciliated cells are also located within the fallopian tubes; the tails of spermatozoa are also structurally the same as cilia.

In recent years a number of patients with immotile cilia have been described. Many had situs inversus, and all had chronic sinusitis, bronchitis, and bronchiectasis. The men also had immotile spermatozoa. Moreover, the disease appears inheritable, usually as an autosomal recessive trait. The abnormality responsible for the lack of ciliary motion was a deficiency of ATPase containing dynein arms. Since then, other ciliary defects resulting in either no motion or random, uncoordinated beating have been described. The term *dyskinetic cilia syndrome* is perhaps the most appropriate name for this collection of disorders.

The clinical manifestations of the dyskinetic cilia syndrome occur in organ systems in which cilia are present. Impaired ciliary clearance in the sinuses and middle ear leads to chronic severe otitis media and sinusitis. Sterility occurs in affected males secondary to ineffective spermatozoal movement. Chronic cough and bronchitis are predominant features; wheezing is also a frequent finding. Bronchiectasis usually occurs in early adulthood.

Treatment is symptomatic and consists of close medical supervision, aggressive antibiotic therapy for pulmonary infections, chest physiotherapy, and bronchodilators. Serous otitis and sinusitis may require drainage and antibiotic therapy as well.

The prognosis for affected individuals is unknown. However, some patients with normal longevity have been reported. The effectiveness of early vigorous medical therapy has not been demonstrated.

Cystic Fibrosis

Cystic fibrosis (CF) is an hereditary disease affecting the exocrine glands.[6] The most important areas involved are the gastrointestinal tract and the lung. The disease is probably inherited as a simple autosomal recessive gene. The risk of another child being born with CF to a couple with one or more affected children is 25% for each pregnancy. Boys and girls are affected in equal numbers.

Sweat analysis reveals high concentrations of sodium and chloride. This abnormality forms the basis for the most important diagnostic test for this disease ("sweat test").

Increased knowledge of the pathophysiology of the intestinal problems, the availability of pancreatic enzyme replacement to improve digestion, vitamin supplements, and a low-fat diet have minimized greatly the problems associated with gastrointestinal involvement.

Progressive pulmonary disease with airway obstruction and recurrent and finally chronic infection is now the greatest threat to life in patients with cystic fibrosis. A comprehensive therapy program, instituted to maintain normal pulmonary hygiene and to provide intensive early treatment of infection, has improved the prognosis, especially for patients diagnosed before extensive lung damage has occurred. Despite these advances, cystic fibrosis is the most common life-threatening chronic lung disease of children, accounting for a substantial percentage of all children hospitalized for pulmonary disease.

Although the pancreas already may be affected severely, the lungs are probably histologically normal at birth. However, the mucus that normally lines the airways and forms part of the mucociliary clearance system of the lung is not cleared normally. This results in patchy obstruction of the small airways with areas of atelectasis and even more prominent areas of overinflation. Stagnation of secretions and bacterial infection follow. A cycle is set up in which a partially obstructed area becomes infected, and the infection causes increased mucus production and inflammatory edema that further compromise clearance of the involved airways (see Fig 3–1). The DNA of dead bacteria and white blood cells markedly increases the viscosity of the mucus and further compounds the problem.

The entire process is patchy and may result in relatively normal areas existing adjacent to severely affected areas. Hemolytic *Staphylococcus aureus* and *Pseudomonas aeruginosa,* along with other gram-negative bacteria cause most of the infection. Eventually, the disease affects all areas of the lungs, with bronchitis, bronchiolitis, bronchiectasis, bronchiolectasis, overinflation, atelectasis, bleb formation, fibrosis, cor pulmonale, and, finally, respiratory insufficiency and death. Bronchiectasis usually is accompanied by bronchial artery hypertrophy and may lead to severe hemoptysis (see below), while overinflation with bleb formation, particularly in the upper lobes, may lead to pneumothorax (see the section on pneumothorax). Both of these are fairly common complications of the disease.

TREATMENT.—Although this section must deal primarily with the treatment of the pulmonary manifestations of cystic fibrosis, it should be obvious that effective treatment of this disease requires a comprehensive approach.[2] Therapy must be directed to the gastrointestinal and hepatic manifestations and psychologic problems as well as to the lung. Preferably, the diagnosis will be made early, before irreversible lung damage has occurred. The treatment then can be prophylactic as well as therapeutic.

Since the basic pulmonary lesion is probably small airway obstruction, any attempt at early treatment must deal with this problem. Mist therapy is used often in an attempt to ensure full humidification or liquefy secretions and make it easier for the normal mechanisms to clear mucus from the lung. Mist tent therapy has never been conclusively shown to be beneficial in cystic fibrosis, and its use is still quite controversial.

Aerosol treatments (see chap. 5) may be used before physical therapy to supply decongestants (phenylephrine), bronchodilators (isoproterenol) or mucolytic agents (acetylcysteine). In general, these treatments are given without positive pressure and before respiratory physical therapy. Aerosols with antibiotics may be given after physical therapy. Aerosol therapy is more generally accepted than is nightly mist although it too lacks convincing experimental support.

Physical therapy (postural drainage with clapping and/or vibrating) is used in an attempt to mobilize and remove viscous secretions (see chap. 7).

Antibiotics, bronchodilators, and other drugs may be used orally or parenterally. Treatment for the specific complications of cystic fibrosis lung disease are used as indicated. Patients with segmental atelectasis frequently are given intermittent positive pressure for several days. In our experience, positive pressure is contraindicated in most cystic fibrosis patients because it tends to increase the overinflation, one of the early and important consequences of diffuse small airway obstruction. Patients with cystic fibrosis treated with positive pressure develop increasing overinflation that may not be reversible even when the positive pressure is discontinued. The extent of the increased overinflation is related to the duration of positive-pressure treatment. Most patients do well with only the simple aerosol.

Pneumothorax, an increasingly frequent event in older patients, may be treated in the conventional manner with chest tube and suction. Almost always, however, pneumothorax becomes a recurring problem and more drastic treatment such as instillation of an irritating agent or thoracotomy with pleural abrasion is eventually necessary. We usually recommend such a definitive procedure as part of the treatment of the initial episode. After this type of therapy, any further recurrence on that side is rare (see the section on pneumothorax).

Hemoptysis, a common complication of bronchiectasis, results from erosion of blood vessels by infection. The bleeding may range from minimal streaking of the sputum to massive, life-threatening hemorrhage. Treatment varies accordingly. Vitamin K is given to ensure adequate formation of prothrombin and normal blood clotting. With normal bleeding no other therapy may be necessary. With more severe bleeding, routine postural drainage may have to be discontinued temporarily and antibiotic treatment intensified. Transfusions may be necessary. Bronchoscopy can be performed to attempt to locate the bleeding site, leading to a possible lobectomy. When more than minimal hemoptysis is present, we usually recommend a 10- to 14-day period of intensive hospital therapy to treat the infection (*S. aureus* and *P. aeruginosa* or other gram-negative organism). Embolization of the bronchial artery system has been used with increasing frequency recently. This technique allows obliteration of the systemic pressure vascular bed, which probably is involved in most episodes of massive hemoptysis. Although the technique is still being improved, it represents a major advance in the treatment of this complication.

Patients with advanced pulmonary disease often develop right ventricular hypertrophy secondary to chronically elevated pulmonary vascular resistance (cor pulmonale). These patients subsequently may develop right-sided heart failure. The basic treatment for this type of heart failure includes intensive efforts to reduce pulmonary infection with increased antibiotics, inhalation therapy, and physical therapy. In addition, specific measures used for treating heart failure include salt restriction, diuretics, and digitalis. The major factors precipitating heart failure in patients with lung disease are hypoxia and acidosis. For this reason, oxygen is indicated in these patients in as high a concentration as possible to raise the oxygen saturation to about 90% without unduly compromising respiratory drive.

Oxygen therapy is used for a variety of reasons in this disease. Supplemental oxygen is useful in patients with severe flare-ups of disease who may not be able to tolerate physical therapy, particularly in the head-down positions. Oxygen therapy for heart failure is indicated as noted above. Patients with anoxic headaches may not be able to tolerate treatments without continuous oxygen. Oxygen is needed for acute exacerbations of chronic illness or, as an emergency lifesaving measure, in patients with newly diagnosed severe lung disease. Finally, oxygen may be needed, particularly at higher altitudes, in the home treatment of an occasional patient with very severe hypoxia but a relatively stable Pa_{CO_2}. Since this is a chronic illness, there is the possibility of long-standing hypercapnia, although this occurs relatively infrequently in ambulatory patients in our experience. Oxygen therapy may be dangerous, and blood gas monitoring is essential, particularly when first used.

Patients with advanced disease or severe acute exacerbations who are in respiratory failure but have indications that substantial improvement can occur (e.g., a patient with moderately severe disease who becomes acutely ill with influenza or a patient with postoperative pain who develops respiratory failure) may need brief respiratory assistance. This is accomplished best with intermittent positive pressure ventilation with added oxygen to give the patient periods of rest or to help during physical therapy. Most severely ill patients may require naso- or endotracheal intubation and continuous respiratory care. Tracheostomy, which greatly reduces the effectiveness of the cough, is usually contraindicated for patients with cystic fibrosis. Patients receiving respirator care usually need to be weaned by gradually decreasing the time spent with assisted respiration and increasing the intervals between respirator support. Serial blood gas measurements are essential during this weaning process.

Pneumonia

Pneumonia is a term for a diverse group of diseases that cause inflammation of pulmonary tissue including the smallest airways and alveoli. It can be a very sharply localized infection, as with classic lobar pneumonia, or a more diffuse disease, as with many viral infections or chemical aspirations. It can be an acute severe disease (e.g., staphylococcal or pneumococcal pneumonia in an infant) or a chronic, smoldering process, as in long-standing infection in cystic fibrosis. It can be a primary disease or can occur secondary to an ongoing chronic illness. Although the general aim of the treatment will be the same in all cases (to reduce infection and inflammatory obstruction as rapidly as possible and minimize the risk of irreversible damage), the specific measures taken will depend in large part on the type of pneumonia, the presence of underlying disease, the condition of the patient, and many other factors.

In any area of inflammation in the lung, ventilation will be compromised by mucosal edema and intra-alveolar and luminal secretions. Local hypoxia will result. Blood entering that portion of the lung will not be oxygenated optimally, and reflex constriction of these vessels will reduce the flow of blood to relatively unaerated lung. Despite this adjustment of blood flow, some blood still will enter the diseased area. This blood will not be oxygenated normally and will mix with blood returning from normal lung. This always results in some disease of arterial Po_2. Carbon dioxide elimination, on the other hand, can be increased in normal areas of lung to compensate for the portion involved with pneumonia. Thus, systemic $Paco_2$ is usually normal unless the pneumonia is very extensive. Usually, with resolution of the inflammation the lung returns to normal. If the initial insult (chemical or infection) is severe, or if the individual's ability to defend against infection is decreased, irreversible damage may occur. Aspiration of hydrocarbon-containing household products and aspiration of gastric contents following vomiting are the most common causes of chemical pneumonia.

TREATMENT.—All patients with pneumonia have hypoxemia and potentially could benefit from oxygen therapy. If the hypoxemia is mild, this therapy may be withheld to spare the patient the inconvenience of a mask or nasal cannulae and to avoid any possible harmful side effects of high oxygen concentrations. Similarly, if the patient has preexisting lung disease and chronic hypercapnia, oxygen therapy may be indicated, although risky, and the patient's blood gases will need close monitoring. The vast majority of infants and young children admitted to the hospital for acute pneumonia will benefit from oxygen therapy. The use of mist therapy for pneumonia is controversial. It seems likely that it does not help resolve the pneumonia directly, but it may guard against dehydration by reducing insensible water loss. In patients receiving oxygen, mist ensures proper humidification. Patients with overwhelming pneumonia may require temporary respirator assistance. Development of empyema, pneumothorax, or other complications also will complicate the treatment. In addition to the supportive inhalation therapy described above, these patients will be receiving specific treatment. This includes antibiotics for bacterial pneumonia and may include corticosteroids for some types of chemical pneumonia. Other supporting measures such as intravenous fluids may also be in progress.

Drowning

Death from drowning occurs either from immediate asphyxia caused by prolonged submersion or from the longer-range metabolic abnormalities associated with the aspiration of either salt or fresh water, or from pneumonia. Occasionally, reflex bradycardia and other arrhythmias may be an important clinical problem of near-drowning.

Aspiration of fresh water may result in extensive absorption of water through the pulmonary epithelium and alveoli, which results in hemodilution, hemolysis, and increased blood volume. In salt water aspiration, hemoconcentration occurs because of transmission of sodium chloride into the blood and water into the alveoli. Cardiac arrhythmias may result from these electrolyte problems as well as from a reflex response to stimulation of the glottis and upper airway.

TREATMENT.—Increasing appreciation of the physiologic differences between fresh water and salt water drowning should not detract from the obvious importance of the immediate institution of emergency resuscitative measures, including clearing of the airway and artificial ventilation. In general, survival from near-drowning depends largely on the duration of asphyxia and the immediacy and quality of resuscitative measures. Preexisting medical problems, particularly if they are respiratory, worsen the prognosis. Victims of near-drowning who reach the hospital are almost invariably past the initial period of resuscitation and have an excellent chance for complete recovery. Their hospital treatment consists of recognition of and attention to electrolyte problems and treatment of aspiration pneumonia and pulmonary edema (from electrolyte imbalance or chemical insult). Medical therapy also may inculde the administration of corticosteroids and antibiotics (to treat pneumonia), digitalis (for heart failure) and bronchodilators. If vomiting is present, continuous nasogastric suction is indicated.

Humidified oxygen may be needed and should be administered as indicated by arterial blood gases. When hypercapnia is present, intermittent positive pressure or continuous respirator therapy (preferably through a nasotracheal tube, although a tracheostomy may be present for other reasons) is necessary. Positive pressure also is used to treat pulmonary edema. If bronchospasm is present, isoproterenol can be administered by aerosol with or without positive pressure to supplement systemic bronchodilators and corticosteroids. Drowning victims with preexisting pulmonary disease who have been on regular medical therapy may need more intensive measures to suppress infection. If there is a reasonable chance that the drowning incident may have been an unsuccessful suicide attempt or a suicide gesture, all medical personnel, including the respiratory therapist, must be alert to conscious interference with therapy by the patient. The prognosis for survival with complete recovery after 24 hours following near-drowning is excellent, and it is likely that infection will be the only remaining problem.

Orthopedic Problems Associated with Respiratory Disease

Skeletal diseases that cause progressive deformity of the thoracic cage or inefficient use of respiratory muscles predispose to gradual restriction of ventilation and impaired cough with resulting infection. Scoliosis is the most commonly encountered disorder in this group. Scoliosis occurs either secondary to an underlying disease (e.g., neurofibromatosis, poliomyelitis) or as an isolated process. The idiopathic type occurs primarily in adolescence and usually in girls. The spinal curvature progresses at an unpredictable rate until all growth centers are closed (at about age 18 years). Minimal scoliosis with slow progression requires no treatment and is not a major health threat. More severe disease may result in life-threatening pulmonary problems and/or permanent respiratory impairment (see chap. 9).

TREATMENT.—Exercises and braces usually are used early in the disease. In rapidly progressive or severe scoliosis, surgery is necessary to fuse the involved vertebrae after obtaining as much correction of the curve as possible. Postoperative pain will further compromise the ventilation and cough in these patients. All patients scheduled for this type of surgical procedure should be evaluated carefully by pulmonary function testing and blood gas determinations before the procedure is performed. The postoperative approach should be explained to the patient. In some of the more severe cases, elective tracheostomy may be required prior to the definitive procedure to allow easier respirator assistance after fusion.

All patients should see and get experience using positive-pressure ventilators before surgery. Breathing exercises also may be very valuable. Postoperative care may include intermittent positive-pressure breathing (IPPB), oxygen administration, intermittent or continuous respirator assistance, and physical therapy. Frequent cultures and prompt antibiotic treatment of infection are also important.

Neuromuscular Diseases Leading to Weakness of Respiratory Muscles

A large number of neurologic and muscular diseases result in progressive weakness of the respiratory muscles. Muscular dystrophy is one example of a progressive muscle disease, and spinal muscular atrophy (Werdnig-Hoffmann disease) is an example of a progressive neurologic disease leading to respiratory complications. The Guillain-Barré syndrome is an example of an acute, self-limited neurologic disease that causes impaired ventilation. In patients with this group of diseases, the vital capacity is reduced gradually and may approach the tidal volume. Exercise tolerance decreases, and eventually the patient becomes dyspneic at rest. Simultaneously, the cough becomes less effective, and retention of secretions and subsequent pulmonary infection occur, accelerating the patient's decline.

TREATMENT.—Medical therapy aimed at the underlying disease will be in progress. Clearly, this will vary with different primary illnesses. In all such patients, treatment and/or prevention of obesity is essential. Antibiotic treatment of any pulmonary infection will be needed.

During acute flare-ups of infection, treatment with antibiotics (systemic and possibly aerosol), aerosol treatment with decongestants and bronchodilators, segmental postural drainage with clapping and vibration, and mist therapy may be indicated. Oxygen should be used for treating acute flare-ups if chronic hypercapnia has not been present. Patients with atelectasis or respiratory failure may need intermittent positive pressure or continuous respiratory assistance.

Since many of these diseases are progressive in nature, and ultimately severe pulmonary problems can be expected, it is often useful to acquaint the patient with the equipment likely to be needed in the future. Practice sessions with IPPB when the patient is relatively well may pay big dividends later when there is severe illness.

Intensive home therapy with aerosols, respiratory physical therapy, and oral antibiotics can be useful for clearing retained secretions and recurrent or persistent infection. Similarly, in patients with recurring atelectasis, IPPB at home may reduce the frequency of hospital admissions. Ultimately, a tracheostomy may be done to allow intermittent suctioning ("button tracheostomy") or to improve ventilation. Patients about to be started on an intensive home treatment program need education concerning the use and cleaning of their equipment.

REFERENCES

1. Behrman, R.E., and Vaughan, V.C. (eds.): *Nelson Textbook of Pediatrics,* Chapter 12 (12th ed.; Philadelphia: W.B. Saunders Co., 1983).
2. Doershuk, C.F., and Stern, R.C.: Cystic fibrosis, in Gellis, S., and Kagan, B.M. (eds.): *Current Pediatric Therapy* (Philadelphia: W.B. Saunders Co., 1978).
3. Heimlich, H.J.: A life-saving maneuver to prevent food choking, J.A.M.A. 234:398, 1975.
4. Newth, Christopher J.L.: Recognition and management of respiratory failure, *Pediatr. Clin. North Am.* 26:617, 1979.
5. Kendig, E.L., Jr., and Chernick, V. (eds.): *Disorders of the Respiratory Tract in Children* (4th ed.; Philadelphia: W.B. Saunders Co., 1983).
6. Wood, R.E., Boat, T.F., and Doershuk, C.F.: Cystic fibrosis: State of the art, Am. Rev. Respir. Dis. 113:833, 1976.

Pulmonary Aspects of Cardiovascular Disease

GORDON BORKAT, M.D.
JEROME LIEBMAN, M.D.

4

A DISCUSSION of pediatric respiratory therapy should include not only a consideration of gas exchange but also a review of the cardiovascular system and its functions. The interrelationships between the two systems often will result in cardiovascular symptoms accompanying or masquerading as pulmonary disease.

This chapter will be devoted to a discussion of basic cardiovascular physiology, including its relationship to the respiratory system, the pathophysiology of symptoms that might be caused by the cardiovascular system, major categories of cardiac problems, and specific examples.

Large numbers of patients with cardiac disease present with pulmonary symptoms. It is important that the respiratory care practitioner be able to recognize the cardiac-related problems so that appropriate management can be initiated quickly.

BASIC CARDIOVASCULAR PHYSIOLOGY

With the use of a schematic box diagram (Fig 4–1), the function of the heart as a four-chambered pump can be easily understood. After the delivery of oxygen to the tissues, the systemic venous blood return to the heart has an oxygen saturation of approximately 70%. The blood enters the right atrium by way of the inferior and superior venae cavae. Flow goes through the tricuspid valve into the right ventricle, which pumps the blood through the pulmonic valve into the pulmonary artery and then to the small blood vessels of the lungs. When blood is in the pulmonary capillary bed, gas exchange with the alveolus occurs. Oxygenated blood returns by way of the pulmonary veins to the left

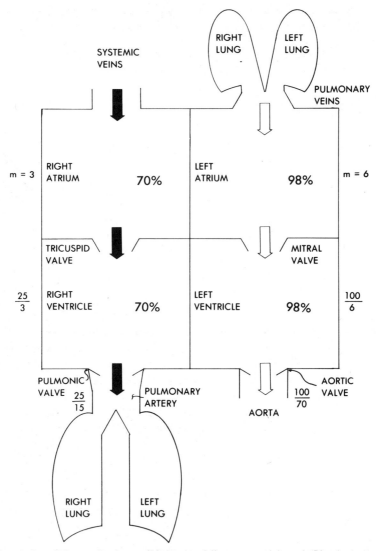

Fig 4–1.—Schematic box diagram of the normal heart. Black arrows = blood of low oxygen saturation (70%); white arrows = blood of high oxygen saturation (98%); m = pressure).

atrium. It then goes through the mitral valve into the left ventricle, which pumps the blood through the aortic valve into the aorta. Arterial blood supplies oxygen to the entire body by way of the systemic capillary bed and then returns to the heart again via the venae cavae.

Hemodynamic abnormalities occur as a result of two basic intracardiac problems. *First,* there can be areas of admixture between blood from the left and right sides of the heart. Mixing can occur through a defect in the walls separating the atria (interatrial septum) or the ventricles (interventricular septum), or by way of a persisting connection between the aorta and pulmonary artery (patent ductus arteriosus). The presence of shunted flow from left to right causes increased pulmonary blood flow. Shunted flow from the right side of the heart to the left side results in an inadequate pulmonary circulation and in undersaturated blood being delivered to the body. *Second*, there can be obstruction to the blood flow. This usually occurs at one of the cardiac valves but occasionally occurs within the arteries or veins.

PATHOPHYSIOLOGY AND MAJOR RESPIRATORY SYMPTOMS

Cardiovascular disease may result in one or more respiratory symptoms or signs.

Tachypnea (rapid respiratory rate) occurs with many cardiac problems. Hypoxemia may cause tachypnea, which is a compensatory and usually futile effort to improve oxygenation of blood for delivery to the tissues. Hypercarbia and acidemia might also result in tachypnea as the patient attempts to increase elimination of carbon dioxide to prevent or correct acidosis.

Wheezing is a high-frequency expiratory sound associated with the forced expulsion of air from the lungs. It might be caused by mechanical or pharmacologic constriction of the lower respiratory tract, or pulmonary venous congestion.

Stridor (a high-pitched inspiratory noise) is usually caused by major mechanical obstruction of the upper airway.

Rales are abnormal respiratory sounds that resemble the crackling sounds produced by air passing through fluid in a tube. This condition can be caused by edema fluid in the lower airways (i.e., bronchioles or alveoli).

Decreased breath sounds may be caused by nonaerated areas of the lung, as with consolidation, or by a large distance between the lung parenchyma and the area of auscultation, as with a pneumothorax or collection of pleural fluid.

Retractions are depressions of the soft tissue areas adjacent to bony tissues and can be seen in three locations: suprasternal notch, intercostal, and subcostal (diaphragmatic). Retractions result from increased inspiratory effort to meet ventilatory needs and reflect use of the accessory muscles of respiration.

CARDIAC PROBLEMS AND RELATED RESPIRATORY SYMPTOMS

Cardiac disease can lead to abnormal respiratory findings through a number of mechanisms, these including increased pulmonary venous and/or capillary pressure, increased pulmonary blood flow and/or pulmonary artery pressure, hypoxemia, acidosis, and mechanical compression of an airway. Each of these might result in one or more respiratory symptoms (Table 4–1).

Increased Pulmonary Venous and Capillary Pressure

When the pulmonay capillary pressure exceeds the intravascular oncotic pressure, there is extravasation of fluid into the alveoli (pulmonary edema). The

TABLE 4–1.—Cardiovascular Mechanisms Causing Respiratory Problems

	TACHYPNEA	RETRACTIONS	WHEEZING	RALES	DECREASED BREATH SOUNDS	STRIDOR
Increased pulmonary venous capillary or pressure	●	●	●	●	●	
Increased pulmonary blood flow and/or pulmonary artery pressure	●	●				
Hypoxemia	●					
Acidosis	●					
Mechanical compression	●	●	●	●	●	●

presence of excess lung fluid causes decreased aeration of alveoli, an increased alveolar-arterial oxygen gradient and a decrease in the arterial oxygen level. These changes are accompanied by a decreased effective lung volume and decreased pulmonary compliance. The respiratory manifestations include tachypnea, retractions, wheezing, rales, and decreased breath sounds.

The cardiac diseases associated with increased pulmonary venous and capillary pressure fall into two groups: left-sided congestive heart failure and specific anatomic obstruction to pulmonary venous return.

In patients with congestive heart failure, the heart is unable to meet the cardiac output needs of the body because of either increased volume and/or pressure work, or primary cardiac muscle disease. As left ventricular pumping becomes ineffective, the end-diastolic pressure increases. In order to continue forward blood flow, the left atrial pressure and subsequently the pulmonary venous and capillary pressure must increase. Pulmonary edema and respiratory symptoms follow. Examples of common cardiac problems that cause congestive heart failure are listed in Table 4–2.

The most common congenital heart lesion that causes congestive heart failure is a ventricular septal defect (Fig 4–2,A). By a few months of age, in patients with this disease, there can be a large flow of blood from the left ventricle to the right ventricle and then out through the pulmonary vascular bed. The total volume-work done by the heart might greatly increase and lead to congestive heart failure. Also common is an endocardial cushion defect, which is a maldevelopment of the central portion of the heart so that there are large ventricular and atrial septal defects (Fig 4–2,B). There also can be an associated insufficiency of the mitral valve so that a portion of the left ventricular blood is pumped back into the left atrium. Congestive heart failure may develop in

TABLE 4–2.—COMMON CARDIAC PROBLEMS AND CARDIAC MECHANISMS CAUSING RESPIRATORY SIGNS

CARDIAC ABNORMALITY	INCREASED PULMONARY VENOUS AND PULMONARY CAPILLARY PRESSURE	INCREASED PULMONARY FLOW AND PRESSURE	ACIDOSIS	HYPOXEMIA	MECHANICAL COMPRESSION
Left-to-right shunts					
Ventricular septal defect	X	X			
Endocardial cushion defect	X	X			
Patent ductus arteriosus	X	X			
Left ventricular obstruction					
Aortic stenosis	X		X		
Coarctation of aorta	X		X		
Primary cardiac muscle disease	X		X		X
Anatomical obstruction to pulmonary venous return					
Hypoplastic left heart syndrome	X		X		
Total anomalous pulmonary venous return	X		X	X	
Decreased pulmonary blood flow					
Hypoplastic right heart syndrome			X	X	
Tetralogy of Fallot				X	
Common mixing chambers					
Common atrium		X		X	
Single ventricle	X	X		X	
Double-outlet right ventricle	X	X		X	
Truncus arteriosus	X	X		X	
Inadequate mixing					
Transposition of the great arteries	X	X	X	X	
Miscellaneous					
Severe cardiomegaly					X
Vascular ring					X

infants a few weeks old. A third common lesion is a patent ductus arteriosus (Fig 4–2,C). The ductus arteriosus usually closes spontaneously soon after birth. However, when it persists, a large amount of blood can flow from the aorta to the pulmonary artery and the pulmonary vascular bed and lead to congestive heart failure because of increased left ventricular volume work. This problem is particularly common in premature infants, and might contribute to prolonging the duration and increasing the severity of the respiratory distress syndrome (see chap. 3).

Obstruction to blood flow through the left ventricle (including aortic stenosis and coarctation of the aorta) results in increased pressure work for the left ventricle, and thus might lead to congestive heart failure. In infants with severe

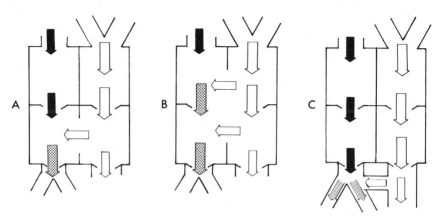

Fig 4–2.—Common problems with left-to-right shunts. **A,** ventricular septal defect. **B,** endocardial cushion defect. **C,** patent ductus arteriosus.

aortic stenosis (Fig 4–3,A), symptoms can be present during the first few weeks of life. Mild cases are often asymptomatic. Coarctation of the aorta is a narrowing of the descending aorta near the entrance of the ductus arteriosus (Fig 4–3,B). If the coarctation is associated with other problems such as ventricular septal defect and patent ductus arteriosus, the left ventricle may do increased pressure work as well as increased volume work, and congestive heart failure often develops in infants by 2 weeks of age.

Obstruction to pulmonary venous return from the lungs can also result in respiratory symptoms. The major examples include the hypoplastic left heart syndrome and total anomalous pulmonary venous return. The former is a maldevelopment of the left ventricle and mitral and aortic valves in the extent that they are too small to support adequate circulation (Fig 4–3,C). Pulmonary venous return is then to a high-pressure left atrium from which there is no easy exit. Pulmonary capillary pressure increases, and pulmonary edema follows. Under normal circumstances, pulmonary venous return is to the left atrium. In total anomalous pulmonary venous return, the pulmonary veins enter the right side of the heart, superior vena cava, or inferior vena cava below the diaphragm (Fig 4–3,D). With any of these conditions, it is possible to have anatomic narrowing and obstruction to flow, thereby raising the pulmonary capillary pressure.

Increased Pulmonary Blood Flow and Pulmonary Artery Pressure

Certain heart problems (with or without associated congestive failure) cause increased pulmonary blood flow and can have associated increased pulmonary artery pressure. Because of decreased pulmonary compliance, tachypnea and retractions can occur.

The major examples include the left-to-right shunt lesions previously mentioned, such as ventricular septal defect, endocardial cushion defect, patent ductus arteriosus and, on rare occasions, an atrial septal defect.

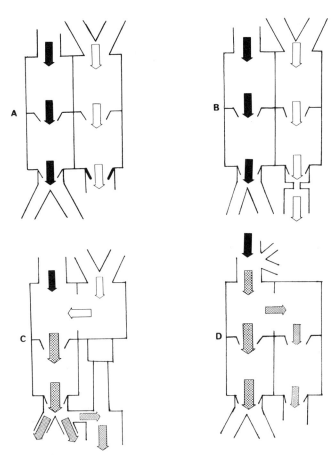

Fig 4–3.—Common problems with obstruction to blood flow on the left side of the heart. **A,** aortic stenosis. **B,** coarctation of the aorta. **C,** hypoplastic left heart syndrome. **D,** total anomalous pulmonary venous return.

Hypoxemia

Hypoxemia occurs when there is a low oxygen content in the blood. This causes cyanosis when there are 5 gm/dl of reduced hemoglobin in the capillaries. In patients with extreme hypoxemia, tachypnea can occur.

Cardiac diseases associated with hypoxemia may be divided into three groups, including those lesions that have decreased pulmonary blood flow, those with common mixing chambers with increased pulmonary blood flow, and those with pulmonary and systemic circulations in parallel with inadequate mixing between the two.

Cardiac problems with decreased pulmonary blood flow include those with obstruction of blood flow to the lungs, causing some flow of blood from the right side of the heart to the left side through an atrial or ventricular septal defect. Blood with low oxygen saturation is now pumped by the left ventricle to the body, causing hypoxemia. A common problem with obstruction to flow is the hypoplastic right heart syndrome, which includes small or absent tricuspid and pulmonic valves (Fig 4–4,A). Since blood cannot go directly to the lungs, it flows from the right atrium to the left atrium across the atrial septal defect. Pulmonary arterial blood is supplied by either a small ventricular septal defect or a patent ductus arteriosus. Another problem is tetralogy of Fallot, which includes pulmonic stenosis (narrowing of the pulmonic valve), a large right ventricle, and a large ventricular septal defect (Fig 4–4,B). Because it is difficult for the right ventricle to eject blood to the lungs through the stenotic pulmonic valve, some flow goes preferentially across the ventricular septal defect to the left ventricle and aorta.

Common mixing chambers occur at the levels of the atria, ventricles, or great arteries. Because of relatively low pulmonary vascular resistance compared to systemic, there is increased pulmonary blood flow. Single ventricle

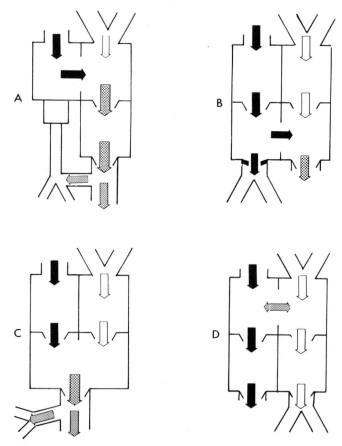

Fig 4–4.—Common problems with hypoxemia. **A,** hypoplastic right ventricle syndrome. **B,** tetralogy of Fallot. **C,** truncus arteriosus. **D,** transposition of the great arteries.

occurs when both the tricuspid and mitral valves empty into a common ventricular chamber from which arise both the pulmonary artery and aorta. In double-outlet right ventricle cases, both great arteries originate from the right ventricle; the only exit from the left ventricle is a ventricular septal defect. Finally, in patients with truncus arteriosus there is only one great artery originating from the heart, being supplied by both ventricles (Fig 4–4,C). Blood supply to both the systemic and pulmonary vascular beds comes from this single artery. In all of these lesions, in addition to the hypoxemia, the increased pulmonary blood flow will often cause congestive heart failure and the respiratory manifestations associated with increased pulmonary venous and capillary pressure.

The final hypoxemic group consists of patients who have transposition of the great arteries, where the right ventricle pumps blood to the aorta and the left ventricle pumps to the pulmonary artery (Fig 4–4,D). Therefore, the pulmonary and systemic circulations are in parallel. Survival and degree of hypoxemia depend on the amount of intermixing that can occur between the two circulations. In addition to the symptoms caused by hypoxemia, there is usually a markedly increased pulmonary blood flow, and the symptoms of congestive heart failure are often present.

Metabolic Acidosis

In patients with metabolic acidosis, respiratory compensation occurs, as manifested by tachypnea. Cardiac diseases cause acidosis in patients who have severe congestive heart failure, severe hypoxemia or a markedly decreased cardiac output. Examples of cardiac problems that cause congestive heart failure and severe hypoxemia have been mentioned previously. Decreased cardiac output exists when there is severe obstruction to flow without associated intracardiac mixing, as with cases of severe aortic stenosis in young infants. It also occurs in patients with primary cardiac muscle disease, those with pericardial effusion and/or bleeding, and many postoperative cardiac patients.

Mechanical Compression

Mechanical compression of the respiratory tract can cause pulmonary symptoms because of obstruction at almost any point in the airway. There can be decreased effective lung volume, decreased pulmonary compliance, or partial or complete airway obstruction. Depending on the site of obstruction, almost any respiratory symptom might be present.

Mechanical compression might be present because of dilated cardiac chambers and great arteries, or abnormal origins and courses of the arteries. Patients with severe congestive heart failure can have enormously enlarged hearts, with compression of the lung and decreased lung volume. Children who have severe mitral insufficiency, with a large percentage of left ventricular volume leaking back through the mitral valve to the left atrium, can have decreased lung volume from the large heart or mechanical compression of the left main-stem bronchus. There are many abnormalities of the great arteries, of which a com-

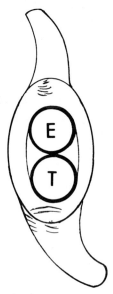

Fig 4–5.—"Vascular ring." Cross-section diagram of double aortic arch encircling esophagus (E) and trachea (T).

mon one is a double aortic arch (Fig 4–5). Abnormal origins of other major arteries can also compress the trachea or a main-stem bronchus. Any time a combination of great arteries completely encircles the trachea ("vascular ring") the extrinsic compression might cause recurrent pneumonia, stridor or wheezing.

TREATMENT OF CARDIAC-RELATED RESPIRATORY PROBLEMS

Respiratory therapy is needed frequently in treating patients after surgery. Almost all children who undergo cardiac surgery will have an endotracheal tube in place and require assisted ventilation while in the recovery room. Some patients who quickly breathe on their own tolerate early extubation and present minimal problems. On the other hand, many children who have congestive heart failure, low cardiac output, or respiratory insufficiency require ventilatory assistance for a prolonged period. Reducing the amount of work required for respiration is an integral part of the management. Additionally, because of operative trauma to the chest and lungs, respiratory effort and effective lung volume might be decreased. Finally, after prolonged endotracheal intubation, mechanical irritation of the upper airway might lead to obstruction and stridor requiring close monitoring and sometimes tracheostomy.

In addition to the many corrective surgical procedures available, there are palliative operations that can markedly reduce symptoms. For certain patients with increased pulmonary blood flow and congestive heart failure, banding of the pulmonary artery might be performed. A small tape is placed around the

TABLE 4–3.—COMMONLY USED CARDIOVASCULAR SURGERY EPONYMS

Blalock-Taussig: Subclavian artery-to-pulmonary artery anastomosis
Waterston-Cooley: Ascending aorta-to-right pulmonary artery anastomosis
Potts: Descending aorta-to-left pulmonary artery anastomosis
Glenn: Superior vena cava-to-right pulmonary artery anastomosis
Edwards: Reposition of the atrial septum to allow right pulmonary veins to drain into the right atrium
Blalock-Hanlon: Removal of a portion of the atrial septum
Rashkind: Creating an atrial septal defect during cardiac catheterization
Mustard: Intra-atrial baffle to direct pulmonary venous blood to the tricuspid valve and body, allowing systemic venous blood to go to the mitral valve and lungs
Senning: Intra-atrial baffle similar to Mustard
Rastelli: Valved conduit from right ventricle to pulmonary artery
Fontan: Conduit from the right atrium to either right ventricle or pulmonary artery
Jatene: Reversal of artery positions for transposition of the great arteries

pulmonary artery to cause partial obstruction that effectively reduces pulmonary blood flow by reducing left-to-right shunting. For patients who are cyanotic because of decreased pulmonary blood flow, many operations are available to improve flow to the lungs. Table 4–3 is a list of the eponyms often used for congenital heart surgery, and includes those that are "corrective" as well as palliative.

In the immediate postoperative period, respiratory failure might occur in patients for a variety of other reasons. In spite of all efforts to evacuate air from the chest, pneumothorax is common. During some shunt procedures, surgical interference with the thoracic duct and chylothorax may result. For almost all procedures, a chest tube for draining residual blood is usually left in place for about 24 hours. Clots might develop and occlude the tube, or massive bleeding (hemothorax) can occur. A great deal of surgery occurs in the area of the phrenic nerve, and damage can result in paralysis of the diaphragm.

On admission to the hospital, some infants with cardiac disease can have severe respiratory manifestations. Impending respiratory failure must be anticipated. Prophylactic endotracheal intubation and ventilatory assistance are often necessary to enable such children to undergo cardiac catheterization and subsequent surgery. Failure to recognize the severity of the patient's condition has led to death during cardiac catheterization or immediately afterward.

Two common problems of premature infants require the combined efforts of all members of the care team for treatment. These are respiratory distress syndrome with patent ductus arteriosus causing congestive heart failure, and persistent fetal circulation (see chap. 3).

Many patients with cardiac diseases can have respiratory manifestations. Respiratory therapists, nurses, and physicians are involved in hospital assessment and management of respiratory problems. When patients have undiagnosed respiratory symptoms, it is important to remember that the primary cause might be cardiac.

SUGGESTED READINGS

Engle, M.A.: Cyanotic congenital heart disease, Am. J. Cardiol. 37:284, 1976.

Liebman, J., Borkat, G., and Hirschfeld, S.: The Heart, in Klaus, M., and Fanaroff, A. (eds.): *Care of the High-Risk Newborn* (2nd ed.; Philadelphia: W.B. Saunders Co., 1979).

Nadas, A.S., and Fyler, D.C.: *Pediatric Cardiology* (3d ed.; Philadelphia: W.B. Saunders Co., 1972).

Rowe, R.D., and Mehrizia, A.: *The Neonate with Congenital Heart Disease* (2nd ed.; Philadelphia: W.B. Saunders Co., 1981).

Rudolph, A.M.: *Congenital Diseases of the Heart* (Chicago: Year Book Medical Publishers, Inc., 1974).

Respiratory Therapy

MARVIN D. LOUGH, R.R.T.
CARL F. DOERSHUK, M.D.

5

THE ABILITY of medical personnel to care for infants and children with pulmonary disease has improved dramatically over the past decade. Two factors responsible for improved care are more formal organization of pediatric respiratory therapy services and the appearance of pediatricians specifically interested in the respiratory management of newborns and older children.

ORGANIZATION OF THE RESPIRATORY THERAPY DEPARTMENT

If the respiratory therapy department has a separate pediatric section, that unit should have as its medical director a pediatrician who is interested in and knowledgeable about respiratory therapy. If the pediatric service is provided as part of the obligation of the general hospital's respiratory therapy department and not as a specific subsection, an interested pediatrician should be a full member of the directing group of physicians.

All of the department personnel should be aware of the special needs of pediatric patients. The respiratory therapy department should be responsible for providing, using, cleaning, and sterilizing the equipment and for the supervision of its maintenance.

The department should have at least one registered respiratory therapist who is especially interested in pediatrics and is willing to continue self-education in the new equipment and methods used in pediatrics. This person should utilize the in-service training program within the department to upgrade the knowledge of the others about pediatric respiratory problems and their care.

The department should have a pediatric specialist, preferably a registered therapist, to supervise the day-to-day activities. Each department member should have the opportunity to attend relevant lectures within the hospital and related meetings in the region. Consideration should be given to mandatory attendance of at least one major respiratory therapy meeting per year with appropriate funding.

The respiratory therapy service should be available on a 24-hour, 7-day weekly basis. Blood gas analysis is integral to the success of ventilatory management. Blood gas determinations are needed around the clock, and usually the best results are obtained when technicians interested in the results make the analysis. Consequently, placing the blood gas unit under the direction of the respiratory therapy department has proved to be an economical and useful operating decision.

Similarly, respiratory therapy technicians are knowledgeable about pulmonary function and can learn the skills of pulmonary function testing rapidly. In our hospital this important service also is staffed by such personnel.

ADMINISTRATION OF RESPIRATORY THERAPY

In treating infants and children, many factors influence the administration of respiratory therapy. The two of primary concern are the size of the infant or child and the psychologic preparation for the therapy to be used.

Size of Patient

The most obvious difference between the child and the adult is size, but the tremendous range of body and organ sizes that exists between infancy and adolescence often is not appreciated. The contrast between a 3-pound premature infant and a 150-pound adolescent is more impressive when it is stated that by weight the adolescent is 50 times the size of the premature infant. Alternatively, the premature infant is only 2% of the size of the 150-pound adolescent.

Less obvious but also important are the differences imposed by the relative immaturity of the overall respiratory mechanism in growing children. The thorax is small, the rib cage relatively soft, the ribs horizontal, and the diameter of the airways relatively smaller. The diaphragm is high and its motion can be impaired by the abdomen. Although respiration is efficient under normal conditions, such factors can make it especially difficult to meet the increased demand imposed by respiratory illness in infancy and childhood.

There are many important differences between the structure of the upper airways of the infant and that of the adult. The nasal passages are narrow, the tongue is proportionally large, the glottis is higher (between the third and fourth cervical vertebrae, compared to the fourth and fifth vertebrae in the adult), the vocal cords slant, and the cricoid ring is relatively small.

The technique by which respiratory therapy is to be administered is determined for the most part by the size of the patient and by the characteristics of the oral airways. Since these factors change considerably from the neonate through childhood, equipment specifically designed to accommodate each age range and size should be used. As patients reach adolescence, adult equipment may be adapted for use.

Psychologic Preparation for Treatment

Following body size and gross anatomic differences, the emotional pattern of the child provides the next most striking contrast to the adult. Dealing with an excited child is one of the most trying experiences a therapist can encounter and the one that is handled with least success. The therapist's successful approach to a child will stem from a fundamental love or understanding of children and a cultivated tolerance of and ability to deal with their eccentricities. Although it is not true that children are "little adults," often many of the childhood needs remain present in adult patients whose emotional needs frequently are unrecognized and unattended.

In children old enough to manifest fear or apprehension, the emotional factor must be cared for with as much concern as the physical condition. Consequently, a sufficient explanation of any treatment to be administered is necessary. When told in simple words exactly what is going to happen, in most instances children, surprisingly, will cooperate in a fashion that older children and adults might well strive to equal. An opportunity to observe the treatment being given to another child is sometimes very helpful. Permitting the child to cry for a short period also can be a part of the treatment preparation. The "don't cry" pressure that is forced upon a child is not necessary and does not represent good judgment. Distressed adults are said to benefit from having a good cry. This same privilege, along with sympathetic reassurance, can be extended to a child who is frightened, apprehensive, or in pain. Once their emotions have been expressed, the therapy often is very well accepted.

The child's reaction to treatment will vary with age. Even a newborn infant requires some type of "explanation" or reassurance about treatment. This is possible by stimulation: auditory, visual, and tactile. A pleasant attitude and cuddling during administration of the treatment can produce a feeling of security in almost any infant. Remember: so little effort, so great the reward.

SELECTION FROM GENERAL EQUIPMENT AND TECHNIQUES

The specific indications for oxygen therapy have been outlined in Chapters 2 and 3. When oxygen is needed, it is of utmost importance that it be administered with maximum efficiency. In order to achieve this goal, one must select a method that will provide the prescribed oxygen concentrations without causing discomfort or harm to the child.

Oxygen Nasal Cannula

Until recently, oxygen therapy via nasal cannula was not tolerated well by infants and young children. The commercially available devices were designed for adults, and the prongs had large external diameters that were uncomfortable, irritating, and, in some cases, dangerous when modified for young children. Since many infants are obligate nose breathers, an adult-size cannula that fits too snugly into the nares of an infant or young child may cause inadvertent CPAP and abdominal distention. At least one manufacturer has developed a cannula specifically designed for infants (Fig 5–1) and young children (Salter Labs No. 1601). Now for the first time, infants and young children can benefit from some of the features of nasal cannula therapy. These include uninterrupted

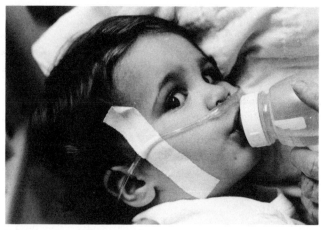

Fig 5–1.—Oxygen nasal cannula specifically designed for infants and young children.

oxygen delivery during mother-infant interaction (bonding), feeding, expectorating, and postural drainage therapy.

One must understand that low-flow oxygen delivered via nasal cannula to a small child does not guarantee low oxygen concentrations. The FiO_2 varies greatly with flow, minute ventilation, and the size of the young child's anatomic reservoir. Because there is such a wide range of oxygen concentrations with the nasal cannula, it is advisable to titrate the gas flow to the child's needs, as demonstrated by arterial blood gases. The lowest flow rate that keeps the PaO_2 in a safe range is the one to use. However, flow rates greater than 5 liters per minute may cause gastric distention and regurgitation. Also oxygen delivered via nasal cannula must be humidified.

Nasal cannula is the therapy of choice for infants going home on low concentrations of oxygen. This type of therapy is easy for the parents to manage as well as providing for patient mobility.

Oxygen Masks

Whenever a more precise concentration of oxygen is indicated, one may select an oxygen mask. Because of the popularity of mask therapy, a variety of oxygen masks are available for infants and children, but it is often difficult to keep a mask on the infant's face. One may wish to consider an oxygen hood as an alternative therapy for infants.

A soft vinyl mask is recommended in order to prevent the pressure necrosis and skin irritation occasionally produced by the more rigid plastic masks. Although the head straps used to hold the mask in place are often uncomfortable, small pieces of cotton placed above the ears will help relieve the pressure and discomfort caused by the strap. The mask should be removed periodically and dried. The patient's face should be dried and powdered to prevent accumulation of moisture that can soften the skin.

TABLE 5–1.—OXYGEN FLOW REQUIRED TO ACHIEVE DESIRED
OXYGEN CONCENTRATION IN MASK THERAPY

OXYGEN FLOW REQUIRED (LITERS/MIN)	OXYGEN CONCENTRATION DESIRED*	
	NONREBREATHING OXYGEN MASK	PEDIATRIC MEDIUM-CONCENTRATION OXYGEN MASK
6–8	40–50%	35–45%
8–10	50–60%	45–55%
10–12	60–95%	55–60%

*Indicates approximate figures.

A sufficient flow of gas (6 to 8 liters/min) must enter the mask to prevent carbon dioxide buildup. Since the space under the mask and around the face is added dead space, the larger adult mask should not be used to administer oxygen to children.

An oxygen hood or tent rather than a mask should be used for comatose infants and children. Since such patients are more prone to vomit, the risk of aspiration may be increased with mask therapy because of obstruction of the flow of vomitus.

There are several types of oxygen masks that meet specific needs. The medium-concentration mask (Fig 5–2) can provide oxygen concentrations from 35% to 60%, depending upon gas flow (Table 5–1). The nonrebreathing mask utilizes a reservoir bag with a close-fitting mask to achieve oxygen concentrations up to 95%.

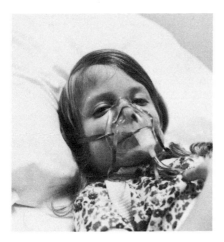 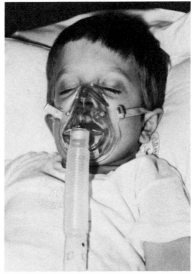

Fig 5–2 (left).—Medium-concentration oxygen mask specifically designed for the pediatric patient.
Fig 5–3 (right).—Venturi-type mixing mask designed to maintain a constant air-oxygen ratio.

VENTURI MASKS

Venturi mixing masks (Fig 5–3) are helpful in providing predictable oxygen concentrations over extended periods of time. This mask is designed to deliver low to moderate concentrations of oxygen incremented from 24% to 50%. The concentration of oxygen is determined by the diameter of the jet orifice, which limits the amount of air entering the large bore tube leading to the face mask. Therefore, the oxygen concentration is predictable as long as no back pressure is created and the patient's peak inspiratory flow does not exceed the total flow of the device. When a patient has an increased inspiratory flow (''gasping'') it may be necessary to increase jet flow, which in turn will increase total flow.

TRACHEOSTOMY MASK

Tracheostomies should be avoided in infants whenever possible because difficulty may be encountered in decannulation. Removal of the tracheostomy tube in infants may be followed by tracheal collapse. Although many hazards are involved in tracheostomy, it can be a lifesaving procedure in treating patients with croup and especially epiglottitis.

Because of the small size of the tracheal lumen, it is rarely possible to use a cuffed tube in children under 3 years of age. Table 5–2 provides the dimensions of two brands of cuffless pediatric tracheostomy tubes.

The child's life depends on a clear cannula. It takes very little secretion to obstruct a small tube. Adequate humidification will prevent or retard thickening of the secretions. Frequent suctioning may be necessary and always should be accomplished with sterile techniques. Indications for suctioning are poor color,

TABLE 5–2.—DIMENSIONS
OF CUFFLESS PEDIATRIC
TRACHEOSTOMY TUBES
(IN MILLIMETERS)

JACKSON SIZE	ID	OD	L
	Shiley		
0	3.1	4.5	39
1	3.4	5.0	40
1.5	3.7	5.5	41
2	4.1	6.0	42
3	4.8	7.0	44
	Portex		
0	3.0	4.5	41
1.5	3.8	5.0	46
3	4.5	6.0	52
3.5	5.3	7.0	55
4	6.0	8.0	59

ID = internal diameter; OD = outside diameter; and L = length; all dimensions in millimeters.

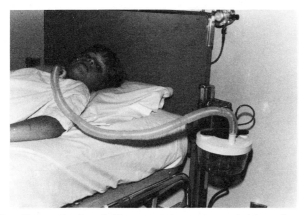

Fig 5–4.—Cascade humidifier and large-bore tubing for delivery of warmed, humidified oxygen to patient with tracheostomy.

retraction of soft tissue around the thoracic cavity, changing vital signs, or noisy breathing. When there is a tracheostomy, a small child's arms may have to be restrained to prevent accidental decannulation.

Selected concentrations of oxygen as well as humidification can be achieved with a tracheostomy mask and a heated humidifer (Fig 5–4). A soft vinyl plastic mask should be used to prevent skin irritation.

The amount of gas flowing through the heated humidifier should be greater than the patient's minute volume to prevent atmospheric air from being drawn in during inspiration. The air and/or oxygen should be warmed to 35 C. It has been our experience that if the gas is warmed to body temperature (37 C), irritation and coughing may result. In order to prevent heat loss from the humidifier to the patient, the tubing should be as short as possible and should have a low heat conductivity.

Oxygen by T-Piece

Oxygen may be delivered directly to the endotracheal tube of a spontaneously breathing child by a T-piece connector. The delivery system should consist of a humidifier, air/oxygen blender, large-bore tubing, a T-piece, and a reservoir tube on the expiratory limb. As with the tracheostomy mask, it is essential that the gas mixture be warmed (35 C) and humidified. Usually, water vapor (not nebulized particles) is all that is necessary to provide adequate humidification. Excessive water delivered by some nebulizers can cause water intoxication in infants. The T-piece and tubing should be supported to prevent unnecessary weight on the endotracheal tube.

Oxygen Tents

For some time the oxygen tent has been the most popular method of providing low to moderate oxygen therapy to infants and small children. With the introduction of masks and cannulae specifically designed for infants and small children, the popularity of this method has diminished somewhat. This form of therapy is still very beneficial for the child who will not keep a mask or cannula in place. The tent most frequently used is referred to as a ''croup tent'' (Fig 5–5).

These tents are designed to be placed on a crib mattress or hung at the head of a youth bed. A cool environmental temperature (6 to 8 F below ambient) is achieved by circulating the canopy atmosphere through ice. High levels of humidity may be attained by means of cold steam atomization. A well-maintained croup tent can provide a canopy atmosphere with up to 50% oxygen. Repeated analysis of tent atmoshpere should be made and recorded.

The following are some of the precautions to be taken in order to maintain adequate oxygen therapy by this method:

1. A tight-fitting canopy must be maintained in order to prevent oxygen leakage. This is sometimes difficult with a restless or uncooperative child. It is worthwhile to mention again that a repeat explanation of the prescribed therapy to the child may prove very helpful. In problem cases it may be useful to permit the mother and/or father to hold the child's hand through a small opening in the zipper of the canopy.
2. The fewer times the tent atmosphere is disrupted by opening the canopy, the better therapy the patient will receive.
3. The smallest tent and canopy should be used to achieve the desired concentration of oxygen while maintaining patient comfort.

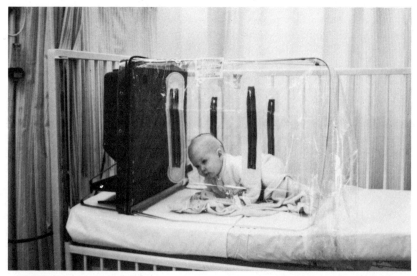

Fig 5–5.—Oxygen tent for delivering an oxygen-enriched, humidified atmosphere to babies and small children. The crib side is down only for the purpose of the picture.

4. Patient comfort always should be of concern. For example, if the ice in the cooling chamber is allowed to melt without being replenished, the canopy atmosphere can increase as much as 8 to 10 F above room temperature.
5. Any device that may produce sparks (toys, games, etc.) should not be given to a child while in a tent.

SPECIALIZED NEWBORN EQUIPMENT

Some pediatric respiratory therapy equipment is designed specifically to care for the newborn patient.

Incubators

During the first month of life there are many critical respiratory problems. These include the respiratory distress syndrome, aspiration pneumonia, and surgical conditions such as tracheoesophageal fistula, diaphragmatic hernia, and omphalocele. Infants with these problems require isolation, warmth, and humidity. The precise control of temperature, oxygen, humidity, and isolation is greatly improved with the use of the incubator (Fig 5–6). One of the most important features of the incubator is the provision for isolation. The plastic hood enclosure isolates the infant from the surrounding environment. Air is passed through a microfilter before entering the incubator. This microfilter is

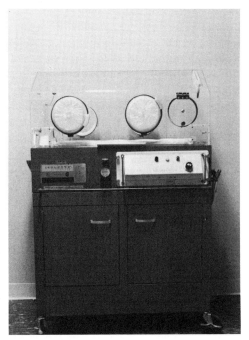

Fig 5–6.—The incubator is used to provide a controlled environment for the newborn infant.

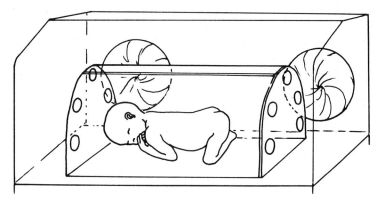

Fig 5–7.—Heat shield in incubator. This plastic shield prevents radiant heat loss from the infant to the colder incubator walls.

effective in removing airborne contaminants down to 0.5 μm in diameter. Due to the slightly positive pressure maintained inside the incubator hood by the air circulation system, there is always a tendency for the air inside the unit to flow to the outside, thus ensuring a high degree of isolation. Good hand-washing techniques to prevent cross-contamination should be mandatory for personnel before entering the incubator.

The circulating air passes through a heating coil to achieve the proper hood temperature, and the infant is warmed by convection. It is often difficult to control the infant's temperature since the heat loss of the infant to the walls of the incubator will vary with the room temperature. If the incubator is placed near a cold window or wall, the infant will radiate even more heat to the cold incubator walls and it will be nearly impossible to maintain the neutral thermal environment. If a plastic heat shield is placed over the infant inside the single-walled incubator (Fig 5–7), the warm incubator air will heat the plastic wall of the shield to the same temperature as the air within the incubator. The infant then will radiate only to the warm inner plastic wall, as radiant waves from the infant (2 to 9 μm) will not penetrate the plastic wall.

High relative humidity is achieved by warm air passing over the water in the humidity reservoir. High relative humidity (75 to 90%) helps in preventing water loss from the skin and respiratory tract. It also may prevent secretions in the respiratory tract from drying.

An enriched oxygen atmosphere may be attained whenever necessary. Some incubators have an oxygen limiter that prevents the oxygen concentration inside the incubator from exceeding 40% (Table 5–3, *top*). Higher concentrations of oxygen can be obtained by placing the red reminder flag in the vertical position, which reduces the air intake and allows oxygen concentrations up to 85% (Table 5–3, *bottom*).

An infant servo-controlled heating module may be used to control the infant's temperature. A highly sensitive thermistor, attached to the infant's ab-

TABLE 5–3.—INCUBATOR OXYGEN THERAPY

RED REMINDER FLAG IN HORIZONTAL POSITION			
Flow of oxygen (liters/min)	4	6	8
Concentration of oxygen	28–31%	32–36%	37–40%

RED REMINDER FLAG IN VERTICAL POSITION			
Flow of oxygen (liter/min)	4–6	8	10	12
Concentration of oxygen	Flow not sufficient for high concentration	70–75%	75–80%	80–85%

domen, serves as the control to provide modulating heat according to the infant's needs. The drawback of servo-controlled incubators is the loss of the patient's temperature as an index of infection.

Mist therapy may be provided to the infant by securing a nebulizer to the inside wall of the incubator. The nebulizer should be cleaned and autoclaved daily and sterile solutions used in order to keep the bacteria count at a minimum.

TRANSPORT INCUBATORS.—The transport incubator (Fig 5–8) is designed to provide a controlled environment under adverse ambient conditions. It is used primarily for transporting high-risk infants from an outside location or between

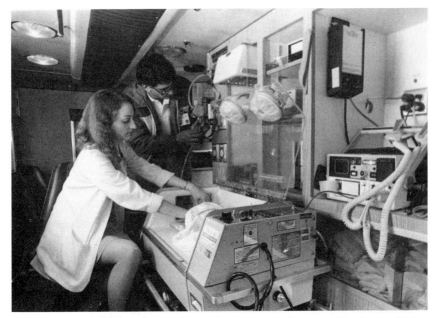

Fig 5–8.—Transport incubator in an intensive care ambulance being readied to transport a high-risk infant from a community hospital.

departments within a hospital complex. A three-way power system permits its operation on 115 volts AC, in motor vehicles with a 12-volt DC power supply, and on the 12-volt DC power pack housed within the unit itself. The operation is essentially the same as the previously described incubator except that it has double-walled construction to minimize the radiant heat loss from the infant. When not in transit, the unit should be plugged into an AC power source to ensure a warm, stable environment and a fully charged DC power pack. An "A," "C" or "E" cylinder of oxygen can be mounted to the support module to provide an oxygen-enriched environment while the unit is in transit.

Hood

In recent years, several observers have suggested that the rigid restriction of oxygen to concentrations of 40% or less for all newborn and premature infants may not be ideal. When administering oxygen to infants, especially when higher concentrations are desired, it is advisable to use a small plastic hood over the head (Fig 5–9) to prevent the wide variations in oxygen concentrations that occur when the incubator is entered. Also, it has been shown that cold oxygen blown on the infant's face will increase oxygen consumption. To avoid this, the oxygen must be warmed to the infant's neutral thermal temperature or to the same temperature as the environment of the incubator. The oxygen must be humidified to minimize water loss and prevent drying of secretions in the respiratory tract. A cascade humidifier with an adjustable heater not only permits hood temperature control but also provides adequate humidification. An oxygen ratio controller (Fig 5–10) can be used effectively to provide precise concentrations of oxygen and air. A total flow of 7 liters/min is required to remove carbon dioxide from the infant hood. After stable conditions have been achieved, hourly checks on both temperature and oxygen should be made and recorded.

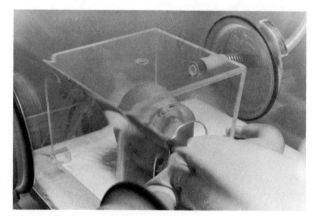

Fig 5–9.—A small plastic hood for administering high concentrations of oxygen to an infant in an incubator.

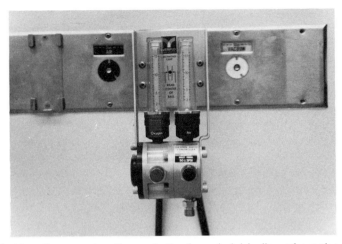

Fig 5–10.—Oxygen-air ratio controller for administration of precise oxygen concentrations.

Continuous Positive Airway Pressure

Continuous positive airway pressure (CPAP), as it relates to the treatment of newborns, has been discussed in Chapter 2. It is also an effective form of therapy for infants and older children with temporary abnormal compliance, ventilation-perfusion ratios or pulmonary diffusion with inadequate ventilation. The equipment and technique are essentially the same as for the newborn, with one exception. Children, unlike newborns, are not obligate nose breathers; therefore, endotracheal intubation is the preferred method of administering CPAP to children beyond the newborn age. Clinical improvement in oxygenation is usually noted with pressures from 2 to 10 cm H_2O. Due to the difference of upper airway resistance in intubated patients, one should extubate whenever the patient is stable at 2 cm H_2O. Berman[5] has demonstrated that Pao_2 values at 2 cm H_2O CPAP are similar to the values obtained after extubation, while Pao_2 values at 0 cm H_2O CPAP were significantly lower. We have made 2 cm H_2O CPAP part of our routine therapy for most children with endotracheal tubes in place

Infant Oxygen Chair

The infant oxygen chair accommodates sick infants up to 8 months of age and provides for enriched and controlled oxygen concentrations (21 to 65%) and humidity or mist therapy (Fig 5–11). The hood raises for easy patient access. A specially designed cassette holder allows for x-ray examination without removing the infant from the chair. Three tilting positions permit patient comfort and treatment of heart failure or respiratory distress.

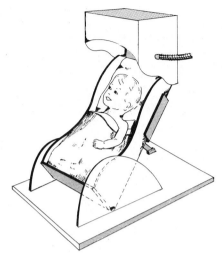

Fig 5–11.—Infant oxygen chair allows for patient comfort and treatment of heart failure and/or respiratory distress.

Radiant Heat Panels

Radiant heat panels are useful for short-term warming in the delivery room and for procedures that require complete access to the infant (Fig 5–12). Since convective and evaporative heat loss are accentuated by radiant heat panels, these units are not widely used for long-term care of small preterm infants. However, patient accessibility makes the unit more attractive for use with the larger infants where temperature homeostasis and caloric conservation are less

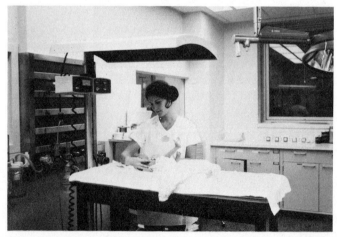

Fig 5–12.—The radiant heat panel provides heat for the infant during examinations and other procedures that expose the infant to ambient room temperatures.

critical. As a safeguard against accidental overheating, the units should only be used in the servo-control mode. The servo probe should be placed at the lower left costal border just below the last rib. Avoid placing the probe over a bony structure or organs that have a high metabolic rate, such as the liver. This will prevent the probe from receiving false signals which may cause under or over heating. False signals may also be sent to the servo-control modula if the infant lays directly on the probe tip, if the probe comes loose, or the probe tip becomes wet.

RISKS AND COMPLICATIONS OF OXYGEN THERAPY

Supplemental oxygen has been demonstrated to cause both pulmonary and systemic toxicity in infants and children. These toxic conditions are manifested by atelectasis, decrease and/or cessation of mucociliary activity, ventilation perfusion mismatch, decrease in the production of surfactant, and severe eye damage (e.g., retrolental fibroplasia). The American Academy of Pediatrics Committee on Fetus and Newborn has made the following recommendations for the safe use of oxygen therapy for the newborns:[2]

1. When an infant born after less than 36 weeks gestation requires supplemental oxygen, the concentration of inspired oxygen should be regulated by measuring arterial oxygen tension.
2. When the measurement of oxygen tension in arterial blood is not available for an infant with generalized cyanosis born after 36 or more weeks gestation, he/she should be given oxygen in a concentration just high enough to abolish the cyanosis.
3. When giving supplemental oxygen, the arterial oxygen tension should be maintained at a level not higher than 80 to 90 mm Hg (the upper level found in "normal" newborn infants). Usually, infants requiring oxygen therapy do not need an arterial Po_2 higher than 50 mm Hg and do well with an arterial Po_2 between 50 and 70 mm Hg. However, even with careful monitoring, arterial Po_2 may reach higher levels in these infants. When this occurs, the inspired oxygen concentration should be lowered promptly. Maintaining an arterial Po_2 between 50 and 70 mm Hg assures adequate tissue oxygenation with the lowest possible alveolar oxygen tension and should minimize the danger of pulmonary oxygen toxicity.
4. The arterial Po_2 in blood obtained from the right radial or temporal arteries will be the same as in retinal artery blood, but frequent sampling from these sites is difficult. Fortunately, the arterial Po_2 of blood obtained from an umbilical arterial catheter with its tip in the abdominal aorta is almost always the same as the Po_2 of blood in the ascending aorta and can be used to regulate the concentration of inspired oxygen. (Exceptions occur when there is systemic hypotension and shock, or when there is persistent pulmonary hypertension.) Arterialized capillary samples have lower oxygen tensions than does arterial blood, especially when the arterial Po_2 is more than 50 mm Hg; and, they should be used with caution.

5. When any infant is in an oxygen-enriched environment, the concentration of oxygen in the environment should be measured with an oxygen analyzer and recorded, or the setting on a reliable oxygen-air mixer should be noted and recorded at least every hour. The performance of the analyzer and oxygen-air mixer should be calibrated and recorded every 8 hours with both room air and 100% oxygen.
6. Except in an emergency, oxygen and compressed air should be warmed and humidified before administration to an infant.
7. An individual experienced in neonatal ophthalmology and indirect ophthalmoscopy should dilate the pupils and examine the retina of all prematurely born infants treated with oxygen at the time supplemental oxygen is discontinued, at discharge from the hospital, and at 4 to 6 weeks after discharge from the hospital.

MONITORING OXYGEN THERAPY

The quality of respiratory care sometimes depends on the tools that we have available to measure the effects of therapy. Recent advances in electronic and computer technology have contributed sophisticated and reliable instruments for monitoring patient care. A degree of sophistication is also required on the part of the practitioner in order to appreciate the value of these monitoring devices.

Although oxygen is precious to life, it can destroy living cells and permanently damage the eyes and lungs when its concentrations become too great. Oxygen is a potent drug and should be administered only when properly ordered and monitored appropriately. One of the most frequently used monitors in respiratory care is the environmental oxygen analyzer. The two types of oxygen analyzers commonly used are the Clark electrode and the Galvanic cell.

GALVANIC CELL.—The galvanic cell monitor, sometimes called a fuel cell monitor, detects a flow of electrical current between two metals, usually silver and lead. These metals are sufficiently electronegative with respect to each other, when immersed in an electrolyte solution, to supply the chemical energy necessary to set the oxygen reduction process in motion at the cathode surface. No external polarizing source (e.g., battery) is required. The signal generated by the cell is proportional to the partial pressure of oxygen and the surface area of the sensor exposed to the environment. The generated signal is displayed on a scale calibrated in percent oxygen. Since the electrical current flow is in part dependent upon the surface area of the cell, accumulated water droplets on the sensor membrane will decrease the surface area and cause inaccurate readings. This device is also affected by changes in the partial pressure of the environment being monitored (e.g., ventilator circuits). The number of molecules at the membrane site will increase as the gas in the ventilator tubing is compressed, thus causing increased diffusion and an increase in the meter reading. Fortunately, the response time of this type of electrode is slow enough to filter out the fluctuations caused by the change in pressure. To be on the safe side, the unit should be recalibrated as part of the pressurized system.

POLAROGRAPHIC ELECTRODE.—The polarographic (Clark electrode) analyzer also detects changes in current between two metals (an anode and a cathode). When the cathode is made slightly negative with respect to the anode, oxygen molecules at the cathode surface undergo electrolytic reduction. The rate at which the oxygen molecules are reduced depends on the density of oxygen molecules diffusing through an oxygen-permeable membrane. When the voltage applied to the cathode is constant, the electrical current produced by the electrochemical reaction is directly proportional to the partial pressure of oxygen within the sensing environment. The partial pressure of oxygen is then displayed as a percentage. This type of electrode is also affected by both changes in partial pressure and humidity.

Both of these analyzers require frequent and careful calibration. Naturally, it would be nice to calibrate the analyzer with a gas approximately the same as the environment about to be analyzed, but this is not always possible. An alternative to "like-gas" calibration is two point calibration using room air and 100% oxygen. After the appropriate warm-up period (usually 1 to 3 min.), the probe should be exposed to 100% oxygen for approximately 1 minute. Adjust the calibration knob until 100% appears. If a small plastic bag or rubber glove is used as a reservoir, care should be taken not to "pressurize" the bag because oxygen analyzers are sensitive to pressure and a calibrating error may occur. This calibrating procedure should be repeated every 8 hours.

Environmental measurements should be made as close to the child's nose or mouth as possible. To prevent cross-contamination, the oxygen analyzers that are used in the premature nursery should not be used in other parts of the hospital, and vice versa. The analyzers used for septic infants in the nursery should not be used for infants considered to be free of infections, such as infants with cardiac disease, failure to thrive, neurologic disorders, or prematurity.

BLOOD OXYGEN MONITORING

During the past decade our knowledge and concern about the toxic effects and associated risks of oxygen therapy have made monitoring of this therapy an absolute must. Our past practice was to periodically withdraw a small sample of arterial blood from an indwelling arterial catheter or from the direct puncture of the peripheral artery and make an analysis for partial pressure of oxygen. These samples, however, yield discontinuous information about the patient's oxygenation, because samples are separated, at best, by several minutes. Several methods of continuously measuring oxygen tension have been developed, including intra-arterial and skin surface electrodes.

The intra-arterial electrode is a polarographic-type built into the tip of a double-lumen catheter (4 or 5 Fr.). One lumen houses the electrode wires and the other is for infusing fluids, blood sampling, and blood pressure monitoring. Conway[6] has reported that the intraarterial electrode has functioned satisfactorily from 10 to 190 hours (mean, 75 hours) in infants. The major drawback to this method of monitoring is that the umbilical artery must be catheterized and that arterial blood samples must be analyzed periodically in order to assess P_{CO_2} and pH.

Another method of continuously monitoring arterial oxygenation is with a catheter oximeter system, which responds to changes in oxygen saturation. The catheter, made from double-lumen polyurethane tubing, is placed in the descending aorta through the umbilical artery. One lumen of the 5 French gauge (1.67 mm) catheter is used for infusing fluids, blood sampling, and measuring blood and intravascular pressures. The other lumen contains the optical fibers and a radiopaque filament. An infrared light, transmitted down one optical fiber, is scattered by the blood and reflected back to the light sensor by a second optical fiber. The signal produced by the light sensor is processed and presented on a digital display and on a strip chart recorder. Most clinicians customarily use PaO_2, not oxygen saturation (SaO_2), as a guide to changes in oxygen therapy and mechanical ventilation. Therefore, one must become familiar with normal or expected saturation ranges and the diagnostic value of this index.

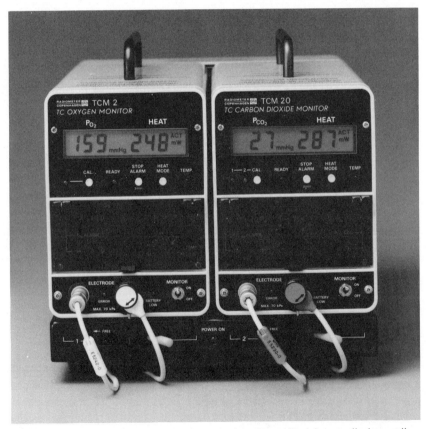

Fig 5–13.—Transcutaneous oxygen and carbon dioxide monitoring units.

In contrast to these relative "invasive" methods of monitoring PaO₂, transcutaneous oxygen monitoring (TCM) has become an important adjunct in assessing and tracking the patient's response to oxygen therapy, mechanical ventilation, continuous positive airway pressure (CPAP), and certain drug therapies. This device (Fig 5–13) employs a heated Clark electrode attached to the skin with a double-sided adhesive ring. Active vasodilation of the cutaneous vessels is achieved by warming the metallic parts of the sensor to a temperature (43 to 45 C) that is higher than normal body temperature. Oxygen diffuses from the arterialized capillary bed through the skin and to the electrode, where an electrochemical reduction of the oxygen takes place. The electrical current produced is converted into a value proportional to the oxygen tension at the electrode membrane interface. This value is displayed on a digital meter and can also be tracked on a strip chart recorder. For optimal results, the electrode should be placed in the infant at an area of good blood flow, usually on the upper part of the chest or the abdomen. If a right-to-left shunt across the ductus arteriosus is suspected, place the electrode in the right upper part of the chest (Fig 5–14), as this area will reflect preductal blood.

The clinical applications of TCM are diverse. The TCM measurements are of particular value in following the immediate effect of changes in oxygen

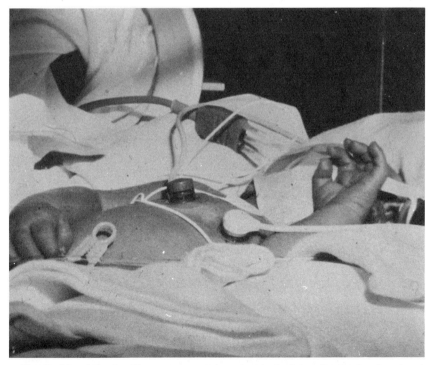

Fig 5–14.—Infant with oxygen and carbon dioxide electrodes in place. Note the oxygen electrode in the upper right-hand portion of the infant's chest, as this area reflects preductal blood values.

therapy and ventilator parameters.[16] Investigators[7, 11] have used TCM to evaluate the adverse effects of routine procedures on preterm infants. Many of the battery-powered devices can be used during the transport of a critically ill infant. TCM has even been used at home in the management of patients with bronchopulmonary dysplasia who are chronically oxygen dependent.[10]

Transcutaneous monitoring was never intended to be a substitute for direct arterial blood measurements. The transcutaneous PO_2 not only reflects the arterial PO_2 but also reflects other physiological parameters such as general circulatory condition, peripheral blood perfusion, skin properties, and anatomic anomalies (shunt, etc.). Therefore, TCM is most helpful when used in conjunction with periodic arterial sampling.

Another noninvasive method of oxygen monitoring that has been gaining popularity over the past couple of years is spectrophotometric oximetry. Unlike TCM, this method does not measure PO_2. Rather, it determines the percentage of the active hemoglobin that is combined with oxygen (SaO_2). This measurement is accomplished by relating oxygen saturation to the transmission of red light through the monitoring sight. Oxygenated blood is much more transparent to red light than is deoxygenated blood; therefore, the optical transmission of infrared light at various wavelengths can be related to oxygen saturation. Although this measurement is not equal to blood PO_2, it is related to the PO_2 by the oxyhemoglobin dissociation relationship and is directly related to the oxy-

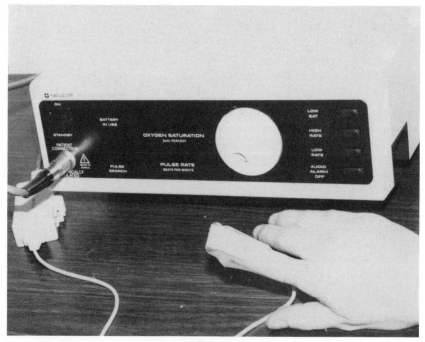

Fig 5–15.—A pulse oximeter with a wraparound adhesive sensor.

gen content of the blood. The Nellcor* pulse oximeter uses a finger sensor, which is a wraparound adhesive bandage. This type of sensor is particularly useful for infants and small children since it can be placed almost anywhere on the patient's body as long as the light emitter and detector are opposite each other (Fig 5–15). This method of monitoring should be verified by arterial blood gases on a routine basis.

AEROSOL THERAPY

It is important not to confuse aerosols with humidity. Humidity represents water in molecular form only, whereas an aerosol is a suspension of particulate water in a gas.

Therapy with aerosols may be given intermittently or continuously over a prolonged period. The purpose of the former is to achieve a pharmacologic effect by delivering small amounts of relatively potent medications, generally in the 1 to 5 μm range, to the respiratory airways. In general, it is felt that the smaller the particle, the further the depth of penetration before deposition occurs. The latter may be helpful in wetting or thinning secretions and decreasing the amount of water that the upper airways must supply to the inspired airstream. Particles larger than 6 μm are almost all deposited in the nose.

Intermittent Aerosol Therapy

Medications administered to children via intermittent aerosol[8, 9] usually fall into one of five categories: (1) bronchodilators, (2) decongestants, (3) antibiotics, (4) mucolytic agents, and (5) corticosteroids. Administration of a nebulized bronchodilator is a standard part of therapy for the patient hospitalized with acute asthma. Isoproterenol (Isuprel) is widely used because of its known effectiveness as a bronchodilator. Recently, isotharine (Bronkosol) has gained popularity for treating children with bronchospasm. It is a little less effective bronchodilator than isoproterenol, but is often used because of its decreased beta$_1$-effect. A dose of 0.01 ml/kg of isoproterenol (1:200) or isoetharine added to a basic solution of normal saline (2 ml) can be used prophylactically as well as therapeutically in the hospital or as part of a home care plan.

Newer, more specific beta$_2$-agonists such as Remiterol and Salbutamol, deserve consideration as alternatives to isoproterenol following published studies that have established dosage and safety. Racemic epinephrine, 0.5 ml of 2% diluted with 3.5 ml of distilled water, has been used effectively as an aerosol or with intermittent positive-pressure breathing in the treatment of children with acute laryngotracheobronchitis and postintubation laryngeal edema. It is felt that the vasoconstrictive action of this drug is what makes it effective and not the bronchodilation. Consequently a bronchodilator such as isoproterenol that does not have the vasoconstrictive action will not relieve the obstruction and may even make the condition worse.

---

*Nellcor Inc., Hayward, Ca.

Phenylephrine (Neo-Synephrine), an effective decongestant with mild bronchodilating properties, is used frequently in conjunction with isoproterenol for simultaneous relief of edema and bronchoconstriction. The rebound effect of the nasal mucosa (paradoxical congestion) observed in patients after a period of phenylephrine nose drop therapy is encountered rarely when phenylephrine is given by aerosol, possibly because the lower airway is less vascular. Young infants may not tolerate phenylephrine given by aerosol and may develop irritation and overinflation.

Most standard antibiotics can be aerosolized. Those that have been used include the penicillins, streptomycin, neomycin, and kanamycin.

A mucolytic or proteolytic agent may be nebulized separately or added to a basic solution. Although enzymatic aerosols have been found to be effective in breaking up the mucoproteins responsible for the viscosity of the sputum, irritation or allergic response of the bronchial mucous membranes usually limits use of these therapeutic agents to short periods of time. Patients with asthma may develop severe bronchospasm when exposed to an aerosol of acetylcysteine. The rotten-egg odor frequently makes it difficult to get children to accept this treatment.

In patients with severe allergy and bronchospasm uncontrolled by the usual methods of therapy, the addition of 0.05 to 0.1 ml dexamethasone (4 mg/ml) to the decongestant-bronchodilator aerosol two or three times a day frequently has replaced or obviated the need for oral steroid therapy. We have not observed the usual systemic side effects of steroid therapy with this dosage schedule, in contrast to the experience of others who have used corticosteroid aerosols delivered from pressurized cartridge-type containers. Because of individualized response of children to these agents, the efficacy should be evaluated by pulmonary function tests before and during a treatment period.

The pressurized-cartridge pocket aerosols should be used sparingly and then only for older children. The coordination of a deep inhalation and a firm squeeze of the cartridge is a difficult maneuver for younger children. An increasing mortality in asthmatics has been associated with the increasing use of the pressurized-cartridge nebulizer. In some countries, this has been correlated with the licensing of extra-strong concentrations of isoproterenol, which increased the likelihood of patient overdosage.[12]

Aerosolized medication should be delivered to infants and children by a simple aerosol system, that is, a nebulizer driven by compressed air or oxygen and a mouthpiece or mask. The flowmeter should be adjusted to aerosolize 2 ml of solution over a 10-min period. A small oil-free compressor can be used to provide aerosol therapy at home (Fig 5–16). The child should be in a seated position and instructed to breathe slowly and deeply through his mouth, briefly holding his breath at the end of inspiration. With proper instructions, even small children can learn the proper breathing pattern. Since the nose can be an efficient filter, greater peripheral deposition usually is achieved when the aerosol is delivered via a mouthpiece, rather than a mask. For infants and young children, a mask is used to ensure aerosol inhalation since mouth breathing

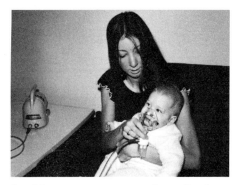

Fig 5–16.—Small, oil-free compressor and medication nebulizer for home aerosol therapy.

cannot be measured and nose clips often are not tolerated. This mode of therapy is much more effective for children than are one or two uncoordinated sprays from the pressurized cartridge, and overusage is controlled far more easily.

Intermittent aerosol therapy is used best in conjunction with other forms of respiratory care, particularly segmental postural drainage to assist the removal of secretions from the respiratory tract.

Prolonged Aerosol Therapy

In general, prolonged aerosol therapy can be achieved by direct inhalation from a nebulizer or by inhalation from a limited compartment such as a mist tent.[8, 9] The goal is to prevent the drying of mucous membranes, including the trachea and major bronchi and/or to add water to secretions to facilitate their removal. In continuous or prolonged mist therapy, 10% by volume USP propylene glycol in distilled water or saline solution (one-quarter to one-half normal) can be used to impair or prevent complete evaporation of particles.

Although at first it was suggested that radioactive aerosols do not deposit in the peripheral airways,[17] later studies using a rapid counter and also the present radionuclide scanning techniques have documented ample deposition.[1, 13, 14, 15, 21] There is sufficient deposition to permit wide use of the latter for diagnostic ventilation testing. Large amounts of aerosol can be visualized directly within the larger bronchi and even in segmental or subsegmental bronchi through a fiberoptic bronchoscope during both oral and nasal breathing.[18, 20] Greater deposition of mist has been noted when using an ultrasonic nebulizer than with a pneumatic nebulizer[19] and when treating patients with cystic fibrosis than control subjects.[4]

EQUIPMENT.—Effective therapy is possible only if adequate equipment is used and kept in good working order. The use of nebulizers, therefore, requires a knowledge of the condition being treated, the site of airway pathology and the nebulizer characteristics.

DIRECT INHALATION.—In the past, this therapy was available only with a pneumatic nebulizer. With the introduction of the ultrasonic nebulizer, which provides a water output of at least 2 ml/min, a mist with more than 50 mg water per liter air can be obtained. This is considerably more water than is required for full humidification at body temperature (44 mg H_2O/liter air). A dilute saline solution (one-quarter to one-half normal) made with distilled water can be inhaled without distress by most patients. Deposition of water in the tracheobronchial tree is enhanced fourfold by mouth breathing. This therapy can be used two to four times a day for 30 to 60 minutes each time. Since the purpose is to mobilize secretions, this therapy should be followed by respiratory physical therapy.

INHALATION FROM A LIMITED COMPARTMENT (MIST TENT THERAPY).—It has been suggested that mist tent therapy might achieve useful deposition of water in the lower airways and/or ensure 100% humidification of the peripheral airways at body temperature.[8, 9]

This therapy requires a nebulizer with a high-volume output (2 ml/min), a small particle (1 to 5 μm) and a dense mist in the tent. Most commercially available ultrasonic nebulizers are suitable for this therapy. Bacterial contamination of nebulizer equipment can be hazardous particularly if *Pseudomonas* contamination occurs. A regular cleaning program at home or in the hospital is mandatory.

Mist tent therapy can be used for treating acute problems in hospitalized patients or for long-term home therapy of chronic conditions such as cystic fibrosis. It can be used successfully for treating cystic fibrosis patients who already have advanced disease; for patients in whom the diagnosis has been made early; it can be added to the treatment program. Mist therapy should be used in conjunction with the other available forms of therapy, including inter-

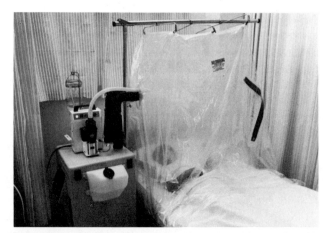

Fig 5–17.—Refrigerated tent in hospital with ultrasonic nebulizer for mist tent therapy. In general, the smaller the canopy size, the easier it is to achieve a dense mist.

mittent aerosol therapy, segmental postural drainage, antimicrobial therapy, and follow-up care at regular intervals at a specialized center.

Mist tents tend to be warmer than the surrounding environment. Consequently, cooling the tent with an ice chest or refrigeration unit (Fig 5–17) or cooling the room with an air conditioner in summer or adding less room heat in the winter are important considerations for patient comfort and acceptance. Even in times of acute illness, no patient should be in continuous mist for more than 18 hours per day as maceration of the skin and a feeling of isolation may develop.

Mist tent therapy with small-particle mist has been used in treating patients with staphylococcal pneumonia, in which thick, tenacious secretions are usually present, and empirically in the treatment of patients with other obstructive airway conditions such as bronchitis, bronchial asthma or bronchiolitis. Criteria for the selection of patients have not been established and the effectiveness of the therapy has not been documented, but it may help provide humidification or reduce insensible water loss.

In the small infant, overhydration can result from intensive use of an ultrasonic nebulizer, especially if a saline solution is nebulized. In patients with considerable retention of secretions, rapid mobilization of secretions may follow initiation of mist tent therapy. Use of segmental postural drainage and suctioning will help the patient clear these secretions. When used intelligently and safely by competent individuals who understand the merits and the hazards, mist therapy can be a beneficial tool for treating patients with obstructive pulmonary disease.

FOG ROOM.—Patients with croup and epiglottitis may be treated with large-particle mist, 10 μm or more in size. The shortcomings of a high-humidity tent were recognized when these patients appeared to have a sense of claustrophobia and confinement. Also, when placed in a tent, patients may become upset by being separated from their mothers and may become more symptomatic because of their anxiety. These difficulties may be overcome by the use of a fog room in which the relative humidity is maintained at 100% and room temperature at 70 to 72 F.[15] In this room, steam is introduced under controlled conditions into the cold airstream of an oversized air conditioner. This results in particles of moisture that are circulated at a rate of 1 air change per minute before being swept from the room and precipitated out as water by the cooling coil of the apparatus. Several children can be treated simultaneously, and the sense of restraint within a tent is avoided. Nursing care often is easier without the interruption of therapy. The child is observed more easily, and the mother can be present to hold and comfort him.[3] Cross-infection is reportedly rare.

INTERMITTENT POSITIVE-PRESSURE BREATHING THERAPY

Intermittent positive-pressure breathing (IPPB), combined with the delivery of a medicated aerosol, is effective in treating children with hypoxia, bronchospasm, pulmonary infection, impaired breathing mechanics, and postoperative complications.

IPPB may be used as a supplement to intermittent aerosol therapy in treating the child with increased airway resistance, decreased muscular strength, atelectasis, ineffective cough, and/or an accumulation of secretions.

IPPB is particularly useful for children with compromised ventilation who are to undergo surgery. The child always should be introduced to IPPB therapy before surgery so that it will be tolerated and nonthreatening following surgery.

The medications previously described for aerosol therapy can be used in conjunction with IPPB to achieve the same pharmacologic effect.

Generally, an IPPB treatment should last for 10 to 15 minutes at a pressure of 10 to 20 cm H_2O. The first treatments should be initiated at low pressures for short periods until the child has adapted to this new experience. Reflex glottic closure that may occur in the uninitiated child when high initial pressures are used can be overcome by lowering the mask pressure and reassuring the child to relax and let the machine do the breathing. Slow, deep breathing and a comfortable position facilitates the diaphragmatic motion in order to prevent hypoventilation and ensure penetration and deposition of the aerosols.

Most IPPB units can be used for treating children over 2 years of age. Steps must be taken to keep mechanical dead space at a minimum. The coordination required to operate the manual Venturi apparatus (Hand-E-Vent, TA-1) makes it unsuitable for use with small children. In order to compensate for the extremely small inspiratory efforts of infants and small children, a breathing unit must be used that provides a means of increasing the sensitivity of the machine. A heated nebulizer, a cascade humidifier, or an ultrasonic nebulizer should be used to provide humidification and/or mist to the mainstream gases.

The usual frequency of treatments is two to four each day, but this may be increased to as often as once every 1 or 2 hours. Care must be exercised in monitoring total medication dosage when frequent treatments are required.

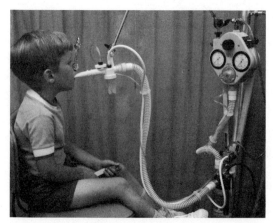

Fig 15–18.—Intermittent positive-pressure breathing via mouthpiece. The child is seated upright in a straight-backed chair. Nose clips help insure delivery of the desired pressure to the lungs. Use of the mainstream humidifier provides for adequate humidification of inspired gas.

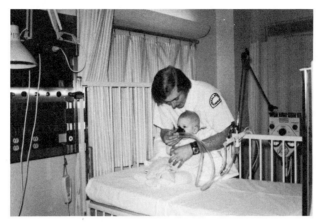

Fig 5–19.—Intermittent positive-pressure breathing via mask. The infant is seated in an upright position while the therapist stands behind to support the back and head of the patient.

Many complications of IPPB appear to stem from the child's adverse reaction to the injudicious use of the equipment. Careful orientation and conditioning of the child are necessary before therapy is begun. He should be permitted to touch the equipment and become aware of what the machine does. The opportunity to observe another child receiving IPPB is also helpful.

Patients older than 4 years of age usually cooperate. Younger patients often do not cooperate until they realize that pain or discomfort is not associated with the treatment. For best results the child should be seated upright in a straight chair (Fig 5–18). The small child or infant should be in a sitting position with back and head supported by the chest and shoulders of the therapist, who stands behind the child (Fig 5–19). This technique provides excellent control of head

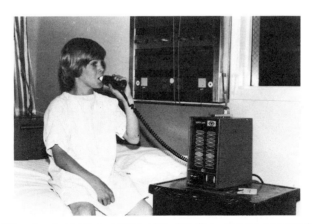

Fig 5–20.—An incentive spirometer for the encouragement of deep breathing. A clown's face lights up when the goal is achieved.

movement. A safeguard against any possible aspiration subsequent to IPPB therapy, which can occur in children in the younger age group, is provided by simple removal of the mask and forward tilting of the child's head by the supporting shoulder. The child may be rocked during the treatment, thus reducing fear and providing assurance that the therapist does not intend harm.

INCENTIVE SPIROMETRY

Incentive spirometry (Fig 5–20) is useful in treating children when a breathing exercise is recommended without an accompanying aerosolized medication. The incentive device has two separate lighted, numbered columns. One column represents an inspired volume goal, which the therapist and patient have selected together; the other column is for display of the patient's effort. On the later column the lights turn on sequentially as the child inspires and attempts to reach the preset inspiratory volume. When the preset inspiratory volume is reached, a clown's face lights up, thus providing a sense of accomplishment for the child. This prophylactic type of therapy is reported to be effective for the prevention of atelectasis during postoperative recovery.

REFERENCES

1. Alberson, P.D., Secker-Walter, R.H., and Forrest, J.V.: Detection of obstructive pulmonary disease, Radiology 111:643, 1974.
2. American Academy of Pediatrics: *Standards and Recommendations for Hospital Care of Newborn Infants,* (6th Ed.; Evanston, IL. 1977).
3. Baker, H.: Five years' experience with a high humidity room, Can. Med. Assoc. J. 72:914, 1955.
4. Bau, S.K., Aspin H., Wood, D.E., and Levison, H.: The measurement of fluid deposition in humans following mist tent therapy, Pediatrics 48:605, 1971.
5. Berman, L.S.: Optimum levels of CPAP for tracheal extubation of newborn infants, J. Pediatr. 89:109, 1976.
6. Conway, M., et al.: Continuous monitoring of arterial oxygen tension using a catheter-tip polarographic electrode in infants, Pediatrics 57:244, 1976.
7. Long, J.G., Phillip, A.G., Lucey, J.F.: Excessive handling as a cause of hypoxemia, Pediatrics 65:203, 1980.
8. National Cystic Fibrosis Research Foundation: *Guide to Diagnosis and Management of Cystic Fibrosis* (Atlanta, 1971).
9. National Cystic Fibrosis Research Foundation: *Source Book in Pediatric Pulmonary Disease* (Atlanta, 1971).
10. Philip, A.S., Peabody, J.L., Lucey, J.F.: Transcutaneous Po_2 monitoring in the home management of bronchopulmonary dysplasia, Pediatrics 65:884, 1980.
11. Speidel, B.D.: Adverse effects of routine procedures in preterm infants, Lancet 1:864, 1978.
12. Stolley, P.D.: Asthma mortality: Why the United States was spared an epidemic of deaths due to asthma, Am. Rev. Respir. Dis. 105:883, 1972.
13. Taplin, G.V., et al.: Early detection of chronic obstructive pulmonary disease using radionuclide lung imaging procedures, Chest 71:567, 1977.
14. Taplin, G.V., Poe, N.D., Isawa, T., and Dore, E.K.: Radioaerosol and xenon gas inhalation and lung perfusion scintigraphy, Scand. J. Respir. Dis. (suppl.) 85:114, 1974.

15. Tovell, R.M., and Little, D.M., Jr.: The utilization of fog as a therapeutic agent, Anesthesiology 18:470, 1957.
16. Tremper, K., Waxman, K., Shoemaker, W.: Use of transcutaneous oxygen sensors to titrate PEEP, Ann. Surg. 193:206, 1981.
17. Wolfsdorf, J., Swift, D.L., and Avery, M.E.: Mist therapy reconsidered, Pediatrics 43:700, 1969.
18. Wood, R.E.: Cystic fibrosis: Current concepts in diagnosis, therapy and prognosis, South. Med. J., in press.
19. Wood, R.E., Boat, T.F., and Doershuk, C.F.: Cystic fibrosis—State of the art, Am. Rev. Respir. Dis. 113:833, 1976.
20. Wood, R.E., Horowitz, J.G., and Doershuk, C.F.: *Tracheal Mucociliary Transport in Cystic Fibrosis,* proceedings of the 7th International Cystic Fibrosis Congress, Paris, 1976.
21. Yeates, D.B., Aspin, N., Bryan, A.C., and Levison, H.: Regional clearance of ions from the airways of the lung, Am. Rev. Respir. Dis. 107:602, 1973.

Mechanical Ventilation

Robert L. Chatburn R.R.T.
Marvin D. Lough, R.R.T.

6

> When Elisha came into the house he saw the child lying dead on his bed. So he went in and shut the door upon the two of them and prayed to the Lord. Then he went up and lay upon the child, putting his mouth upon his mouth, his eyes upon his eyes, and his hands upon his hands; and he stretched himself upon him, the flesh of the child became warm. –*II Kings 4:32-35*

SINCE THIS EARLY DESCRIPTION of mouth-to-mouth resuscitation of a child, humans have sought to improve ventilatory techniques. Many complicated and sophisticated mechanical ventilators have since been developed, although most are designed for the adult patient and only a few are specifically designed for pediatric use.

The requirements for a pediatric ventilator are quite challenging because of the special problems presented by infants and small children. Infants have a higher metabolic rate, a larger surface area in relation to weight, relatively smaller airway diameter, much smaller tidal volume, high respiratory rate, and higher airway resistance than do older children and adults (Fig 6–1).

These anatomical and physiologic differences necessitate a respirator that can deliver small but accurate volumes against the high resistance of relatively small airways and against lungs that often have a low compliance. This chapter describes many of the devices used in mechanical ventilation and makes recommendations for their clinical use.

MECHANICAL VENTILATING DEVICES

Several pieces of equipment are essential in the delivery room and newborn nursery. One of the most important is a resuscitation tray. Numerous devices are available for application of positive pressure by bag and mask. Figure 6–2 shows the equipment used in our delivery room and premature nurseries.

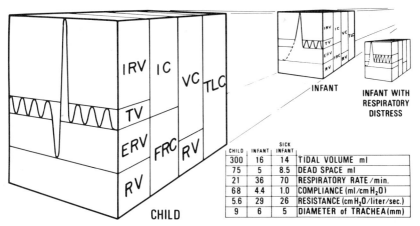

CHILD	INFANT	SICK INFANT	
300	16	14	TIDAL VOLUME ml
75	5	8.5	DEAD SPACE ml
21	36	70	RESPIRATORY RATE /min.
68	4.4	1.0	COMPLIANCE (ml/cm H_2O)
5.6	29	26	RESISTANCE (cm H_2O/liter/sec.)
9	6	5	DIAMETER of TRACHEA (mm)

Fig 6–1. —Lung characteristics of a 6-year-old, a normal infant, and an infant with respiratory distress syndrome. The challenges a respirator must meet in order to ventilate either the child or the infant as compared to the adult are tremendous. More significant, the demands for effective ventilation of the sick infant are even greater. (Adapted from Cook, C.D.: *Respiration and Metabolism of Newborn Infants*, exhibited at the VIIIth International Congress of Pediatrics, Copenhagen, 1956.)

When the need arises for artificial ventilation by bag and mask, the mask should be applied to the infant's face with care taken to ensure a small but definite leak around the mask to act as a "pop-off" that will prevent excess pressure delivery and carbon dioxide accumulation. Also, the flow around the mask results in the delivery of continuous positive airway pressure that can be varied by the size of the leak around the face of the infant. Hustead and Avery[19] suggest that pressures of 35 cm H_2O for intervals of 1 to 2 seconds are safe and may be required. Gruber and Klaus[15] recommend pressures as high as 65 cm H_2O when breathing by bag for infants with the respiratory distress syndrome.

Hospital divisions that care for children of all ages should have additional resuscitation apparatus on the tray (Fig 6–3). This tray also should provide resuscitative equipment for visitors and hospital personnel.

Bag and mask ventilation is frequently underrated as a means of treating acute respiratory failure in both children and adults. Although its use is common as an immediate resuscitative measure, this technique has definite advantages in many circumstances. Frequently, conditions exits under which intermittent supportive assistance will suffice for respiratory insufficiency. Endotracheal intubation and/or tracheostomy should be used only when continuous supportive measures are necessary. The trauma usually associated with the latter procedures often can be avoided by a skilled therapist using a bag and mask. The deciding factors should be the frequency with which assistance is needed. The bag and mask obviate the need for a tube in the airway, per-

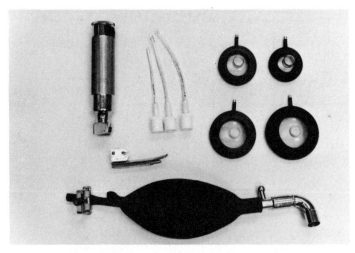

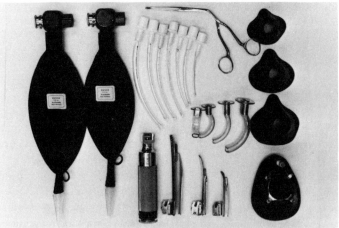

Fig 6–2 (top).—Emergency resuscitation tray for the premature intensive care nursery.

Fig 6–3 (bottom).—Emergency resuscitation tray for children, adolescents, and adults.

mitting normal clearance of pulmonary secretions and allowing the patient to cough effectively.

Mask and Bag Equipment

The two types of bags commonly used for ventilation of infants and children are flow-inflating and self-inflating.

FLOW-INFLATING BAGS.—Anesthesia equipment manufacturers provide a variety of 0.5-liter and 1-liter thin rubber anesthesia bags that are suitable for use with children. This type of bag utilizes a flow of gas, usually an oxygen-air mixture. Pressure and inflation of the bag are varied by adjusting either the gas flow or a resistance valve. A manometer should be placed in the system for visual indication of applied pressure.

SELF-INFLATING BAGS.—Unlike the flow-inflating bag, the self-inflating bag does not require a gas source. The recoil characteristics of this bag allow for reinflation following manual deflation. This is an advantage when a source of compressed gas is not available during an emergency. This bag is also useful for supporting ventilation during the transportation of patients from one location to another. Table 6–1 lists some characterisitics of commonly used self-inflating bags. Some of the problems associated with self-inflating bag and mask systems are (a) oxygen concentrations vary and are sometimes unknown; (b) the "feel" for bagging is lost due to the recoil characteristics of the bag; and (c) the safety release valve often is limited to less than 40 cm H_2O. Varying oxygen concentrations can be remedied by adding a reservoir to the system.

Bag and mask ventilation is useful only when one can establish and maintain an adequate airway. When controlled or prolonged assisted ventilation becomes necessary, a tracheal airway should be established. Complications arising from the use of bag and mask therapy include pneumothorax, pressure necrosis from the mask, and dependence on assisted ventilation. The incidence of these complications may be minimized by careful attention to nursing care and the technique of bagging, and frequent checking for the opportunity to wean the patient from bag and mask therapy.

ARTIFICAL AIRWAYS

The anatomy of the pediatric airway is an important consideration when choosing an artificial airway. In an infant, the trachea is most narrow below the vocal cords at the level of the cricoid cartilage. This cartilage is the only complete tracheal ring and serves as an anatomic cuff when an artificial airway is used. The endotracheal tube selected should fit snugly to permit more adequate ventilation, but too much pressure may cause trauma to the cricoid region. The resulting edema narrows the airways internally and may cause postextubation stridor, which may be severe. Patients who have convulsions or move actively

TABLE 6–1.—CHARACTERISTICS OF SELF-INFLATING BAGS
FOR INFANTS AND CHILDREN

BAG	APPROXIMATE VOLUME (FULL)	OXYGEN RESERVOIR	MAXIMUM $FiO_2(\%)$	PRESSURE RELIEF
Hope	730	Sleeve	100	40 cm H_2O
Penlon	250	Tube	100	Fixed leak
Ambu	500	Tube	100	None
Laerdal				
Infant	240	Tube	100	35 cm H_2O
Child	500	Tube	100	35 cm H_2O
AIRbird	500	Tube	90	None
Hudson	600	Tube	100	None

TABLE 6–2.—GUIDE TO CHOICE OF ENDOTRACHEAL TUBES

AGE	FRENCH SIZE	INTERNAL DIAMETER (mm)	ORAL LENGTH (cm)	NASAL LENGTH (cm)	SUCTION CATHETER (FRENCH)
Premature	12	2.5	8	11	6
Newborn	14	3.0	9	12	6
6 mo	16	3.5	10	14	8
1 yr	18–20	4.0–4.5	12	16	8
2 yr	22–24	5.0–5.5	14	17	8
2–4 yr	24–26	5.5–6.0	15	18	10
4–7 yr	26–28	6.0–6.5	16	19	10
7–10 yr	28–30	6.5–7.0	17	21	10
10–12 yr	30–32	7.0–7.5	20	23	10
12–16 yr	32–34	7.5–8.0	21	24	12

during their intubation are at risk of more severe complications (e.g., vocal cord paralysis, granulation, and subglottic stenosis).

Table 6–2 provides data to assist in determining the inside diameter (ID) and length of endotracheal tubes suitable for use in treating infants and children. To prevent an increase in resistance, the 15-mm male connector must be as large as, if not larger than, the internal lumen of the endotracheal tube. For description of an intubation procedure, see Chapter 8.

Once the tube is in place, it must be properly secured. This is accomplished by drying the upper lip and cheeks and painting them and the exterior of the endotracheal tube with tincture of benzoine. After the benzoine has become tacky, a piece of ½-in. adhesive tape should be placed on the right cheek, drawn across the upper lip and pressed firmly to the skin. It is then wrapped firmly around the tube (two revolutions) in a counterclockwise direction and secured to the left cheek. The process is repeated beginning on the left cheek. Common adhesive tape rather than waterproof adhesive tape should be used. A nasotracheal tube is secured in the same manner.

The position of the tube within the airway should be confirmed by chest x-ray film in order to avoid accidental intubation of the right or left bronchus.

Endotracheal tube suctioning is a potentially dangerous but necessary procedure. Suctioning requires two people; one should hyperventilate the patient with an anesthesia bag and then stabilize the endotracheal tube while the other person performs the actual suctioning. Apnea and bradycardia are sometimes associated with suctioning and can be prevented by prior hyperventilation. Turning the patient's head to the right or left during the suctioning will help direct the catheter and ensure that both the right and left main-stem bronchi are cleared. See Chapter 8 for a detailed suctioning procedure.

Extubation in most instances is an elective procedure and should be done in a controlled manner. The nasal and oral pharynx should be suctioned to clear the airway of any material that might be aspirated when the tube is removed.

The endotracheal tube should be removed at end inspiration since the next respiratory maneuver will be an exhalation, which will minimize the risk of aspiration. A racemic epinephrine aerosol (1:8 dilution) may be helpful if stridor occurs following extubation.

POSITIVE-PRESSURE VENTILATION

Acute respiratory failure in infants and children can often be reversed if recognized early and treated appropriately. Therefore, the success of a mechanical device in replacing the lost function can have an enormous impact on the mortality and morbidity of these children.

The ultimate goal of mechanical ventilation is to provide effective gas exchange with minimal circulatory impairment and minimal trauma to the lung. This requires that a ventilator move gas into the lungs, hold it there for a predetermined amount of time, and release it to a present baseline. Most ventilators cause this to happen by altering the pressure in the airways relative to atmosphere. Infant ventilators are often referred to as being of the "volume" or "pressure" type. These designations refer to the fact that certain ventilators are designed to be used primarily in either the volume-limited or pressure-limited mode, although any given machine can generally be made to do both. The term *limited* as opposed to cycling, means that some variable (e.g., pressure or volume) rises to a preset value during inspiration and is held or limited at that value until inspiration is terminated by the cycling variable (Fig 6–4). Both types of ventilators will produce a tidal volume, but the principle used to do so may affect which is selected and the results obtained.

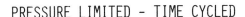

PRESSURE LIMITED - TIME CYCLED

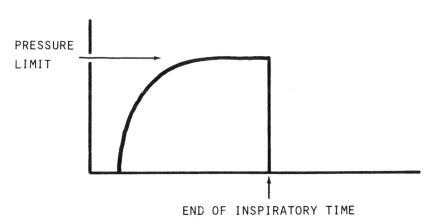

END OF INSPIRATORY TIME

Fig 6–4.—Distinction between "limiting" and "cycling." In this illustration a pressure limit (determined by a pressure relief valve) is reached early in inspiration, but termination of gas pressure and flow does not occur until passage of a preset time interval (time-cycled).

Volume-Limited Ventilation

Volume-limited ventilation is different from pressure-limited ventilation in terms of how the ventilator is used clinically. During volume-limited ventilation, the ventilator is adjusted to provide the desired tidal volume and inspiratory flow rate. Most ventilators operated in this mode deliver the tidal volume at a nearly constant flow rate, which produces the characteristic inspiratory waveforms shown in Figure 6–5. Changes in the lung mechanics are reflected by changes in proximal airway pressure while the volume delivered remains

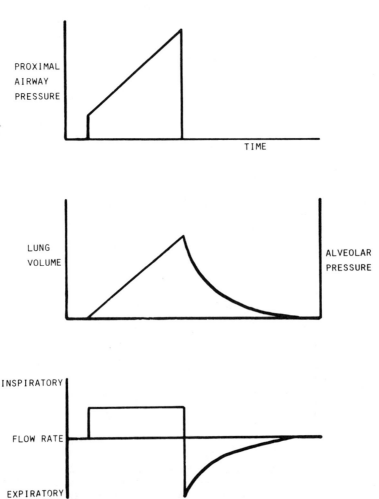

Fig 6–5.—Characteristic waveforms produced by an idealized constant-flow, volume-limited ventilator.

relatively constant. Thus, airway pressures depend upon the tidal volume, flow rate, airway resistance, and respiratory system compliance. In fact, changes in the patient's pulmonary mechanics, which reflect the severity of the disease, can be monitored and quantified by observing these pressure changes.

It must be recognized, however, that only a few volume ventilators designed specifically for infants and children are available today. One of these, the Bourns LS-104-150, was designed in 1964 and is no longer manufactured. The design requirements for infant volume ventilators are strict. The unit must be capable of small but very predictable tidal volumes, low flow rates, and variable $I:E$ ratios, and be able to respond to the more rapid and shallow respiratory efforts of infants and small children. Because of the technical difficulties in meeting these criteria, a whole new class of infant pressure ventilators has evolved, having no correlates in adult therapy.

Theory of Pressure-Limited Ventilation

The basic goal of pressure-limited ventilation is to mechanically support some fraction of the patient's minute exhaled volume. By definition, minute exhaled volume is the product of tidal volume and respiratory rate,

$$\dot{V}_E = V_T \times f \tag{1}$$

when $\dot{V}_E$ = minute exhaled volume, V_T = tidal volume, and f = respiratory rate or frequency. This mathematical relationship may be expressed graphically (Fig 6–6).

In this type of diagram any three parameters connected by straight lines are mathematically interrelated such that if any two are known, the third can be calculated. Thus, in Figure 6–6, if V_T and f are known, $\dot{V}_E$ can be derived using equation 1. These variables are easily understood and convenient to quantify when using volume-cycled ventilators. However, during pressure-limited ventilation the delivered volme is not preset. Rather, it is a product of complex interrelationships between ventilator controls and lung characteristics. In many clinical situations, such as pediatric or neonatal ventilation, it is often difficult or impractical to actually measure tidal volumes. Therefore, it is important to have a thorough understanding of the factors that determine tidal and minute volumes. This knowledge can then be applied to any specific ventilator in order to satisfy patient needs under a variety of clinical situations.

The goal of this section is to develop an operational diagram that describes the variables that are common to pressure-limited, time-cycled ventilators. Ventilator manufacturers, in their quest to be unique, use various combinations

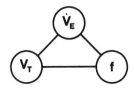

Fig 6–6.—The mathematical relationship among V_T, f, and $\dot{V}_E$ can be symbolically diagrammed as a triad. If any two variables are known, the third can be calculated.

of controls to obtain the same basic function. For example, some models may have a control to directly set a calibrated inspiratory time (e.g., Sechrist, Healthdyne, Bear Cub) while on others, inspiratory time is indirectly set with the rate and $I{:}E$ ratio (e.g., Bourns BP200). For this reason, knowledge of a general operational diagram will facilitate understanding of the available infant ventilators. It is also necessary to be familiar with at least some part of this diagram in order to use a specific ventilator under conditions of varying lung compliance and resistance.

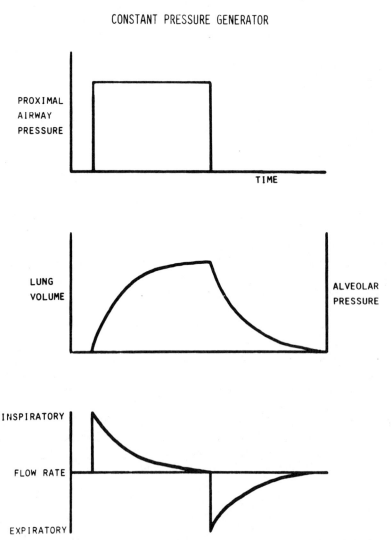

CONSTANT PRESSURE GENERATOR

Fig 6–7.—Characteristic waveforms of an idealized pressure-limited, time-cycled infant ventilator.

For delivery of a tidal volume during mechanical ventilation, there must be a positive-pressure difference between the airway opening and the lungs, and this pressure difference must exist for a long enough time to generate flow into the lungs. During pressure-limited ventilation, proximal airway pressure rises rapidly to some preset level and is maintained at that level for the duration of the inspiratory time (Fig 6–7). Alveolar pressure also rises as volume is delivered to the lungs. The flow rate at which this volume is delivered decreases as alveolar pressure approaches proximal airway pressure and stops when the two pressures are equal. The inspiratory flow rate, and hence the tidal volume, at any point in time depends on two factors: the magnitude of the pressure difference between the airway opening and the lungs and the mechanical properties (i.e., resistance and compliance) of the respiratory system.

Pressure-limited ventilators generate nearly rectangular airway-pressure waveforms. Thus, in clinical terms, the pressure difference between the airway opening and the lungs, created by the ventilator, can be thought of as the difference between peak inspiratory pressure (PIP) and positive end-expiratory pressure (PEEP). For any given value of compliance of the respiratory system, tidal volume (V_T) is proportional to the pressure difference generated by the ventilator (i.e., PIP-PEEP), assuming that there is enough time for airway pressure to equilibrate with the lung pressure. With this in mind, Figure 6–6 can be expanded to include the relationship among PIP, PEEP, and tidal volume (Fig 6–8). The pressure difference, PD, is connected to V_T by a dotted line because it is not the only variable that determines the delivered tidal volume.

The clinical significance of the compliance and resistance of the respiratory system is that for a set pressure difference created by the ventilator, the compliance and resistance of the respiratory system will determine the tidal volume delivered in a given inspiratory time. This relationship is often conceptualized in terms of a time constant. The time constant is a measure of the time necessary to deliver a given volume with a given pressure difference. It is defined by the equation

$$T_C = R \times C \qquad (2)$$

where T_C = time constant (seconds), R = resistance (cm H_2O/ml/sec), and C = compliance (ml/cm H_2O)

Technically, 63.2% of the total volume (i.e., the potential tidal volume after equilibration of lung pressure with mouth pressure) is delivered during the first time constant. During the next time constant, 63.2% of the remaining volume is delivered. This process continues during each time constant. After a period of time equal to three time constants, over 95% of the total volume is delivered. For practical purposes, volume delivery is complete after five time constants (Fig 6–9). Furthermore, it also takes five time constants for passive exhalation to occur.

In practice, the quantitative value of the time constant for a patient's lungs is generally unknown; however, clinical observations can give a qualitative estimate of lung compliance and resistance. The simplest and most direct

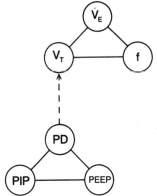

Fig 6–8.—Tidal volume is proportional to the pressure difference, PD, between PIP and PEEP (i.e., PD = PIP − PEEP)

method is to measure the pressure generated during hand ventilation. Breath sounds, chest rise, blood gases, and other clinical observations can all be used to form a dynamic concept of the condition of the patient's pulmonary system. Once this concept has been formed, predictions can be made about the tidal volume that can be delivered with a given ventilator setting and qualitatively explained in terms of time constants. The success of such treatment will be depend upon one's experience and accuracy in forming a clear idea of the patient's condition and a thorough understanding of the ventilator capabilities.

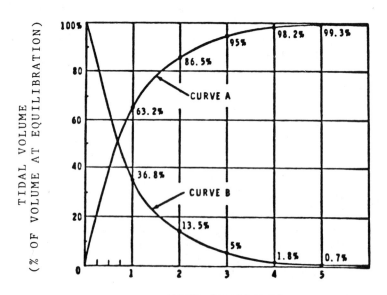

TIME CONSTANTS

Fig 6–9.—Graph of tidal volume as a function of time. Tidal volume is expressed as a percentage of the potential volume that would be delivered if lung pressure equilibrated with proximal airway pressure. Time is expressed in time constants. Curve A represents passive inspirations during pressure-limited ventilation. Curve B represents passive expiration during any type of ventilation.

At this point, the diagram in Figure 6–8 can be elaborated upon to include all of the factors that determine tidal volume (Fig 6–10).

The diagram in Figure 6–10 shows that the time constant, pressure difference, and inspiratory time (T_I) all have a direct effect on tidal volume. These variables are related by an exact mathematical equation,[9] however, they cannot be grouped in triads, so they are connected to V_T by dotted lines. While the time constant and the pressure difference play a large part in determining tidal volume, Figure 6–10 shows that inspiratory time is also an important factor. If the time constant of the lungs is such that the time necessary to deliver a given tidal volume is equal to or longer than the set inspiratory time, then a decrease in inspiratory time will decrease the tidal volume. For example, suppose the compliance and resistance of the respiratory system were 2.0 ml/cm H_2O and 50 cm H_2O/liter/sec, respectively (common infant values). The time constant would be 0.1 seconds, and it would take about 0.5 seconds (five time constants) for the alveolar pressure to equilibrate with proximal airway pressure. If PIP = 25 cm H_2O and PEEP = 5 cm H_2O, then the pressure difference would be 20 cm H_2O. Since volume equals pressure times compliance, the maximum tidal volume at equilibration would be 40 ml. However if T_I is less than 0.5 seconds, the actual delivered volume will be less than 40 ml. Similarly, if expiratory time is less than 0.5 seconds, there will not be enough time to exhale completely, and alveolar PEEP will be higher than proximal airway PEEP.

On some ventilators, such as the Sechrist, inspiratory time and expiratory time can be set directly. Such models have no control knobs for rate and $I:E$ ratio because these parameters are automatically set as a result of inspiratory and expiratory times. To facilitate understanding of these relationships, the term *total cycle time* will be used. Total cycle time (TCT) is defined as the time from the beginning of one inspiration to the beginning of the next, or the sum of the inspiratory and expiratory times. It is also related to ventilator frequency (bpm):

$$\text{TCT} = T_I + T_E = \frac{60 \text{ seconds}}{f} \tag{3}$$

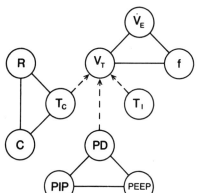

Fig 6–10.—This diagram includes all of the variables that affect tidal volume. The variables T_C, PD and T_I are joined to V_T by dotted lines because these variables are not related in groups of three as are the other variables.

If the inspiratory and expiratory times are set at 1 and 2 seconds, respectively, the total cycle time will be 3 seconds. By rearranging equation (3), the resultant respiratory rate is found to be 20 bpm:

$$f = \frac{60 \text{ seconds}}{TCT} \tag{4}$$

$$f = \frac{60}{3} = 20$$

By adding the parameter of $I:E$ ratio, the diagram will be complete. The $I:E$ ratio is related to inspiratory time and expiratory time by definition

$$I:E = T_I:T_E = T_I/T_E \tag{5}$$

The ratio may also be expressed as a fraction

$$I:E = \frac{I}{E} \tag{6}$$

This is the basis for considering one $I:E$ ratio to be greater or less than another (e.g., $1:2 > 1:10$ because $1/2 > 1/10$). In the above equation, I and E can be expressed using either of the following conventions:

$$I = T_I/T_E \text{ (example } 2:1)$$
$$E = 1$$

or

$$I = 1$$
$$E = T_E/T_I \text{ (examples } 1:3, \ 1:0.5)$$

On some ventilators such as the Bourns BP200, the inspiratory and expiratory times are established indirectly as the result of the rate and $I:E$ ratio settings. The rate setting determines the total cycle time, and the $I:E$ control divides it into inspiratory and expiratory times. Under these conditions, inspiratory time can be calculated using the equation

$$T_I = \frac{60}{f} \times \frac{I}{I + E} \tag{7}$$

It is often desirable to maintain the same inspiratory time while changing the respiratory rate. This requires an adjustment of $I:E$ ratio as described by the equation

$$\frac{I}{E} = \frac{T_I}{TCT - T_I} = \frac{T_I}{(60/f) - T_I} \tag{8}$$

The operational diagram can now be completed (Figure 6–11). It will cover all variables of pressure-limited, time-cycled mechanical ventilation that affect minute exhaled volume. The shaded circles represent variables that may be controlled directly by ventilator settings.

The operational diagram shown in Figure 6–11 includes the control variables

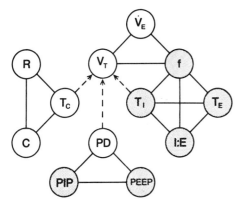

Fig 6–11.—The complete operational diagram for pressure-limited, time-cycled infant ventilation. Shaded circles represent variables directly controlled by ventilator settings.

found on all infant ventilators (i.e., PIP, PEEP, T_I, T_E, $I:E$, and f). Of course, any given ventilator will have controls for only a few variables with, perhaps, a display of those variables that are indirectly affected. For example, the Bear Cub has direct controls for T_I and f and digital displays for the resulting T_E and $I:E$ ratio. One control variable that has not been included in Figure 6–11 is flow rate (i.e., the continuous flow rate through the ventilator delivery circuit). Besides providing for the patient's spontaneous inspiratory demands, the continuous flow rate may affect the tidal volume by influencing the shape of the airway pressure waveform. For example, by adjusting the flow rate on a typical infant ventilator, one may obtain triangular, "shark-fin," or rectangular waveforms. However, the previous discussion of pressure-limited infant ventilation assumed a flow rate that produced a rectangular waveform and hence flowrate was not included in the operational diagram.

The operational diagram is concerned with the mechanical support of minute ventilation, which is defined in terms of arterial carbon dioxide tension. However, oxygenation is just as important a consideration as is ventilation. What is needed at this point is some concept of how changes in the ventilator settings affect oxygenation as well as ventilation. One useful index, mean airway pressure ($\bar{P}_{aw}$), takes into consideration changes in the pattern of ventilator breaths and correlates well with arterial oxygen tension. That is, ventilator changes that increase mean airway pressure, within reasonable limits, will generally increase oxygenation, assuming that cardiac output is not adversely affected. Mean airway pressure may be defined as the average pressure that exists at the airway opening over one respiratory cycle ($T_I + T_E$).[26] The factors that affect $\bar{P}_{aw}$ are the shape of the airway pressure waveform, PIP, PEEP, and the proportion of the respiratory cycle devoted to inspiration. During pressure-limited, time-cycled infant ventilation, this relationship can be expressed by the equation

$$\bar{P}_{aw} = \frac{K \times (PIP - PEEP) \times T_I}{T_I + T_E} + PEEP$$

$$= \frac{K \times (PIP - PEEP) \times I}{I + E} + PEEP \qquad (9)$$

where $\bar{P}_{aw}$ = mean airway pressure (cm H_2O), PIP = peak inspiratory pressure (cm H_2O), I = numerator of I:E ratio (dimensionless), E = denominator of I:E ratio (dimensionless), K = waveform constant (dimensionless). This constant reflects the shape of the airway pressure waveform. For an ideal rectangular waveform, K = 1.0; for a triangular waveform, K = 0.5. Under clinical conditions, K varies with flow rate and T_I, ranging in value from 0.89 to 0.98.[14]

Mean airway pressure may be estimated using the above equation, but more commonly, it is measured using electronic[1] or pneumatic[11] devices. It is interesting to note that from equation 9, we see that mean airway pressure is not affected by changes in ventilator frequency as long as the airway pressure waveform *(K)* and the I:E ratio remain constant.

In summary, the level of mechanical support during pressure-limited ventilation of infants results from complex interactions between the ventilator and the patient's respiratory system. Understanding these relationships, and hence, development of rationales for specific ventilator setting changes, can be facilitated by the use of an operational diagram such as the one shown in Figure 6–11. Such a diagram illustrates the interdependence of ventilator control variables and their effects on minute ventilation.

Application of Pressure-Limited Ventilation

The primary application of infant pressure ventilators and pressure-limited ventilation in general is the support of preterm neonates, especially those with respiratory distress syndrome (RDS). This mode of ventilation evolved from studies by Reynolds[27] and others, who suggested that it resulted in adequate ventilation of infants with lung disease (decreased compliance) at lower peak inspiratory pressures. Unfortunately, this mode may also result in a higher mean airway pressure if care is not taken to optimize ventilator settings. Therefore, clinical experience is invaluable, as the proper application of pressure-limited ventilation is often more an art than a science.

To further complicate matters, the ventilator management of an infant with RDS usually differs from that of an infant with persistent pulmonary hypertension, and both may be quite different from an infant with meconium aspiration. In addition, there is no commonly accepted protocol for optimizing ventilator variables, so techniques and philosophies differ from hospital to hospital. Nevertheless, it is possible to develop a logical approach to this mode of therapy based on theory, experience, and studies on actual patients. We shall describe one such system designed for the treatment of infants with RDS.[7] While this algorithm is relatively specialized and by no means universally accepted, it can be used as a basis for understanding the principles of pressure-limited ventilation.

The algorithm presented here provides a rapid and consistent means of arriving at ventilator management decisions based on blood gas interpretations. While additional clinical observations are important in ventilator management, blood gas analysis plays a key role in assessing the efficacy of mechanical support. This system of optimizing ventilator settings is aimed at providing the best gas exchange at the lowest mean airway pressure and FiO_2 in order to reduce lung injury. The algorithm is based on the accumulated clinical experience of respiratory therapists and physicians at our institution, on lung model experiments, and on other previous studies. This flow chart is intended to help the clinician "fine tune" ventilatory support once mechanical ventilation has been initiated and the patient is out of immediate danger.

USING THE FLOW CHART

The flow chart illustrated in Figure 6–12 is composed of two types of symbols, diamonds and squares. Diamond-shaped symbols express the fact that a decision must be made about a specific condition. One or two lines enter each diamond, or "decision symbol," and two lines emerge from it. Emerging lines are labeled with decisions, such as YES or NO. These lines indicate the direction to be taken, based on the decision made about the information written inside the symbol. Square symbols indicate the type and direction of a particular ventilator-setting change. Table 6–3 lists other symbols and abbreviations used in the flow chart and in the text.

We make several assumptions concerning use of the algorithm: (1) that mechanical ventilation has been initiated at appropriate settings (suggested settings to begin ventilation are f = 20 to 30 breaths/min, PIP = 20 to 25 cm H_2O, PEEP = 3 to 5 cm H_2O, and $I:E$ = 1:2 to 1:1); (2) that significant metabolic acidosis has been corrected; (3) that complications such as pneumothorax and endotracheal tube misplacement or obstruction have been ruled out; (4) that the infant has uncomplicated RDS without significant components of persistent pulmonary hypertension, sepsis, etc.; (5) that other observations, such as chest movement and breath sounds, are being made continuously and are being integrated into clinical decisions. In addition, it is necessary to define normal limits of blood gas values. Table 6–4 lists suggested normal limits determined by the patient's postnatal age. The distinction of age is based on the assumption that infants ventilated for more than 72 hours may have incurred some degree of compensated respiratory acidosis[5] and may have either a stable or improving lung condition.

To use the algorithm, begin with a blood gas analysis. Look first at the arterial CO_2 tension. Based on your decision about this value, you will be directed to areas of the flow chart primarily concerned with oxygenation or ventilation. Increasing or decreasing ventilator support, even the weaning of a patient to CPAP, is automatically incorporated into the various pathways. After each ventilator-setting change you are directed to begin again with a blood gas analysis. Of course, transcutaneous blood gas determinations may be substituted, assuming good correlation with arterial blood gas values has been established. Also, you may elect to repeat the assessment of the patient before you enter the flow chart again. The legend for Figure 6–12 gives an example of the use of the algorithm.

The magnitude of each ventilator change will depend on how far out of

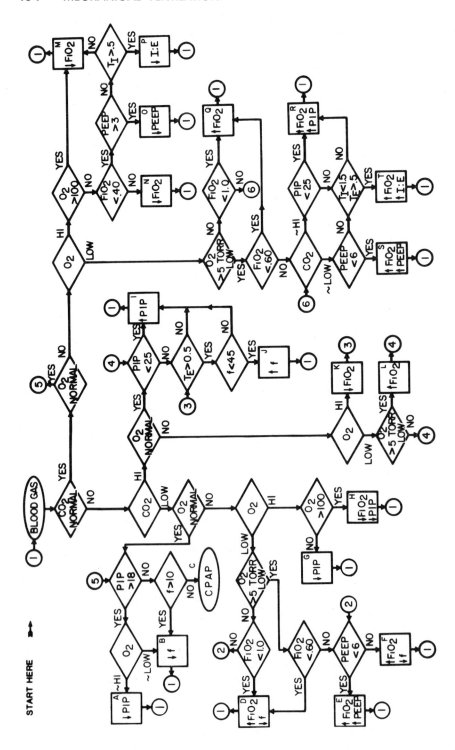

normal range the patient's blood gas values are, assuming that factors such as endotracheal tube placement and breath sounds have been considered. In general, we recommend frequency changes in the range of from 2 to 10 breaths/min; PIP changes from 2 to 3 cm H_2O; and PEEP changes from 1 to 2 cm H_2O. A given change in $I:E$ will have a variable effect depending on the frequency of ventilation and on inspiratory time and tidal volume. The usual change in either I or E is about 0.25 to 0.50 (e.g., a change from 1:1 to 1:1.5 would be a change of 0.50 in E). The magnitude of a change in FiO_2 depends on the patient's PaO_2. If the PaO_2 is extremely outside the normal range, changes in FiO_2 from 0.05 to 0.10 are appropriate. If the PaO_2 is relatively close to the normal range, increments of 0.02 to 0.03 are more common. While indices such as $P(a/A)O_2$ and PaO_2/FiO_2 are sometimes used to adjust the FiO_2,[12, 22] it is usually difficult to predict what the PaO_2 will be in a neonate when a given change in FiO_2 is made. FiO_2 adjustment, like other aspects of ventilator management, usually requires that clinical experience play an important role in decision making.

Fig 6–12.—Flow chart illustrating the algorithm used to optimize pressure-limited mechanical ventilation of infants with RDS. Diamond-shaped symbols call for decisions, while squares indicate types and directions of ventilator-setting changes. You enter the algorithm at the top of the chart, where BLOOD GAS appears in an oval, indicating that you need a set of blood gas values to get started. The line leaving the BLOOD GAS oval takes you to the CO_2 NORMAL diamond. Here you answer the question, "Is the arterial CO_2 tension normal?" If the CO_2 is not normal, you follow the NO line and reach the CO_2 diamond. But if at the CO_2 NORMAL diamond your answer is yes and you move to the O_2 NORMAL diamond, you then answer the question, "Is the arterial O_2 tension normal?" If it is normal, you follow the YES line from the O_2 NORMAL diamond upward, reaching a circled numeral 5. That circled 5 indicates that you should find another circled 5 on the chart—one that directs you into a diamond. There is only one circled 5 pointing into a diamond, and you find it in the upper left portion of the chart. It directs you to a diamond labeled PIP>18. You are now being asked, "Is the positive inspiratory pressure greater than 18 cm H_2O?" You answer that question, and if the PIP is greater than 18, you follow the YES line to the O_2 diamond. On the other hand, if the PIP is not greater than 18, you follow the NO line to the f>10 diamond. If the PIP is not greater than 18 and you reach the f>10 diamond, you now are being asked, "Is the rate greater than 10/min?" If it is not, then the NO line directs you to an oval containing the expression CPAP, which indicates that you can try to wean the patient from mechanical ventilation to CPAP. On the other hand, if the rate (f) is greater than 10, the YES line from the f>10 diamond directs you to the ↓ f square. This square instructs you to reduce the rate (f), after which you move out of the ↓ f square, going left to the circled numeral 1. Reaching that numeral tells you to find the circled numeral 1 that points into a symbol. There is only one circled 1 pointing into a symbol, and you find it just to the left of the BLOOD GAS oval, where you originally entered the flow chart. So now you obtain another blood gas analysis and enter the algorithm again. (The text discusses starting ventilator settings, conditions and complications that make use of the algorithm invalid, and the concept of normal blood gas values.)

TABLE 6–3.—Abbreviations and Symbols Used in the Flow Chart
and in the Text

CO_2	Arterial carbon dioxide tension (mm Hg)
O_2	Arterial oxygen tension (mm Hg)
FiO_2	Fraction of inspired oxygen
PIP	Peak inspiratory pressure (cm H_2O)
$\overline{P}_{aw}$	Mean airway pressure (cm H_2O)
PEEP	Positive end expiratory pressure (cm H_2O)
CPAP	Continuous positive airway pressure without mechanical ventilation (cm H_2O)
$I:E$	Ratio of inspiratory to expiratory time
f	Ventilator frequency (breaths/min). Unless otherwise specified, a change in frequency should be accompanied by a change in $I:E$ to maintain the same T_I so that tidal volume remains constant.
T_I	Inspiratory time (sec)
T_E	Expiratory time (sec)
HI	The variable in the decision symbol is above normal range.
LOW	The variable in the decision symbol is below normal range.
$\approx$HI	The variable in the decision symbol is at the high end of normal.
$\approx$LOW	The variable in the decision symbol is at the low end of normal.
$\uparrow$	Increase
$\downarrow$	Decrease
$>$	Greater than. . .
$<$	Less than. . .
Torr	mm Hg

It should be remembered that many uncontrollable factors may influence ventilation and perfusion and the resulting gas exchange of a neonate, and that a given maneuver sometimes produces an unexpected and difficult-to-explain result. Therefore, the algorithm, though based on sound reasoning, can give less than optimal results in certain situations. At such times the clinician must rely on personal experience and intuition in the absence of other relevant clinical data.

SPECIFIC RATIONALES

In this flow chart each square symbol, which contains a recommended ventilator change, is labeled with a letter in the upper right-hand corner. The letter corresponds to a specific line of reasoning that justifies the change. We prefer to limit ventilator changes to no more than one per blood gas result. When two simultaneous changes have been recommended, one relates to FiO_2. The limits for the ventilator settings in this algorithm (e.g., f up to 45 breaths/min, PEEP up to 6 cm H_2O) represent our usual clinical practice in the management of the uncomplicated patient, but may have to be changed according to other protocols in the management of some complicated patients. The following is an explanation of the specific rationale corresponding to each square-symbol letter:

A. Decreasing PIP will decrease tidal volume and should increase $PaCO_2$. If you have arrived here or at B via 5, then the ventilator changes represent weaning procedures, with the hope that the infant's spontaneous respirations will help maintain normal gas exchange. It should be noted that infant ventilators are designed to be used primarily in the IMV mode. Changes in $\overline{P}_{aw}$ have been shown to be directly related to oxygenation. The reduction in $\overline{P}_{aw}$ caused by the lowering of PIP is appropriate, as PaO_2 is relatively high.

B. Ventilation is reduced by a decrease in frequency. Compared to a decrease in PIP, the decrease in frequency should have less potential for lowering PaO_2 because it has little or no effect on lung volume.

C. When the ventilator settings have been reduced to PIP<18 and f<10, the infant may be given a trial of CPAP with the ventilator through the endotracheal tube. The FiO_2 may be raised slightly to help compensate for the increased work of breathing when IMV is stopped.

D. Ventilation is decreased by a decrease in frequency rather than a decrease in PIP, for the same reason as in B. However, the low oxygenation necessitates a concomitant increase in FiO_2.

E. If the FiO_2>0.60 and PaO_2 is very low (more than 5 mm Hg below the lowest acceptable value), it is better to make a ventilator-setting change that substantially increase $\overline{P}_{aw}$. Therefore, if PEEP is less than 6 cm H_2O, it can be increased, and a concomitant temporary increase in FiO_2 may be in order. Increasing PEEP in this situation has two effects: first, it increases $\overline{P}_{aw}$, which should improve oxygenation; second, it should reduce the tidal volume and increase $PaCO_2$.

F. Ventilation is decreased by a frequency decrease, rather than a decrease in PIP, as explained in B. In contrast to D, here the reduction in frequency should be made while the $I:E$ is maintained or slightly increased (as long as T_I<1.5 seconds). If the $I:E$ is held constant, $\overline{P}_{aw}$ and hence oxygenation will not decrease along with the frequency. On the other hand, an increase in Paw achieved by increasing the $I:E$ may improve oxygenation. As in E, a temporary increase in FiO_2 might be necessary to assure adequate oxygenation.

G. Lowering PIP will decrease tidal volume and should increase $PaCO_2$. This, in conjunction with the decrease in $\overline{P}_{aw}$, should decrease PaO_2.
Note: if the PIP is relatively low (<23) compared to f (>20), it would probably be better to decrease f instead, as in H, to prevent atelectasis.

H. PIP is decreased for the same reason as in G. In addition, the FiO_2 should

TABLE 6–4.—SUGGESTED NORMAL LIMITS
OF BLOOD GAS/pH VALUES FOR USE
WITH THE ALGORITHM

	AGE OF INFANT	
	≤72 hours	>72 hours
pH	7.25–7.45	7.25–7.45
$PaCO_2$ (mm Hg)	35–45	45–55
PaO_2 (mm Hg)	50–80	50–80

be immediately reduced, as a high PaO_2 has been implicated in the etiology of retrolental fibroplasia.

I. Increasing PIP increases the tidal volume and should decrease $PaCO_2$. A change in PIP rather than in frequency at this point illustrates our philosophy that this form of ventilation is truly IMV, favoring relatively large tidal volumes and low rates. We have arbitrarily set an upper limit of 25 cm H_2O on PIP (and thus limited tidal volume), although at times we are forced to exceed this limit (see J and T). The increase in $\bar{P}_{aw}$ consequent to increasing PIP could also increase oxygenation.

J. Once the upper limit of PIP has been reached, ventilation is increased by means of frequency. However, an arbitrary limit on frequency has been set at 45 breaths/min. When this limit has been reached, further increases in ventilation should be made by raising PIP above 25 cm H_2O. Notice that a further limitation of frequency is that T_E must be at least 0.5 second because time constants for the lungs of preterm infants may range approximately from 0.05 to 0.14 second. This means that lung pressure may require as much as 0.5 to 0.7 second to equilibrate with mouth pressure. Maintaining T_E at 0.5 second reduces the risk of alveolar gas trapping.

K. The FiO_2 is reduced because of the high PaO_2. At the same time, either PIP or frequency is increased based on decisions starting with an evaluation of T_E. An alternative approach at this point would be simply to decrease the PEEP, assuming it is greater than 3 or 4 cm H_2O. This would at once increase the tidal volume (decreasing $PaCO_2$) and decrease $\bar{P}_{aw}$ (decreasing PaO_2). If the PaO_2 is much greater than 100 mm Hg, a concomitant decrease in FiO_2 may be necessary to avoid the risk of retrolental fibroplasia.

L. Increasing FiO_2 is probably the surest way to increase PaO_2. In addition, since $PaO_2 > 5$ mm Hg below normal and $PaCO_2$ is above normal, a change in PIP or f is indicated. If $PaO_2 < 5$ mm Hg below normal, however, a change in ventilation only, especially by an increase in PIP, might bring oxygenation into the normal range.

M. If the PaO_2 is too high, the FiO_2 should be immediately reduced, as in H.

N. The FiO_2 is reduced before PEEP is lowered, as maintenance of PEEP might also allow a substantial reduction in FiO_2. The upper limit of PEEP is 6 cm H_2O, so the algorithm would not lead to an instance in which the FiO_2 is too low while the PEEP is too high.

O. Given that the FiO_2 is relatively low, the next consideration should be given to PEEP. This block allows for the reduction of PEEP, the lower limit of which we have set at 3 cm H_2O. In addition to decreasing $\bar{P}_{aw}$ and thus, it is hoped, PaO_2, this maneuver may increase the tidal volume, which would eventually allow a reduction of PIP.

P. If PEEP has already been reduced, $\bar{P}_{aw}$ may be lowered by decreasing the $I:E$. Maintaining T_I at 0.5 second helps to ensure delivery of adequate tidal volume.

Q. When oxygenation is low, an FiO_2 increase is the most direct way of increasing PaO_2. If $FiO_2 > 0.60$ and PaO_2 is very low, an increase in $\bar{P}_{aw}$ is indicated (R, S, T).

R. An increase in PIP is recommended because it should improve ventilation as well as oxygenation. A concomitant increase in FiO_2 might be necessary if the PaO_2 is too low.

S. If PEEP is relatively low, it may be increased independently of PIP to improve oxygenation. The possible slight decrease in tidal volume should not be a problem, as the $PaCO_2$ is in the the low range of normal. As in R, a concomitant increase in FiO_2 might be necessary.

T. Once PIP is at 25 cm H_2O, an increase in the $I:E$ may be used to increase $\overline{P}_{aw}$ and consequently improve oxygenation. Note that an $I:E$ increase should be considered only when T_I is less than 1.5 seconds and T_E is greater than 0.5 second. If one of these conditions is not met, it would be better to increase PIP above 25 cm H_2O, our recommended upper limit, as well as to increase FiO_2 if it is less than 1.0.

Readers should remember that the flow chart represents our own philosophy of ventilator management, which is by no means universally accepted. For example, some researchers advocate higher frequency and lower pressures in order to prevent barotrauma. Until long-term controlled studies show an advantage of high-frequency ventilation over conventional techniques, we prefer to use rates lower than 60 breaths/min. We believe that this algorithm represents what can be considered "conventional" therapy for preterm neonates. This approach can be of great benefit as a learning aid for those inexperienced in neonatal ventilation, as well as a guide for consistent care in neonatal intensive care units. Such consistency is especially important if control groups are to be defined in studies comparing conventional ventilation to other forms of treatment.

CHARACTERISTICS OF PEDIATRIC VENTILATORS

The following ventilators are commonly used in pediatric respiratory therapy.

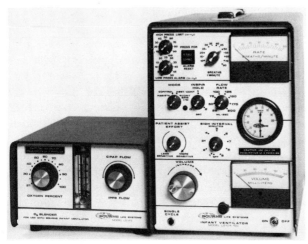

Fig 6–13.—The Bourns LS-104 respirator.

Bourns LS104–150

The Bourns LS104–150 (Fig 6–13) is an electrically operated volume, pressure, or time-cycled ventilator. This machine is one of the most versatile units available for ventilating infants and small children up to 3 years old. Although it is no longer in production, many are still in use today and can be purchased in some areas as reconditioned units. This ventilator will deliver constant tidal volumes from 5 to 150 ml at flow rates of 25 to 200 ml/sec (1.5 to 12 liters/min). Ventilators used for infants must have the ability to generate low inspiratory flow rates. For example, with a typical tidal volume for a neonate of 18 ml at a respiratory frequency of 40 breaths/min, delivery of the required tidal volume requires a flow of only 2 liters/min with an inspiratory:expiratory $(I:E)$ ratio of $1:2$. For a typical adult with a tidal volume of 500 ml and a respiratory frequency of 16 per minute, the ventilator must deliver a flow of 24 liters/min at the same $I:E$ ratio.

The LS104-150 is used primarily in the volume-limited mode (assist, control, assist/control, or IMV) and is volume- or pressure-cycled. It can, however, be used in the pressure-limited mode, in which case it is considered to be time-cycled and produces the characteristic rectangular pressure waveform. In this mode, the peak pressure limit is adjusted by means of a pop-off valve located on the rear panel of the ventilator. Once the pop-off is set, the duration of the pressure hold becomes a function of the tidal volume and the inspiratory flow rate. Thus, during the inspiratory phase, airway pressure rises to the preset limit, at which point the excess pressure is vented to the atmosphere.

Some models of the LS104-150 are equipped with an inspiratory-hold control, allowing the ventilator to be volume-limited and time-cycled. This control makes it possible to create a plateau pressure that can be used to calculate airway resistance and static respiratory system compliance. Note that a pressure plateau is different from a pressure hold (Fig 6–14).

When the ventilator is used in the assist mode, it is triggered within 35 msec in response to an inspiratory effort producing a pressure drop as small as 0.05 cm H_2O. In the control mode, the ventilator operates at frequencies from 0.5 to 80 breaths/min. Sighs, if used, can be interjected at intervals of 1 to 9 minutes. However, the sigh volume is automatically set at twice the tidal volume. This often produces high peak inspiratory pressures on infants with low compliance and thus it is frequently not used.

The ventilator can supply positive end-expiratory pressure (PEEP) from 0 to 20 cm H_2O and can compensate for small leaks in the delivery circuit (such as around the uncuffed endotracheal tubes generally used for infants and small children). The leak compensation valve, labeled ''sensitivity control,'' is located on the exhalation manifold on the back of the machine. It's function is often a source of confusion. In the assist mode, the machine senses the patient's inspiratory effort by comparing the pressure in the delivery circuit to the pressure in the PEEP venturi chamber. When the patient begins inspiration, the pressure in the delivery circuit drops relative to the pressure in the venturi

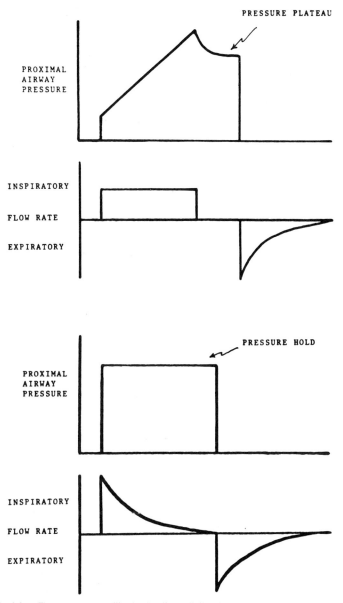

Fig 6–14.—These curves illustrate the distinction between a pressure plateau and a pressure hold. A pressure plateau is generated by delivering a preset volume and delaying the opening of the exhalation valve until all airflow in the lungs has ceased. Once volume delivery from the ventilator has stopped, airway pressure drops from its peak value to the plateau pressure as gas is redistributed within the lungs. A pressure hold is characterized by a rise in inspiratory pressure to some peak value, which is deliberately sustained for the duration of the inspiratory time.

chamber, and the ventilator is triggered into the inspiratory phase. This happens because normally, the circuit is isolated from the PEEP chamber by a one-way valve. Any leaks in the delivery circuit also drop the pressure, making the ventilator self-triggered. To correct this, the leak compensation valve, when opened, creates a flow of gas from the PEEP venturi into the delivery circuit to effectively "feed" the leak and maintain PEEP. If the valve is opened when there is no leak, more patient effort is required to trigger inspiration, so the ventilator is less "sensitive."

CONTROL VARIABLES
FiO_2: 21–100%, Requires LS145 O_2 blender
Frequency: 0.5–80 bpm
I:E ratio: 2:1–zero
Inspiratory pressure limit: 0–100 cm H_2O
CPAP/PEEP: 0–20 cm H_2O
Flow rate: 25–200 ml/sec
Tidal volume: 5–150 ml
Inspiratory hold: 0–2 sec
Sigh interval: 1–9 min or off
Patient assist effort: -0.05 to -1.0 cm H_2O

ALARMS
Low inspiratory pressure
High inspiratory pressure
Apnea

SPECIAL FEATURES
Manual breath button
Rate and volume meters
Variable relief valve

Servo 900C

The Servo 900C ventilator (Fig 6–15) is classified as a pneumatically powered, electronically controled, volume-, time-, or pressure-cycled ventilator. It can be used to ventilate adults, children, and infants. Sigh volumes are automatically set at twice the tidal volume and should be used cautiously on infants with low compliance. Special accessories are available for use with children and infants. These include small-bore patient tubes (10 mm ID), child size cuvette for the CO_2 analyzer, and a humidifier with approximately 30 ml of dead space, all aimed at decreasing compressible gas volume.

CONTROL VARIABLES
FiO_2: 21–100%, optional blender
Frequency: 10–120 bpm
Inspiratory time: 20–80%
Inspiratory pressure: 0–100 cm H_2O
PEEP: 0–50 cm H_2O
Minute volume: 0.4–40 liters

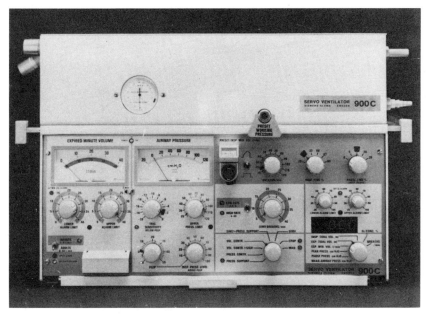

Fig 6–15.—The Siemens Servo ventilator 900C.

Sigh rate: 1 per 100 breaths
Sigh volume: twice tidal volume
Trigger effort: − 20 to 0 cm H_2O
Pause time: 0–30%

ALARMS
High inspiratory pressure
Low inspiratory pressure
High volume
Low volume
Loss of power
Apnea
Inadequate air and/or oxygen pressure

SPECIAL FEATURES
Square-wave, sine-wave, or decelerating flow patterns
2-minute alarm delay
Adaptable for anesthesia

Bear 5

The Bear 5 (Fig 6–16) is controlled and monitored by microcomputers. With this new technology, Bear has been able to expand the capabilities of this ventilator to ventilate infants, young children, and adults. This unit is classified as a pneumatically powered, electronically (microcomputer) controled, volume-,

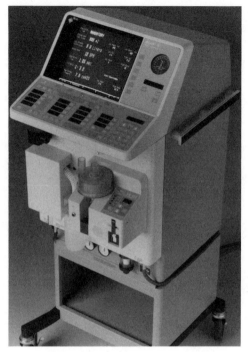

Fig 6–16.—The Bear 5 ventilator.

time-, or pressure-cycled ventilator. A time-cycled mode that operates identically to the CMV/IMV mode on the Bear Cub or BP200 makes the unit useful in the newborn intensive care. The fact that sigh volume and rate are adjustable over a wide range makes it attractive for ventilating infants and young children with low compliance. The microcomputer also provides a graphic display of real time pressure, flow, and volume on a CRT. The ability to visualize these parameters in real time may assist the operator when making decisions about inspiratory pause, demand versus continuous flow, and pressure-supported ventilation.

CONTROL VARIABLES
FiO_2: 21–100%
Frequency: 0–150 bpm
Inspiratory time: 0.10–3.0 sec
Inspiratory pressure: 0–150 cm H_2O
PEEP: 0–50 cm H_2O
Tidal volume: 50–2000 ml
Sigh rate: 2–60 SPH
Sigh volume: 65–3000 ml
Assist sensitivity: 0.5–5 cm H_2O

Inspiratory pause: 0–2 sec
Pressure support: 0–72 cm H_2O

ALARMS
Inadequate air and/or oxygen pressure
Low inspiratory pressure
High inspiratory pressure
Low exhaled volume
High exhaled volume
Low PEEP
High PEEP
Low mean airway pressure
High mean airway pressure
Low rate
High rate

SPECIAL FEATURES
Square, sine, accelerating, decelerating waveforms
Static compliance and resistance monitoring
CRT-based
Self-diagnostics

Babybird 2

Unlike its predecessor, the original Babybird, the Babybird 2 is electronically rather than pneumatically controlled. This facilitates the setting of frequency and inspiratory time and makes the ventilator similar in configuration to other infant ventilators on the market. This machine is time-cycled, pressure-limited, and delivers continuous flow IMV or CPAP. This machine was designed to be used with an additional monitor (e.g., Bird Model 9900), since it has only a few monitoring features as part of the ventilator.

CONTROL VARIABLES
FiO_2: optional, separate unit
Frequency: 2 150 bpm
Inspiratory time: 0.1–3.0 sec
Inspiratory pressure limit: 0–80 cm H_2O
Flow rate: 0–25 lpm
CPAP/PEEP: 1–30 H_2O

ALARMS
Inadequate air and/or oxygen pressure
Electrical power failure
Incompatible timer setting: indicates that the set frequency and inspiratory time are incompatible with 0.2-sec minimum expiratory time.
Inspiratory time failure: indicates that the inspiratory time has exceeded 4.25 sec.
Patient overpressure: indicates that the relief pressure setting has been violated

SPECIAL FEATURES

Manual breath button: provides a single breath independent of control settings during CPAP or IMV

Relief pressure: permits adjustment of maximum circuit pressure from 30–80 cm H_2O; if violated, triggers audible and visual alarms and immediately reduces circuit pressure to zero

Bear BP-200

The BP-200 (Fig 6–17) is classified as a continuous flow, time-cycled, pressure-limited ventilator that operates in the IPPB/IMV or CPAP mode. This unit requires an additional monitor (e.g., Pneumogard 1200) since it does not have an alarm for loss of pressure in the delivery circuit or a visual display of mean airway pressure.

CONTROL VARIABLES

FiO_2: 21–100% internal blender

Frequency: 1–60 bpm on the models, 1–150/min on new or modified units

$I:E$ ratio: 4:1–1:10

Inspiratory pressure limit: 10–80 cm H_2O

CPAP/PEEP: 0–20 cm H_2O. There is no mechanism to prevent inadvertent system PEEP at high frequencies and flow rates.

Flow rate: 0–20 lpm

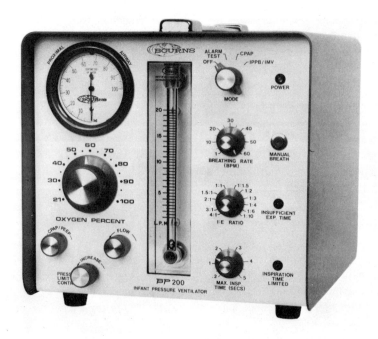

Fig 6–17.—The Bourns BP-200 respirator.

Maximum inspiratory time: 0.2–5.0 secs. The inspiratory time set with this control takes precedence over that set by the frequency and $I:E$ ratio controls. Thus, the clinician can adjust settings in terms of frequency and inspiratory time instead of frequency and $I:E$ ratio if desired.

ALARMS
Power failure

Inadequate air and/or oxygen pressure

Insufficient expiratory time: If the set combination of frequency and $I:E$ ratio results in an expiratory time of less than 0.45–0.55 sec.

SPECIAL FEATURES
Manual breath: When the ventilator mode selection switch is turned to CPAP, the manual breath pushbutton allows delivery of one mechanical breath at the inspiratory time determined by the current settings of frequency and $I:E$.

Bear Cub

The Cub (Fig 6–18) is classified as a continuous flow, time-cycled, pressure-limited ventilator that will deliver IMV or CPAP. The main functional difference between the Cub and its predecessor, the BP-200, is that the Cub is designed to be used primarily as a nonconstant pressure generator,[9] whereas the BP-200 is more of a constant-pressure generator at normal flow rates.

CONTROL VARIABLES
FiO_2: 21–100% internal blender

Frequency: 1–150 bpm

Inspiratory time: 0.1–3.0 sec

Inspiratory pressure limit: 0–72 cm H_2O

CPAP/PEEP: 0–20 cm H_2O. The exhalation manifold is designed to prevent inadvertent system PEEP at high frequencies and flow rates.

Flow rate: 3–30 lpm

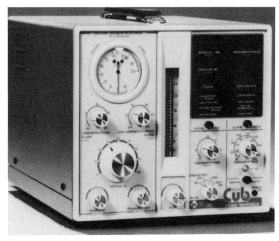

Fig 6–18.—The Bear Cub infant ventilator.

ALARMS

Low inspiratory pressure: OFF–50 cm H_2O

Loss of PEEP/CPAP: OFF–20 cm H_2O

Prolonged inspiratory pressure

Ventilator inoperative: includes failure to cycle, electrical power failure, high/low inspiratory time, panel control malfunction, prolonged solenoid on time, timing circuit failure

Inadequate air and/or oxygen pressure

Excessive inverse $I{:}E$ Ratio: activated if $I{:}E > 3{:}1$

Rate/time incompatibility (visual only): indicates that the set frequency and inspiratory time are incompatible with 0.25 sec minimum expiratory time.

Alarm silence (visual alert): 30 sec

Adjustable alarm loudness: 65–75 dB

SPECIAL FEATURES

Manual breath button: permits delivery of a single breath during CPAP only

Proximal airway pressure analog output jack: BNC type connector, 10 mv/cm H_2O scale, 0–100 cm H_2O range.

Digital displays: inspiratory time, expiratory time, $I{:}E$ ratio, frequency, mean airway pressure

9 VDC output jacks: Two 9VDC, 200 mA, 3-pin female connector; protected by a ½ A fuse

Proximal airway line purge: Gas flows steadily through the proximal airway line from the ventilator to the patient circuit to remove condensation and ensure accurate pressure measurements.

Test mode: tests the integral rechargeable nickel cadmium battery, visual indicators, and digital display segments.

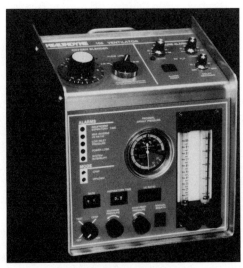

Fig 6–19.—The Healthdyne Model 105 infant ventilator.

Healthdyne Model 105

The Healthdyne 105 (Fig 6–19) is classified as a continuous flow, time-cycled, pressure-limited ventilator that operates in a CPAP or IMV mode. One very valuable feature of this unit is that it can be used for transporting patients as well as in the intensive care unit. A small power pack will operate the electronics of the machine for up to 4 hours of continuous use.

CONTROL VARIABLES
FiO_2: 21–100% internal blender
Frequency: 1–150 bpm
Inspiratory time: 0.1–4.9 sec
Inspiratory pressure limit: 1–85 cm H_2O
CPAP/PEEP: 0–20 cm H_2O; requires separate exhalation manifold. There is no mechanism to compensate for inadvertent system PEEP at high frequencies and flow rate.
Flow rate: 3–60 lpm

ALARMS
High patient circuit pressure
Low patient circuit pressure
Apnea during CPAP
Insufficient expiratory time
Maximum inverse $I:E$ ratio
Inadequate air and/or oxygen pressure
Electrical power failure
System failure
Alarm delay: 0–90 seconds

SPECIAL FEATURES
Manual breath button: permits delivery of a single breath during CPAP or IMV
Rechargeable battery: (optional, 8 volts DC)
Proximal airway line purge: Gas flows steadily through the proximal airway line from the ventilator to the circuit to remove condensation and ensure accurate pressure measurements.
Dual flow meters: Two independent flowmeters provide an accumulative flow rate in excess of 60 lpm, which allows ventilation of neonates as well as older children and some adults.
Test mode: provides an electronic test of visual and audible alarms system.

Sechrist Model IV-100B

The Sechrist IV-100B (Fig 6–20) ventilator delivers continuous flow for IMV and/or CPAP. It is time-cycled and pressure-limited.

Control Variables
FiO_2: 21–100%
Inspiratory time: 0.1–2.9 sec

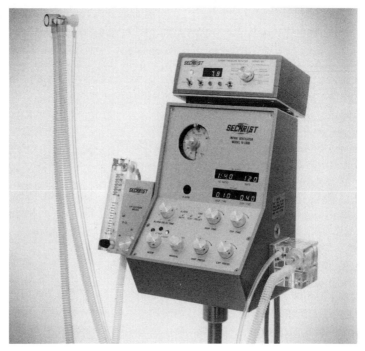

Fig 6–20.—The Sechrist Model IV-100B infant ventilator with an airway pressure monitor on top.

Expiratory time: 0.3–60.0

Inspiratory pressure limit: 7–70 cm H_2O

CPAP/PEEP: 0–15 cm H_2O. The exhalation manifold is designed to prevent inadvertent system PEEP at high frequencies and flow rates.

Flow rate: 0–32 lpm, flush 40 lpm

Alarms

Low patient circuit pressure

Apnea during CPAP

Fail to cycle

Inadequate air and/or oxygen pressure

Prolonged inspiration

Electrical power failure

Alarm delay: 3–60 sec

Alarm mute: 25 sec

SPECIAL FEATURES

Test: initiates self-test sequence, which activates alarm signals and a count sequence to display all numbers

Time preset: Pushing this button when the mode selector is in the CPAP position allows the operator to observe the settings of the inspiratory and expiratory times before switching to the VENT mode and to make adjustments if desired.

Interchangeable exhalation manifolds: allows ventilation of infant and pediatric patients as well as scavenging of anesthetic gases.

Waveform control: allows adjustment of proximal airway pressure waveform from rectangular to quasisinusoidal or "shark fin."

Proximal airway line purge: Gas flows steadily through the airway line from the ventilator to the patient circuit to remove condensation and ensure accurate pressure measurement.

Manual breath button: Inspiration occurs as long as the button is pushed. Inspiratory pressure is limited to the setting of the inspiratory pressure control.

Star

The Star infant ventilator (Fig 6–21) is a time-cycled, pressure-limited ventilator that will deliver IMV or CPAP. The ventilator includes a comprehensive monitoring system. The electronics are microprocessor controled.

CONTROL VARIABLES
FiO_2: 21–100%
Frequency: 1–150 bpm
Inspiratory time: 0.1–3.0 sec
Inspiratory pressure limit: 8–90 cm H_2O
CPAP/PEEP: 0–24 cm H_2O
Flow rate: 2–40 lpm

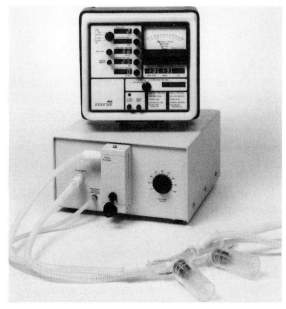

Fig 6–21.—The Star infant ventilator.

ALARMS

Low inspiratory pressure: 0–60 cm H_2O

Low PEEP/CPAP: 4 cm H_2O below operator set point

Prolonged inspiratory pressure

Air leak: activates when demand flow exceeds 8lpm for 15 seconds

Ventilator inoperative: alarm activates when the ventilator is not performing as specified

Inadequate air and/or oxygen pressure

Electrical power loss

Rate/time incompatability: indicates that the set frequency and inspiratory time are incompatible with 0.3 sec minimum expiratory time

Alarm silence (visual alert): 60 sec

SPECIAL FEATURES

Manual breath button: permits delivery of a single breath at any time

Analog output jack: proximal airway pressure

Digital displays: flow rate, inspiratory time, expiratory time, I:E ratio, frequency, mean airway pressure

Microprocessor controlled: as future clinical requirements are proven to be desirable, they can be added to the ventilator via software updates

RS-232 computer connectors: when connected to personal computers, ventilator information can be collected, reviewed, and displayed in trend or numerical form

Continuous or intermittent demand flow during CPAP or IMV

PRACTICAL POINTS OF VENTILATOR MANAGEMENT

The following aspects of ventilation require special attention.

Humidification

There is little disagreement about the need for warming and humidifying the gases during mechanical ventilation. There is, however, reasonable doubt about the degree of heat and humidification necessary to augment this function. At one time, the maxim was that inspired gas should be 100% saturated with water vapor at 37°C. Yet, recent studies have shown that during normal breathing, the nose heats the inspired gas to only 31° to 32°C at a relative humidity of 95%. Providing inspired gas at higher temperatures during mechanical ventilation may cause patient discomfort.

Humidifiers, especially those designed for infant ventilators, have undergone a tremendous technical evolution over the past few years. The earliest designs were simply "pass-over" humidifiers, which were heated by thermostatically controlled hot plates or heating elements. These simple devices have been refined to reduce compliance and include alarms. Most are made with modular components to facilitate cleaning. Simple thermostatically controlled humidifiers are designed to maintain constant water temperature and, if other factors remain unchanged, constant gas temperature and relative humidty. In practice, however, factors such as the flow rate of the gas and environmental temperature are variable and affect the temperature and relative humidity that reaches the patient. In addition, as the water is consumed from the reservoir, the compliance of the ventilator delivery circuit increases and may affect the tidal volume.

To address these problems, manufacturers have developed humidifiers with temperature probes that can be placed at the proximal airway. The probe provides a feedback signal that allows the humidifier to automatically adjust its heat output to maintain a constant inspired gas temperature. Automatic water feed systems have also been incorporated to keep a constant water level in the humidifier. These changes in design represent another step in humidifier evolution, but problems remain. In fact, making humidifiers more efficient caused the biggest problem: "rainout." Rainout, or condensation of water along the delivery circuit, is inevitable since the gas delivered by the humidifier is highly saturated at a temperature well above room temperature. As the gas travels through the circuit to the patient, it is cooled, and the water condenses in the tubing. Large amounts of water in the circuit can cause inadvertent tracheal lavage, fluctuating pressure readings, occlusion of pressure gauge lines, and "phantom" adventitious breath sounds.

The simple solution to the condensation problem is to maintain the temperature of the gas as it travels the length of the delivery circuit. This has been accomplished by placing heating wires inside the circuit and using a temperature probe at the proximal airway to control the amount of heat delivered by the wires. The temperature probe of the humidifier is placed at the outlet of the humidifier to regulate the temperature of the gas going into the delivery circuit. Now, if the heating wires are adjusted to maintain this temperature, condensation will be eliminated. Disposable ventilator circuits with heating wires such as those made by Isothermal Systems Inc. can be used with existing humidifiers.

One last point should be made concerning the clinical application of ventilator humidifiers. The temperature probes used in these devices respond relatively slowly to sudden changes in temperature. That is, if the gas flowing through the ventilator circuit suddenly changes from 32°C to 37°C, the probe requires several seconds to record and display the fact. If the temperature should suddenly go back to 32°C, the probe cannot follow this change and ends up reading an average temperature somewhere between the two extremes. This is exactly what can happen in some modes of ventilation, such as assist-control. To understand why, you must visualize what happens to the ventilating gas during one respiratory cycle.

Consider a typical humidifier with a temperature probe at the proximal airway but no heating wires in the circuit. The gas that makes up the tidal volume comes from two locations: from inside the circuit tubing and from the space over the water in the humidifier. During the expiratory phase, the gas in the circuit is cooling while the gas in the humidifier is heating. During the inspiratory phase, the temperature probe at the proximal airway is first exposed to the cooler gas that was in the tubing and then to the warmer gas from the humidifier. Thus, the probe is exposed to an oscillating gas temperature, but the total cycle time is typically so short that the probe cannot respond fast enough to record the actual instantaneous temperatures. The clinical significance is that the temperature you set using the temperature probe is actually an average temperature and the patient may be inspiring gas at 3° to 5°C above the set temperature. Consequently, the patient may experience discomfort with what appears to be a ''normal'' inspiratory gas temperature. This is another argument for using temperatures below 37°C in some modes of ventilation. The problems is avoided, however, when using a continuous flow IMV mode (e.g., most infant ventilators) as the temperature of the gas flowing by the temperature probe is relatively constant.

Weaning from the Ventilator

Psychological preparation is definitely the first step in the weaning process. The child should be given an explanation, in words appropriate for age, of exactly what is going to happen and in what sequence. Continuing reassurance by supportive personnel should be maintained. Early in the weaning process it is important that a respiratory care practitioner with whom the child has an established rapport is at the bedside to allay the child's fears.

The most popular method of weaning an infant or child from a ventilator is intermittent mandatory ventilation. This technique has the advantage of allowing a gradual transition from machine control to ventilator independence. At first the frequency of the mandatory breaths is just a little less than the child's respiratory rate. During recovery, the mandatory breaths are spaced progressively further apart, until they are discontinued entirely.

The second method of weaning is to permit the patient to breathe spontaneously for short periods of time. The length of time can be increased gradually, while ensuring that the patient does not become fatigued. Humidified gas should be provided during the weaning process. Weaning by this method is sometimes assisted by applying continuous positive pressure to the airway whenever the patient is off the respirator. The CPAP then can be gradually decreased until the patient can breathe without assistance.

Still a third method of weaning for patients with chronic lung disease is to switch the respirator to the assist mode, allowing the patient to trigger the respirator at his own rate. The trigger sensitivity can be decreased gradually, while the patient is encouraged to provide greater effort until he is able to ventilate adequately without the assistance of the ventilator. Ventilators with assist/control features are very helpful for this weaning process. Should the patient have apnea, the assist/control mode will take over a predetermined rate and continue ventilation until the apneic period is ended.

The next stage in this weaning process occurs when the inspired oxygen can be kept below 50% and the peak inspiratory pressure is less than 30 cm H_2O. The patient is then allowed to breathe without ventilator assistance for progressively longer periods until the respirator can be discontinued completely. CPAP can be used with this method during the progressive periods when the patient is off the respirator.

Weaning children from a ventilator is frequently a long and difficult process. Frequent blood gas analysis will help make the procedure easier and quicker. Whenever possible, the ventilator should remain at the bedside until the child is satisfied that he can breathe without assistance from the machine.

Monitoring the Ventilator

Continuous monitoring of the ventilated infant or child is an essential aid for clinical management. The monitoring devices used for the ventilator patient differ only slightly from those that are standard for all intensive care patients (e.g., ECG, blood pressure, apnea). The need for a device to detect the malfunction or failure of the ventilator is essential. Most ventilator manufacturers build in systems that provide digital readouts of airway pressure variables during mechanical ventilation. Parameters such as peak, mean, and baseline pressure are continuously monitored, and the operator can define alarm limits for each displayed value. For those ventilators without adequate monitoring devices, sophisticated monitors, such as the Pneumogard 1230A (Novametrix Medical Systems Inc.), are available. It displays values and provides alarms for airway temperature, peak inspiratory pressure, CPAP/PEEP, and FiO_2. In addition, there is a digital readout for frequency, $I:E$, duration of positive pressure, mean airway pressure, and a separate transducer that measures esophageal pressure. The unit also has a built-in strip chart recorder for airway pressure or esophageal/central venous pressure waveforms. A smaller version of this device, the Pneumogard 1200, has displays and alarms for peak, mean, and CPAP/PEEP pressures only along with readouts for frequency, $I:E$ ratio, and duration of positive pressure.

While ventilator monitors are impressive, educational, and, in some situations, indispensable, they are also expensive. It can be argued that the value of a monitor may vary inversely with its cost. It is possible to have a monitor that is more expensive than the ventilator it is monitoring. Ultimately, the alert therapist, physician, or nurse is still the best monitoring system.

Psychologic Care

Doctors Klaus and Kennell[20] have documented the importance of an early relationship between the neonate and parents, and suggest that separation between them should be avoided whenever possible and minimized when unavoidable. It is crucial that the intensive care staff do whatever is necessary to facilitate this relationship. Take time to explain the ventilator to the parents and encourage them to participate, in some way, in their infant's care. Be sensitive to the symptoms of grief and make sure the parents don't feel "left out." If necessary, provide special ventilator tubings so that the mother can hold, rock, and feed the infant outside the incubator. The whole idea is to send a healthy baby home to some very attached parents.

When the older child is placed on a mechanical ventilator he is deprived of one of his most important functions, his ability to speak. Whenever a child cannot speak he will exhibit other forms of communication; anxiety, fear, and stress are often expressed in the form of negative behavior. Being able to recognize and to react appropriately to this type of behavior can reduce the child's frustration. Explaining the necessary procedures to the child and assisting him with communicaton will generally increase his tolerance for frustration and decrease the negative behavior.

Tubing Support

The Angel frame can be used to support the ventilator tubing, thus helping to prevent accidental decannulation (Fig 6–22). Infants will require folded or wrapped diapers on either side and at the top of their heads to decrease mobility and take up space between the head and frame. The respiratory tract can be suctioned by raising the tube support and disconnecting the endotracheal tube adapter.

HIGH-FREQUENCY VENTILATION

The term *high-frequency ventilation* (HFV) loosely covers a variety of new and controversial techniques of respiratory assistance having the common characteristic that the patient's gas exchange needs are supported by ventilators that operate at higher than normal frequencies. The rationale for using high frequencies is that they allow the use of smaller tidal volumes, which in turn generate lower airway and intrathoracic pressures than does conventional ventilation. By using smaller volumes and pressures, one hopes that cardiovascular impairment and pulmonary barotrauma will be reduced.

Just what "higher than normal" frequencies are, though, has not been generally agreed upon. The only definite classification that currently exists is the

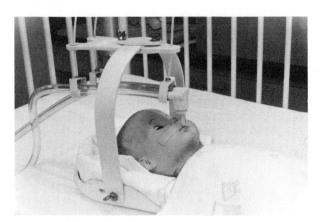

Fig 6–22.—The Angel frame for tubing support during mechanical ventilation.

one imposed by the Food and Drug Administration. The FDA considers frequencies above 150 breaths/min to be experimental and prohibits the sale of ventilators that are capable of frequencies in excess of this limit. Actually, any attempt to classify the new modes of HFV on the basis of frequency alone is confusing because the frequency ranges reported by investigators using various techniques overlap. A more meaningful classification scheme is based on how the ventilator is designed, similar to the way conventional ventilators may be characterized (e.g., in terms of input-power source, cycling-control variable, waveform, and modes of operation). According to this system, there are currently four major types of HFV: (1) high-frequency positive-pressure ventilation (HFPPV), which is essentially the use of a conventional volume or pressure-limited ventilator modified by the use of a delivery circuit with minimum compressible volume; (2) high-frequency oscillation (HFO), in which a mechanism forces gas in and out of the airway, usually with a quasisinusoidal pressure waveform; (3) high-frequency jet ventilation (HFJV), characterized by the delivery of short, rapid bursts (jets) of gas to the airway through a small-bore tube or cannula (usually less than 2 mm in diameter); and (4) high-frequency chest-wall compression (HFCWC), employing some type of device that vibrates the chest wall externally, causing gas to oscillate in the airways.

Reports of HFV in children have been limited. In 1977, Heijman et al.[17] reported the successful use of HFPPV in infants during plastic surgery and in a few neonates with RDS. The use of HFV in infants with RDS has generated a great deal of interest because a reduction of ventilating pressures could possibly result in a reduction of morbidity and mortality associated with pulmonary barotrauma in this population. Marchak et al.[21] and Frantz et al.,[13] using HFO on infants with RDS, achieved adequate gas exchange at lower peak inspiratory pressures (PIP) and smaller airway pressure swings. However, mean airway pressure was not reduced. Pokora et al.[25] reported similar findings using HFJV. Conventional ventilation at rapid rates (a form of HFPPV) has also been used,[2, 18] although not enough data has been reported to make adequate conclusions about safety and efficacy.

Carlo et al.,[4] have successfully used short term HFJV on infants with severe RDS. Using a crossover study design, premature infants requiring ventilation for RDS were switched from conventional pressure-limited ventilation to HFJV (250/min at the same inspired oxygen concentration) for periods of 1 to 3 hours. HFJV resulted in a reduction of average peak inspiratory pressure from 29 ± 3 cm H_2O to 20 ± 4 cm H_2O with no change in end-expiratory pressure. This resulted in a reduction in average mean airway pressure from 14 ± 3 to 10 ± 2 cm H_2O. There was a slight decrease in $PaCO_2$ (39 ± 4 to 34 ± 4), but PaO_2 did not change (Fig 6–23). A typical pressure recording from this study is shown in Figure 2–13, illustrating the difference in airway pressure waveforms between CV and HFJV. These data indicate that short-term HFJV provides adequate gas exchange in infants with RDS at lower peak and mean airway pressure than does CV. In addition, this study highlighted some of the technical difficulties associated with jet ventilation.

These difficulties lie in two main areas, humidification and airway pressure

Fig 6–23.—This figure compares ventilatory pressure and blood gas tensions on conventional ventilation (CV) versus high-frequency jet ventilation (HFJV). Results are expressed as mean ± standard deviation; *$p < 0.001$, † $p < 0.05$. The pressures and blood gases during HFJV are those obtained at the time $PaCO_2$ was most comparable to that during the initial period of CV.

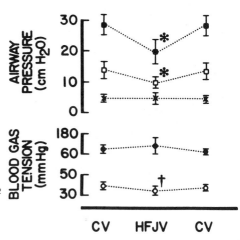

measurement. Humidification is a problem during HFJV because of the relatively high pressures used to deliver the jet gas to the patient (typically 3 to 50 psi). Conventional humidifiers are not built to withstand such pressures. Some researchers have relied on heating and humidification of a blow-by or CPAP gas in the hope that it would be entrained with the jet gas. The problem with this approach is that entrainment decreases as downstream (respiratory system) impedance increases. In fact, with small (3-mm ID) endotracheal tubes used in infants with RDS, there may be no entrainment at all, and the patient will receive cold, dry gas. To avoid this, some researchers have described the use of an infusion pump to inject water directly into the stream of gas from the jet ventilator. The result is that a relatively cool aerosol is delivered to the airways. While this technique has been widely used, there have been recent reports[23, 24, 25] describing tracheal damage and obstruction that may have been caused by inadequate jet-stream humidity. In addition, when this technique is applied to preterm infants, complications may arise due to fluid overload, electrolyte imbalance, and reduction of body temperature. The ultimate goal of a HFJV humidifier is to provide temperature and humidity comparable to that in conventional systems. Such a device has been reported[10] and is illustrated in Figure 6–24. This figure shows a schematic representation of a jet ventilator and the associated delivery circuit used in this institution. The jet ventilator consists of a variable pressure regulator, a solenoid valve, and a timing circuit (controlling the frequency and $I:E$ ratio of the valve). The jet humidifier consists of a chamber with two compartments. One chamber preheats the gas before it reaches the ventilator. An infusion pump injects water droplets into the jet gas as it leaves the ventilator and flows through the second chamber of the humidifier. Here the droplets are vaporized, and the temperature and humidity of the effluent gas is comparable to that of conventional humidifiers. The jet gas is then delivered to the patient through small-bore (⅛'' ID) low-compliance tubing. To maintain the temperature of the gas, the jet tubing is situated within the bias flow circuit. The bias flow gas provides for the patient's spontaneous

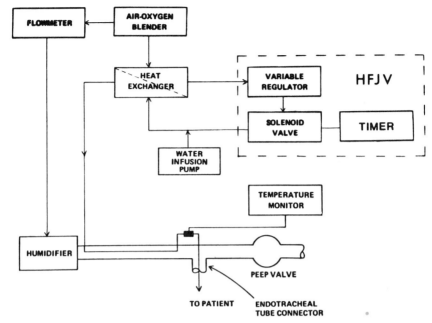

Fig 6–24.—This schematic diagram illustrates the high-frequency jet venti-lator used in this study, including the heating and humidification system. The gas delivered by the variable pressure regulator is preheated by a heat ex-changer before it reaches the solenoid valve. Water is then added to the jet gas distal to the solenoid valve using an infusion pump. The mixture of gas and water droplets passes back to a second chamber of the heat exchanger and then to the injector cannula (14 gauge) via a small-bore tubing, which is situated within the positive end-expiratory pressure (PEEP) circuit. The heated PEEP gas helps maintain the temperature of the jet gas.

respirations and allows independent control of end-expiratory pressure. This gas is conditioned by a conventional humidifier. The jet gas is delivered to the patient's endotracheal tube through a special adaptor, which contains a 14-gauge stainless steel injector cannula.[6]

Because of the use of a "jet injector" and the possibility of a variable amount of entrained gas, delivered volumes are difficult to estimate. Thus, airway pressure measurements are used to make ventilator changes. However, the higher frequencies used during jet ventilation in conjunction with the fact that airway pressures are generated distal to the point of jet injection make airway pressure measurement a more complicated matter than simply attaching a pressure gauge to the Y-adapter of the delivery circuit. Airway pressure must be measured at some point inside the endotracheal tube (such as at the distal tip), and this point must be far enough away from the jet injector to prevent errors due to the high-velocity jet flow.[16] This requires the use of some type of long, narrow catheter, but systems composed of long, narrow pressure moni-toring lumina attached to standard pressure transducers may have severely limited frequency responses. The limited frequency response may be recognized by either an attenuation of the measured pressure signal[8] or by resonance that would make the measured waveform amplitude appear larger than it really is.[3] These problems lead to inaccurate airway pressure measurements, which in turn make it difficult to compare HFJV to CV. Thus, any research comparing some form of HFV to CV in terms of airway pressures must include documentation that the entire pressure-measuring system (not just the pressure transducer) is accurate for the pressure waveforms used.

HFV appears to offer some advantages over CV in a variety of clinical situations. Nevertheless, more long-term controlled studies will be necessary before its safety and efficacy are proven and specific indications for its use have been identified.

REFERENCES

1. Banner, M.J., Gallagher, T.J., and Bluth, L.I.: A new microprocessor device for mean airway pressure measurement, Crit. Care Med. 9:51, 1981.
2. Bland, R.D., Kim, M.H., Light, M.J., and Woodson, J.L.: High-frequency mechanical ventilation in severe hyaline membrane disease: An alternative treatment? Crit. Care Med. 8:275, 1980.
3. Boynton, B.R., Mannino, F.L., Meathe, E.A., Kopitic, R.J., and Friederichsen, G.: Airway pressure measurement during high frequency oscillatory ventilation, Crit. Care Med. 12:39, 1984.
4. Carlo, W.A., Chatburn, R.L., Martin, R.J., Lough, M.D., et al.: Decrease in airway pressure during high-frequency jet ventilation in infants with respiratory distress syndrome, J. Pediatr. 104:101, 1984.
5. Carlo, W.A., Martin, R.J., Versteegh, F.G.A., Goldman, M.D., Robertson, S.S., and Fanaroff, A.A.: The effect of respiratory distress syndrome on chest wall movements and respiratory pauses in preterm infants, Am. Rev. Respir. Dis. 126:103, 1982.
6. Chatburn, R.L., McClellan, L.D., and Lough, M.D.: A new patient-circuit adapter for use with high frequency jet ventilation, Respir. Care 28:1291, 1983.
7. Chatburn, R.L., Carlo, W.A., and Lough, M.D.: Clinical algorithm for pressure-limited ventilation of neonates with respiratory distress syndrome, Respir. Care 28:1579, 1983.
8. Chatburn, R.L., Carlo, W.A., Primiano, F.P., Jr., and Lough, M.D.: Airway pressure measurement during high frequency ventilation, (Abstract) Respir. Care 28:1336, 1983.
9. Chatburn, R.L., Primiano, F.P., Jr., and Lough, M.D.: Mechanical ventilation, in Lough, M.D., Chatburn, R.L., and Schrock, W.A. (eds.): *Handbook of Respiratory Care.* (Chicago: Yearbook Medical Publishers, 1983).
10. Chatburn, R.L., and McClellan, L.D.: A heat and humidification system used for high frequency jet ventilation, Respir. Care 27:1386, 1982.
11. Chatburn, R.L., Lough, M.D., and Primiano, F.P., Jr.: Modification of a ventilator pressure monitoring circuit to permit display of mean airway pressure, Respir. Care 27:276, 1982.
12. Cohen, A., Taeusch, H.W., and Staunton, C.: Usefulness of the arterial/alveolar oxygen tension ration ratio in the care of infants with respiratory distress syndrome, Respir. Care 28:169, 1983.
13. Frantz, I.D., III, Werthammer, J., and Stark, A.R.: High frequency ventilation in premature infants with lung disease: Adequate gas exchange at low tracheal pressure, Pediatrics 71:483, 1983.

14. Gilenski, J.A., Marsh, H.M., and Hall, R.T.: Calculation of mean airway pressure during mechanical ventilation in neonates, Crit. Care Med. 12:642, 1984.
15. Gruber, H., and Klaus, M.: Intermittent mask and bag therapy, J. Pediatr. 76:194, 1970.
16. Heard, S.O., Banner, M.J., and Jaeger, M.J.: Airway pressure measurement during high frequency jet ventilation, (Abstract) Crit. Care Med. 12:262, 1984.
17. Heigman, L., Nilsson, L., and Sjostrand, U.: High frequency positive pressure ventilation (HFPPV) in neonates and infants during neuroleptal analgesia and routine plastic surgery, and in postoperative management, Acta Anaesth. Scand. Suppl. 64:111, 1977.
18. Heigman, K., and Sjostrand, U.: Treatment of respiratory distress syndrome: A preliminary report, Opusc. Med. 19:235, 1974.
19. Hustead, R.F., and Avery, M.E.: Observation of mask pressure achieved with the Kreiselman infant resuscitator, N. Engl. J. Med. 265:939, 1961.
20. Klaus, M.H., and Kennell, J.H.: *Maternal-Infant Bonding*, (St. Louis: C.V. Mosby Co., 1976).
21. Marchak, B.E., Thompson, W.K., Duffty, P., et al.: Treatment of RDS by high-frequency oscillatory ventilation: A preliminary report, J. Pediatr. 99:287, 1981.
22. Maxwell, C., Hess, D., and Shefer, D.: Use of the arterial/alveolar oxygen tension ratio to predict the inspired oxygen concentration needed for a desired arterial oxygen tension, Respir. Care 29:1135, 1984.
23. Meeuwis, H., Vaes, L., and Klain, M.: Long term high frequency jet ventilation in a 3-year old child, Crit. Care Med. 11:309, 1983.
24. Ophoven, J.P., Mammell, M.C., Gordon, M., and Boros, S.J.: Tracheobronchial histopathology associated with high-frequency jet ventilation. Crit. Care Med. 12:829, 1984.
25. Pokora, T., Bing, D., Mammel, M., and Boros, S.: Neonatal high frequency jet ventilation, Pediatrics 72:27, 1983.
26. Primiano, F.P., Jr., Chatburn, R.L., and Lough, M.D.: Mean airway pressure: Theoretical considerations, Crit. Care Med. 10:378, 1982.
27. Reynolds, E.O.R.: Pressure waveform and ventilator settings for mechanical ventilation in severe hyaline membrane disease, Int. Clin. Anesthesiol. 12:269, 1974.

Bronchial Hygiene

JAN S. TECKLIN, M.S., L.P.T.

7

Respiratory physical therapy includes several evaluative and therapeutic procedures. Bronchial hygiene is one area of respiratory physical therapy that is truly an interdisciplinary effort. Physical and respiratory therapists, nurses, and physicians are likely to become involved with some aspects of bronchial hygiene.

This chapter will not attempt to discuss the entire scope of respiratory physical therapy. Rather, it describes the evaluation and treatment of disorders that result in impaired bronchial hygiene in the child. In recent years there has been a great deal of clinical research regarding the effects of bronchial hygiene procedures in children. These data will be discussed where they apply.

When developing a treatment plan aimed at improving bronchial hygiene, the therapist should begin by carefully reviewing the patient's chart. A review of the patient's most recent chest x-ray films may also be helpful. Next, the therapist should proceed with a detailed chest assessment, primarily to identify areas of pain and/or areas of retained secretions. Finally, the child's ability to produce a strong, effective cough should be noted.

CHART REVIEW

Reviewing the child's hospital chart can provide an excellent background of the current illness and any medical history. The information collected may include:

Initial onset of symptoms (including secretions)
Severity of symptoms
Progression of disease process
Home treatment
Medical/surgical history
Family medical history
Socioeconomic history

Based on this information, the therapist may start to define the child's bronchial hygiene problem and begin to develop an individualized care plan.

CHEST ASSESSMENT

The four aspects of chest assessment are inspection, palpation, percussion, and auscultation.

INSPECTION

The therapist should observe the patient's posture, sitting position (children with lung disease will often sit leaning forward), symmetry of chest movement, breathing pattern, and splinting (caused by pain). General observations may include cyanosis, shortness of breath when speaking, nasal flaring, fingernail clubbing, and skin condition (i.e., dehydration, signs of cachexia). Auditory inspection of breathing may produce helpful clues. Audible noise on expiration including wheezing, rhonchi-like sounds, and gurgling often indicate moderate to excessive amounts of secretions in the larger airways. Inspection of the child's mucus is a very important part of the initial and subsequent assessments. The therapist should note the amount, color, and viscosity of the secretions produced, as well as the presence of malodorous secretions or blood. Factors or situations that appear to stimulate coughing should also be recorded.

PALPATION

Palpation involves a trained sense of touch to obtain clinical information about the movement of the chest and the underlying tissue. The most effective way to palpate for fremitus is by comparing corresponding areas of each lung, e.g., right middle lobe to lingula. Tactile fremitus may provide information about areas in which secretions are present. Vocal fremitus is a normally occurring vibration that can be palpated when the patient says "ninety-nine." Lung pathology commonly reduces the vocal fremitus in the overlying area of the thorax. Hence, vocal fremitus is often markedly reduced or absent in areas of atelectasis or pneumonia. Another type of fremitus, rhonchal fremitus, typically identifies the turbulence of airflow passing around secretions in a partially obstructed bronchus.

PERCUSSION

Percussion provides information about lung density. Disorders that increase the relative amount of air in the thorax (hyperinflation, pneumothorax) will result in a hyperresonant percussion note. Conversely, consolidation or filling of the lung with fluid or secretions will commonly produce a dull percussion note. Since secretions can result in either hyperinflation or consolidation, percussion may be useful in helping the therapist determine whether excessive pulmonary secretions exist.

AUSCULTATION

Auscultation may be the most useful of the four assessment modalities in iden-tifying and localizing areas of poor bronchial hygiene and retained secretions. Pulmonary specialists differ with regard to the terminology used in ausculta-tion. A discussion of lung sounds, per se, is beyond the scope of this chapter. Waring presents a useful and functional description of some commonly encoun-tered adventitious lung sounds:

> Rales are discontinuous, non-musical, crackling or bubbling, soft or loud, inspiratory or expiratory, palpable or impalpable sounds produced by air bubbling through fluid in the lungs or more commonly by the snapping open of approximated airway walls. A rhonchus is a continuous, musical, soft or loud, usually expiratory, usually non-palpable sound produced by air moving with velocity past a fixed obstruction in the airway.[19]

Waring further divides rales into fine, medium, and coarse. The implication is that fine rales are produced more peripherally and coarse rales more centrally within the tracheobronchial tree. Rhonchi are further categorized as sibilant— soft and high-pitched—or sonorous—loud and low-pitched. Rhonchi are con-sidered primarily as indicators of larger airway obstruction. Using the above descriptions, it appears that rhonchi are indicative of excessive excretions within the airways, and rales may indicate secretions or fluid in the smaller airways. Bronchial or tubular breath sounds are commonly heard in areas of lung consolidation, and decreased breath sounds may be heard over hyperin-flated lungs. Each of these latter two situations may be secondary to secretion retention.

COUGH ASSESSMENT

Coughing is a reflex response to irritation of sensory receptors within the res-piratory epithelium, and a therapeutic tool that can occasionally be enhanced or improved. The physician's diagnostic evaluation of the child's cough focuses upon the nature of events which stimulate coughing and the characteristics of the cough. The therapist's evaluation should be more concerned with the effec-tiveness of the cough in expelling secretions; therefore, the therapist assesses the voluntary, active cough, and the physician is usually more concerned with the reflex, symptomatic cough.

When assessing the child's ability to cough, the therapist must identify the components of a successful coughing effort. These components include 1) a deep inspiration and 2) a coordinated glottic closure followed almost immedi-ately by 3) a strong contraction of the expiratory muscles (mainly the abdomi-nals) 4) then a sudden opening of the glottis 5) producing an expulsive expira-tion. This extraordinarily high linear velocity of airflow, thought to approach 500 miles per hour, propels secretions or other debris into the pharynx, where the material can be easily expectorated or swallowed. The cough is often taken for granted until its effectiveness is diminished or absent.

Because their abdominal muscles are poorly developed and because they may lack the ability to coordinate several complicated muscular tasks simultaneously, the infant and toddler commonly do not cough well on a voluntary basis. When this relative lack of ability to cough impedes the child's improvement, other, more invasive methods to remove secretions are occasionally considered. Among these methods are tracheobronchial aspiration and bronchoscopy (see Chapter 8). The latter method is especially important in very serious or emergency situations.

OTHER ASSESSMENT TECHNIQUES

Additional means of patient assessment for bronchial hygiene may include examining the chest x-ray film, speaking with the nursing staff, and questioning the patient. Specific chest x-ray findings may alert the therapist to the possibility that secretions are responsible for the abnormal finding. Segmental or lobar atelectasis, pneumonia, areas of hyperinflation, abscesses, and bronchiectasis are associated with excessive secretions. These changes are usually not difficult for the experienced therapist to recognize. Since each of the above disorders is commonly caused by secretions or results in secretions, each should be considered a potential indication for bronchial hygiene.

It is always useful to speak with the patient's primary care nurse prior to assessing or treating the child. The nurse can provide valuable information about the medical condition, level of cooperation and understanding, and emotional state. Often the child can offer useful information regarding where secretions seem to be located, how coughing is most easily performed, and what situations will stimulate cough. When the therapist communicates with the patient, it is necessary to approach the child on his or her own level. This does not mean being childish or using "babytalk;" rather, it means speaking in phrases that the child is likely to comprehend.

INDICATIONS FOR BRONCHIAL HYGIENE

There are several general situations in which bronchial hygiene may be useful. When a child has an increase in the amount of bronchopulmonary secretions or the secretions are particularly viscous, or when the natural secretion removal mechanisms are not operating well, bronchial hygiene techniques may be useful. The last of the three situations needs some clarification. Normally, secretions are constantly transported up the tracheobronchial tree by the coordinated motion of the cilia, which line the respiratory epithelium. The normal individual has the ability to eliminate large collections of secretions by coughing. Several common situations arise in which these mechanisms are rendered less effective.

Any patient who is intubated or has a tracheostomy will have lost a large portion of the ability to cough. The ciliary transport of mucus is impaired if the tube is cuffed. Therefore, such a patient will probably benefit from periodic bronchial hygiene treatments. If the patient also has a primary pulmonary disorder, bronchial hygiene becomes critical and may be needed every 3 to 4 hours.

Another group of patients who need periodic bronchial hygiene are those with respiratory muscle weakness or paralysis. This is especially true when the abdominal muscles are involved since they are largely responsible for coughing. Patients whose cough is ineffective, for whatever reason, will require tracheobronchial aspiration to assist in the removal of secretions. Specific conditions that commonly necessitate bronchial hygiene include atelectasis, bronchopneumonia, bronchiectasis, bronchitis, cystic fibrosis (CF), and asthma (when secretions are prevalent).

Treatment

Bronchial hygiene should never be a rote, mechanical, step-by-step procedure. Each treatment session must be carefully planned in advance based upon the findings of the initial evaluation and subsequent changes in the patient's condition. No two treatments should be identical. Bronchial hygiene treatments may include many therapeutic modalities. While it is unusual for a patient to receive every modality during each treatment, it is common for the therapist to employ several modalities in most treatments.

Positioning

There are two major therapeutic implications for placing a child with respiratory disease in one or more specific positions. First, toddlers and infants who have relatively large abdominal viscera can be placed in a seated or semirecumbent position to provide for easier diaphragmatic excursion. In this position, gravity pulls the viscera down, which allows the diaphragm to descend more easily on inspiration. Second, several investigators have shown that repositioning a patient can have major changes, either detrimental or beneficial, in the patient's arterial blood gas values.[15, 5] This is particularly true for patients with unilateral lung disease.[16] Although these investigators did not study pediatric patients, it appears that the mechanisms at work in adults may apply to some pediatric disease states as well.

Positioning for gravity-assisted bronchial drainage is a time-honored, if not completely scientifically supported, treatment for patients with excessive pulmonary secretions. The treatment is based on the principle that once secretions are identified in the tracheobronchial tree, the patient can be positioned to employ the effects of gravity to drain those secretions toward the pharynx. This treatment modality is based on tracheobronchial and pulmonary segment anatomy. Once secretions have been identified in one or more lung segments, the patient is positioned to place the segment uppermost with the bronchus leading from the segment in as close to a vertical position as is possible, or practical.

The drainage positions for a child or an infant do not vary from those used for adults. A child has the same anatomic arrangement of airways, and therefore the obstructed lung segments can be drained as they are in the adult. The

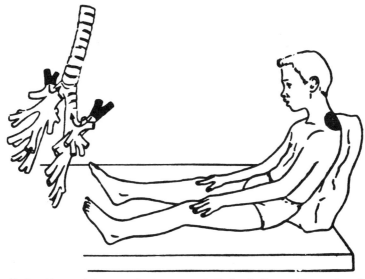

Fig 7–1.—Upper lobes, apical segment. Patient sits and leans back on a pillow at a 30-degree angle against the therapist. Clap between the clavicle and the top of the scapula on each side.

positions for drainage of the pulmonary segments are shown in Figures 7–1 thru 7–9 for children and Figures 7–10 and 7–11 for infants. For toddlers, the only equipment needed for drainage is the therapist's lap or shoulder. When only positioning is to be used during the treatment, the child should be positioned to allow for drainage and should remain in the position for 15 to 20 minutes. At the end of this time the child should either be asked to cough, or if coughing is not possible, tracheobronchial aspiration may be performed.

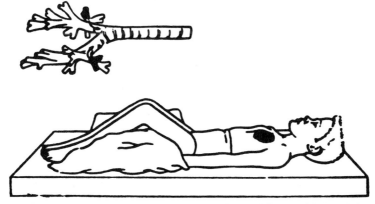

Fig 7–2.—Upper lobes, anterior segment. Patient lies on his back in a flat position. Clap between the clavicle and nipple on each side.

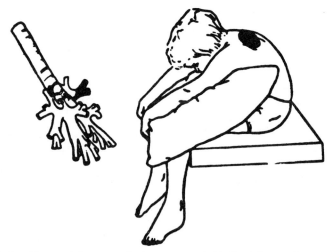

Fig 7–3.—Upper lobes, posterior segment. Patient leans forward over a folded pillow at a 30-degree angle. Clap over the upper back on both sides.

It is important for the child to be comfortable during treatment. Pillows between the knees or for support behind the thorax may be helpful. Flexion of the hips and knees will help reduce the tension of the abdominal muscles, which, in turn, will ease diaphragmatic descent. The Trendelenberg and prone positions are not tolerated well in severely ill patients. In the former position, the diaphragm must overcome the weight of the abdominal contents, which now push directly on the inferior aspect of the major inspiratory muscle. In the

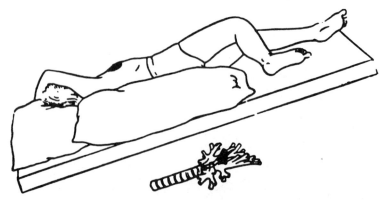

Fig 7–4.—Right middle lobe, lateral segment, medial segment. Bed is elevated 14 inches (about 15 degrees). The patient lies head down on the left side and rotates ¼ turn backward. The knees should be flexed. Clap over the right nipple. In females with breast development or tenderness, use cupped hand with heel of hand under armpit and fingers extending forward beneath the breast.

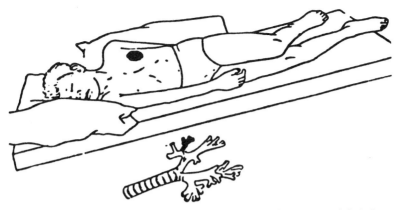

Fig 7—5.—Lingular segment, left upper lobe, superior segment, inferior segment. Patient in a head-down position on the right side and rotated ¼ turn backward. Clap over the left nipple.

latter position, the child's body weight restricts anterior expansion of the thorax.

Although the Trendelenberg and prone positions may be uncomfortable for some patients, they are usually not dangerous except in a few situations. Crane[2] suggests that infants with congestive heart failure, intracranial surgery or hemorrhage, untreated tension pneumothorax, apnea and bradycardia, persistent fetal circulation, and severe respiratory failure should not be placed in Trendelenberg. She also states that infants with indwelling chest tubes, nasal prongs, or untreated pneumothorax should not be placed in prone position. It is certainly difficult to argue with these precautions, but they should be considered ''rela-

(Text continues p. 202)

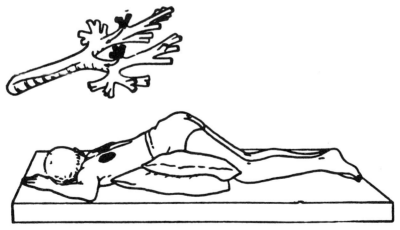

Fig 7—6.—Lower lobes, superior segment. Patient lies on abdomen with two pillows under the hips. Clap over the middle part of the back at the tip of the scapula on either side of the spine.

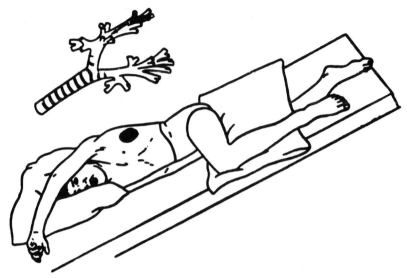

Fig 7–7.—Lower lobes, anterior basal segments. The foot of the bed is elevated 18 inches (about 30 degrees). The patient lies on side with pillow under the knees. Clap over the lower ribs just beneath the axilla.

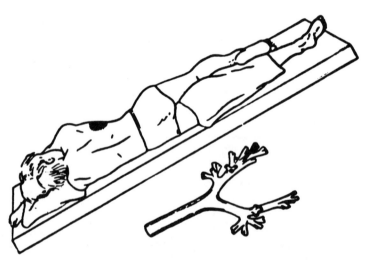

Fig 7–8.—Lower lobes, lateral basal segments. The foot of the bed is elevated 18 inches (approximately 30 degrees). The patient lies on abdomen, head down, and rotates ¼ turn upward from a prone position. The upper leg is flexed over a pillow for support. Clap over the uppermost portion of the lower ribs.

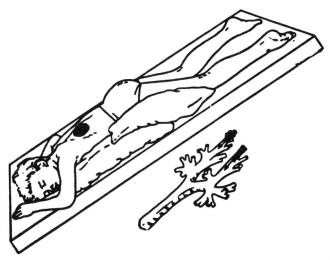

Fig 7–9.—Lower lobes, posterior basal segments. The foot of the bed is elevated 18 inches (about 30 degrees). The patient lies on abdomen, head down, with a pillow under the hips. Clap over the lower ribs close to the spine on each side.

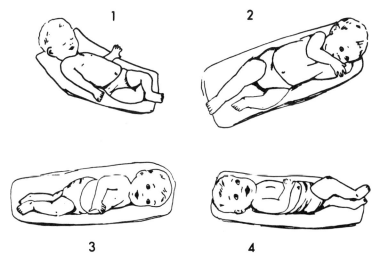

Fig 7–10.—Positions for chest physiotherapy. **(1)** The anterior segment of the upper lobes is drained in a supine position at a 30-degree upright angle. **(2)** Drain the apical segment of the right lung while the infant lies on his left side at a 30-degree upright angle. **(3)** The posterior segment of the right upper lobe is drained in a prone position with the right side elevated 45 degrees. **(4)** Drain the anterior segment of the upper lobe in a supine position.

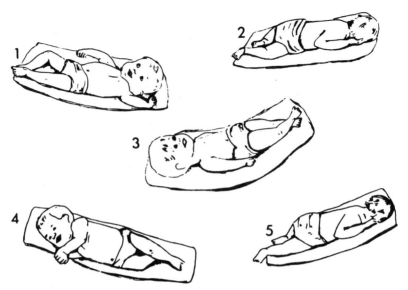

Fig 7–11.—**(1)** The right middle lobe is drained at a 15-degree, head-down angle with a 45-degree rotation to the left. To drain the lingula, rotate to the right. **(2)** The superior segment of the lower lobes drains in a prone position. **(3)** Drain the anterior basal segments of the lower lobes at a 30-degree angle, head-down position. **(4)** The basal segments of the lower lobe are drained at a 30-degree, head-down position while the infant is lying on the side. **(5)** The posterior basal segments of the lower lobes are drained at a 30-degree, head-down prone position.

tive.'' Similar precautions should be used for positioning older children who are acutely ill. Children with status asthmaticus, increased intracranial pressure, and severe acute congestive heart failure should not be placed in a head down position. However, simply having a chest drainage tube in place should not be considered a complete contraindication for lying prone. Similarly, intubation and tracheostomy are not contraindications for the prone position. If the drainage position requires the child to be placed in the prone position, the therapist and nurse must attempt to position the child properly while being extremely cautious not to put pressure on the endotracheal or tracheostomy tube, or on the chest drainage tube.

Few studies have examined only the effects of positioning on measures of bronchial hygiene. Wong et al. studied the effects on mucociliary tracheal transport rates of gravity drainage in subjects with CF. They found marked improvement in tracheal transport rates when subjects with poor or absent tracheal transport were placed in a 25-degree Trendelenberg position.[20]

Percussion

Chest percusison, when used for bronchial hygiene, is a rhythmical clapping of the chest wall, using a cupped hand technique, in the area of the thorax that corresponds to the segment of lung for which drainage is being provided. Many therapists prefer manual chest percussion while others prefer to use various cuplike devices or implements, and still others prefer to use electrically or pneumatically powered mechanical percussion devices. The cuplike devices were recently described and pictured by Crane.[2] A mechanical percussor is shown in Figure 7–12. Two recent studies have shown no differences between manual percussion and mechanical percussion.[9, 14]

Percussion is commonly used when secretions are very thick or tenacious and when the child is having a difficult time expectorating them. Manual percussion should be applied to the chest wall at the appropriate site for at least 1 minute. In children who have very thick and copious secretions, such as occurs with CF, 3 to 5 minutes of percussion in each drainage position is commonly suggested.[18]

Percussion should be neither painful nor injurious. When working with children, especially young children, one should remember that a great amount of force can be applied with percussion. It is possible to bruise the thorax and to fracture ribs. Therefore, it is advisable to use one or two layers of towelling over the chest wall when percussing the chest of a child. Although the towelling may diminish slightly the effect of percussion, it is better to err on the side of safety rather than risk chest wall injury. When percussing the chest of a small child one may wish to use one of the percussion cups. The cups come in various sizes, and smaller ones may be applied more specifically to a particular area of a small chest.

Percussion may be contraindicated in a number of situations because of its vigorous nature. Active hemoptysis is a major contraindication since percussion may dislodge a clot that is forming at the site of bleeding. Platelet deficiencies or other clotting problems (such as inhibition of platelet function by penicillin-related antimicrobials) may be a relative contraindication because of the increased susceptibility of the child to bleeding and bruising. Flail chest, major

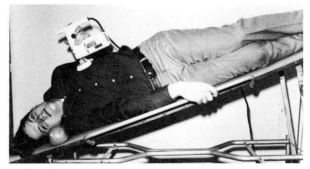

Fig 7–12.—Mechanical percussor. Using this device, the patient may perform a postural drainage treatment independently, including both percussion and vibration. Assistance may be required for the posterior basal and superior segments of the lower lobes.

chest trauma, thoracic reconstruction surgery, osteoporosis, and other conditions in which obvious harm could follow percussion are additional contraindications. Although percussion may not be indicated, positioning and other modalities to help loosen and remove secretions may be useful. Percussion should not be administered directly over fresh incisions or over a chest tube, but percussion should be used in other areas of the chest in children who have had surgery involving the thorax. It may be helpful to discuss respiratory care modalities with the attending surgeon.

Numerous investigators have demonstrated the therapeutic efficacy of positioning for drainage and percussion. Finer and colleagues[7] published two studies that examined the effects of bronchial hygiene techniques in neonates. Their first study showed a major improvement in PaO_2 when percussion was added to positioning for drainage. The latter study examined bronchial hygiene as a measure to prevent postextubation atelectasis. The group of infants who received bronchial hygiene had a significantly lower incidence of postextubation atelectasis and had a lower incidence of reintubation.[11]

Another use for percussion has been identified by Burrington and Cotten.[1] They successfully used percussion to loosen aspirated foreign bodies in children. Their regimen included first localizing the object via chest x-ray films and then positioning the child to drain the appropriate segment or lobe. Five deep inhalations of a bronchodilator were followed by vigorous chest percussion and active coughing by the child. The foreign body was removed with this regimen in 24 of 28 children. One child suffered cardiorespiratory arrest during the procedure, and some workers believe that this may totally contraindicate this therapy for foreign bodies. However, Law and Kosloske[13] also studied bronchial hygiene techniques as a means for removing foreign bodies from the tracheobronchial tree. They compared a regimen similar to that used by Burrington and Cotten with bronchoscopy. The latter study found only 12 of 49 foreign bodies were removed with percussion. However, bronchoscopy successfully removed 24 of 26 objects. In addition, 32 of the 37 patients, in whom percussion had failed, were successfully treated with bronchoscopy. Law and Kosloske suggested immediate bronchoscopy for foreign body aspiration only in a respiratory emergency. Inhalation of a bronchodilator, positioning, percussion, and coughing were suggested for the first 24 hours in nonemergency aspirations. If bronchial hygiene was unsuccessful, bronchoscopy would follow.

Bronchial drainage with percussion was studied by two different investigators working with children who had asthma. Kang et al.[11] compared bronchial drainage with percussion to drainage alone in a group of children with chronic lung disease including five asthmatics. Three of the five with asthma had an increase in forced expired volume in 1 second (FEV_1) was greater than $> 15\%$ when percussion was added to the treatment program. Huber et al.[10] studied two groups of children with moderately severe asthma. One group was treated with bronchial drainage positioning and percussion, while the other group served as a control. The treated group showed a mean improvement in FEV_1 of 10.5%, whereas the control group had a slight overall decrease in FEV_1.

Bronchial hygiene has been studied and examined more extensively in children with CF than in any other patient population. The results of the studies have been recently reviewed.[18] For patients with CF and asthma who have moderately severe disease and produce sputum, bronchial hygiene is clearly beneficial in the short-term treatment. There is a major improvement in removal of secretions when positioning for drainage is accompanied by percussion. Also, both small and large airway obstruction is significantly reduced.[17] What remains to be shown is whether these short-term benefits have any role in improving survival, or at least retarding the decline of pulmonary function.

Vibration

Manual or mechanical chest vibration is another technique that can be used either in conjunction with percussion or in its place. Vibration is a more difficult technique to learn than percussion. Vibration is appropriate in many instances in which percussion is either contraindicated or may be too vigorous for the patient's comfort. There are very few clinical situations in which any form of vibration is contraindicated. Vibration is particularly appropriate for the child who has had recent chest trauma or thoracic surgery.

Vibration is commonly applied during the expiratory phase of deep breathing or the expiratory phase of a ventilator breath. It is performed by placing one or both hands on the thorax in the area which corresponds to the segment in which secretions are found. As the child exhales, a very quick, fine tremulous vibration is generated by a rapidly alternating contraction and relaxation of all muscles from the shoulders to the hands. One way of evaluating your vibrating skill is to apply vibration to the chest wall of a normal individual while he says "aaah." You should be able to hear the fine, rapid vibration as it interrupts the sound coming from the person's larynx. Vibration may be very difficult to master. It is a much more subtle technique then percussion. Therefore, many novices who attempt vibration feel that they are not being effective and prematurely discontinue their attempt to learn.

Vibration is thought to work in two or three different ways. It is thought to "squeeze" secretions proximally in the tracheobronchial tree after those secretions have been loosened by percussion. However, vibration alone appears to be able to loosen and help transport secretions as an aid to bronchial hygiene. Many patients report that vibration assists in stimulating a good voluntary cough. Whatever the mechanism, it seems clear that manual and mechanical ventilation are useful techniques.

Chest "shaking" is a skill that is similar to vibration. Shaking, however, is much more vigorous and not all children can tolerate it. The difference between vibration and shaking is largely a difference in degree. Vibration is a finer, more delicate technique. Shaking is a coarse, more vigorous technique that is probably most appropriate for patients with particularly tenacious secretions.

As noted above, vibration and shaking are commonly employed as an adjunct to percussion. Usually, percussion is applied for 1 or more minutes. Following the percussion, the child is asked to breathe deeply for several respiratory cycles during which vibration or shaking is applied during the expiratory phase. Following the application of these or any manual techniques, voluntary coughing should be encouraged. Tracheobronchial aspiration may be done.

A problem arises in using manual chest vibration in the young child or infant who is acutely ill. It is not uncommon for these children to have a respiratory rate of 50 or 60 breaths per minute. It is often impossible to coordinate manual vibration with the expiratory phase of breathing in patients with such a rapid respiratory rate. Therefore many therapists prefer mechanical vibrators for young children and infants. A common device used is an electric toothbrush with the brush tip replaced with a pad or rubber stopper which is then applied directly to the chest wall. At least two studies have examined the use of mechanical vibration for the infant. Crane et al.[3] found no statistically significant differences between percussion and vibration when examining their effects on $TcPO_2$. Curran and Kachoyeanos[4] compared percussion with a padded nipple to vibration with an electric toothbrush in several neonates. There was greater improvement in PaO_2, color, and breath sounds when mechanical vibration was used. One word of caution is in order. One must exercise care when using any electric motor around high concentrations of oxygen. Any electrical device being used in an oxygen-rich environment should be evaluated by the hospital biomedical engineering staff or the safety committee prior to use.

Deep Breathing

Current respiratory therapy curricula often do not provide sufficient instruction in muscle function, assessment, and training for the respiratory therapist to be expected to appropriately develop any muscle training or reeducation regimen for the patient. However, deep breathing is a means of improving secretion removal and thereby improving bronchial hygiene. Deep breathing should be employed by the patient during any bronchial hygiene procedure. It may be especially beneficial for the child during positioning for drainage. The deep breathing will help move air past the obstructing secretions, and the mechanical drag of the expiratory flow of air is probably helpful in further loosening and draining those secretions.

Secretion Removal

Although the above procedures of positioning for gravity-drainage, percussion, vibration and shaking, and deep breathing are all important elements in a regimen of bronchial hygiene, the most important element is the ultimate removal of the loosened secretions. This is best accomplished by coughing. In situations in which the infant or child is unable to or simply refuses to cough, it may be necessary to employ other means for secretions removal. The most commonly used technique is aspiration of secretions from the airway by means of a suction catheter.

Coughing can be improved in a number of ways. One of the most important considerations in achieving an effective cough is proper positioning. Yamazaki et al.[21] showed that a sitting position resulted in a stronger cough force than the supine position. These investigators also determined that manual pressure over the thorax or abdomen increased the cough force. Many young children actually find coughing difficult in any position other than sitting. However, they may find it more difficult to cough with the externally applied pressure around the thorax or over the abdomen. Children often comment that the added pressure makes it impossible for them to cough. Nonetheless, the therapist may want to try adding external pressure to help a child who has a weak cough. Another critical aspect of a good cough is the depth of the inspiratory effort prior to the cough. This is often the easiest aspect for the therapist to improve in an ineffective cough. The use of incentive spirometry provides good objective information when training the child to inhale deeply prior to trying to cough.

Another part of coughing, the expiratory muscle contraction, is one that is easily improved in a cooperative, alert child. Expulsive expiratory exercises, such as occur when expiring against resistance, can provide resistive exercise for the appropriate muscles of expiration. Blow bottles, although not commonly used for postoperative care, can be used for this type of expiratory strengthening exercise.

Any type of forced expiratory maneuver is painful for the postoperative patient. One technique that appears useful in moving secretions but is not as painful as coughing is "huffing" or "huff coughing." Although no data exist to support the use of huffing in patients who have had surgery, there are published anecdotal reports of its usefulness.[12] Huffing is a forced expiration with an open glottis, and is similar to an extended clearing of the throat.

Tracheobronchial aspiration is another mechanism for removing secretions from the child's airway when cough is impossible or ineffective. This has been described in detail elsewhere (see Chapter 8).

In summary, this chapter has been organized to provide the respiratory therapist with a logical approach to bronchial hygiene in children. Major emphasis was placed upon assessment of the patient. Individualized treatment regimens will provide the most effective and least tiring respiratory care. The initial assessment of the patient is obviously important in developing the plan for bronchial hygiene. As important is each subsequent reevaluation. Basic information has been provided about the major modalities of treatment including positioning, percussion, vibration, and cough. It is important to consider each of these used singly or in combination with the goal of improved bronchial hygiene.

REFERENCES

1. Burrington, J.D., Cotten, E.K.: Removal of foreign bodies from the tracheobronchial tree, J. Pediatr. Surg. 7:119, 1972.

2. Crane, L.D.: Physical therapy for neonates with respiratory dysfunction, Phys. Ther. 61:1764, 1981.
3. Crane, L.D., Zombek, M., Krauss, A.N., et al.: Comparison of chest physiotherapy techniques in infants with HMD (Abstract), Pediatr. Res. 12:559, 1978.
4. Curran, C.L., Kachoyeanos, M.K.: The effects on neonates of two methods of chest physical therapy, Matern. Child. Nurs. J. 4:309, 1978.
5. Douglas, W.W., Rehder, K., Beynen, F., et al.:Improved oxygenation in patients with acute respiratory failure: The prone position, Am. Rev. Respir. Dis. 115:559, 1977.
6. Downes, J.J., Goldberg, A.I.: Airway management, mechanical ventilation and cardiopulmonary resuscitation, in Scarpelli, E.M., Auld, P.A.M., Goldman, H.S. (eds.): *Pulmonary Disease of the Fetus, Newborn, and Child.* (Philadelphia: Lea & Febiger, 1978).
7. Finer, N.N., Boyd, J.: Chest physiotherapy in the neonate: A controlled study. Pediatrics 61:282, 1978.
8. Finer, N.N., Moriartey, R.R., Boyd, J., et al.: Post-extubation atelectasis: A retrospective review and a prospective study, J. Pediatr. 94:110, 1979.
9. Hartsell, M., Traver, G., Taussig, L.M.: Comparison of manual percussion and vibration vs. mechanical vibration alone on maximal expiratory flows, Cystic Fibrosis Club Abstracts, 1978.
10. Huber, A.L., Eggleston, P.A., Morgan, J.: Effect of chest physiotherapy on asthmatic children (Abstract), J. Allergy Clin. Immunol. 53:2, 1974.
11. Kang, B., Rogers, W.L., Niederhuber, S.S., et al.: Evaluation of postural drainage with percussion in chronic obstructive lung disease (Abstract), J. Allergy Clin. Immunol. 53:2, 1974.
12. Kigin, C.M.: Chest physical therapy for the postoperative or traumatic injury patient. Phys. Ther. 61:1724, 1981.
13. Law, D., Kosloske, A.: Management of tracheobronchial foreign bodies in children: A reevaluation of postural drainage and bronchoscopy, Pediatrics 58:362, 1976.
14. Maxwell, M., Redmond, A.: Comparative trial of manual and mechanical percussion techniques with gravity-assisted bronchial drainage in patients with cystic fibrosis. Arch. Dis. Child. 54:542, 1979.
15. Piehl, M.A., Brown, R.D.: Use of extreme position changes in acute respiratory failure, Crit. Care Med. 4:13, 1976.
16. Remolina, C., et al.: Positioned hypoxemia in unilateral lung disease, N. Engl. J. Med. 304:523, 1981.
17. Tecklin, J.S.: Physical therapy for children with chronic lung disease, Phys. Ther. 61:1774, 1981.
18. Tecklin, J.S., Holsclaw, D.S.: Cystic fibrosis and the role of the physical therapist in it's management, Phys. Ther. 53:386, 1973.
19. Waring, W.: The history and physical examination, in Kendig, E.M., Chernick, V. (eds.): *Disorders of the Respiratory Tract in Children.* (Philadelphia: W.B. Saunders Co., 1977).
20. Wong, J.W. Keens, T.G., Wannamaker, E.M., et al.: Effects of gravity on tracheal transport rates in normal subjects and in patients with cystic fibrosis. Pediatrics 60:146, 1977.
21. Yamazaki, S., Ogawa, J., Shohzu, A., et al.: Intra-pleural cough pressures in patients after thoracotomy, J. Thorac. Cardiovasc. Surg. 80:600, 1980.

Diagnostic and Therapeutic Procedures in Pediatric Pulmonary Disease

ROBERT E. WOOD, PH.D., M.D.

8

THE AIRWAY

ANAEROBIC METABOLISM is quite inefficient; thus adequate ventilation and gas exchange are among the most fundamental requirements for human life. Although cardiovascular function may continue for many minutes after interruption of ventilation, the establishment of adequate gas exchange is always the first priority in resuscitation and life support. Initially, the major efforts should be directed toward achieving ventilation rather than establishing an artificial airway. Thus, mouth-to-mouth respiration or bag and mask ventilation (with a tight-fitting face mask) should be the first step in resuscitation.

Establishment of Artificial Airways

GENERAL PRINCIPLES REGARDING INTUBATION

1. Establishment of an artificial airway should be attempted only when the patient is in a relatively stable condition (that is, when ventilation and adequate oxygenation have been achieved) or if ventilation *cannot* be achieved without the use of an artificial airway (e.g., with anatomic airway obstruction).
2. Prior to beginning intubation, make certain that all necessary equipment is

at hand and in good working order, including proper laryngoscope and blade(s), endotracheal tubes, and adaptors.

3. The procedure should be performed by the most capable individual present, with due regard to the urgency of the situation and requirements for teaching. Techniques for emergency intubation should be learned by observing an expert rather than by trial and error.

4. The tube used for establishing the airway should be sufficiently large to provide for adequate ventilation of the patient but must be small enough so that the larynx and upper airway are not damaged by the tube.

5. No force should be used to pass the tube into the trachea.

6. A patient who is struggling often does not need intubation *at that moment;* simply clearing the mouth and pharynx of foreign material and providing an oral airway may be sufficient.

EQUIPMENT NEEDED FOR INTUBATION

1. Laryngoscope with appropriate size blade. There are various types of laryngoscope blades, but the type used is probably less important than the skill with which it is used. The size of the blade should correspond to the size of the patient.

2. Endotracheal tubes of appropriate size (see Table 6–2).

3. Suction catheters of appropriate size (see Table 6–2).

4. Endotracheal tube adapters of appropriate size. The adapter should have a standard 15-mm taper and should be the same nominal size as the endotracheal tube. With smaller tubes (<4.5 mm), it is useful to use an adapter a half-size larger than the tube. This makes suctioning easier, since there is often a slight narrowing at the point of insertion of the adapter into the tube.

5. Anesthesia bag with oxygen.

6. Suction line and vacuum source.

7. Tape and other supplies for immobilizing the tube.

OROTRACHEAL INTUBATION

It is not always necessary to visualize the larynx for successful intubation. However, direct inspection of the larynx prior to intubation not only facilitates intubation but provides useful diagnostic information and assures that the pharynx and upper airway are clear of foreign material. The patient should be in a supine position and hyperventilated with oxygen (if possible) prior to intubation. The patient's head should be tilted back no more than 20 to 30 degrees and the head and chin brought forward. The laryngoscope is held in the *left* hand and the blade gently inserted along the right side of the tongue. Be careful not to traumatize the lips, teeth, or gums. The tip of the laryngoscope is then placed at the base of the tongue (in the vallecula, between the base of the tongue and the epiglottis). The laryngoscope and blade are then *lifted* straight upward to bring the tongue and mandible out of the line of vision. Any foreign material or excessive secretions should be cleared before proceeding with intubation.

The endotracheal tube is held in the right hand and should be passed into the larynx under direct vision. If the glottis cannot be seen, then the tube will more often go into the esophagus than down the airway. Note that in the infants the larynx is located higher in the neck and more anteriorly than in adults and is thus more difficult to visualize. An assistant may apply gentle pressure on the anterior neck to help bring the larynx into view. It is often helpful to stiffen the tube by cooling it in ice. Only under the most unusual conditions should a stylet be used, and then the tip of the stylet must not extend beyond the tip of the tube. If force is required to advance the tube, either the tube is not in the airway or the tube is too large for the airway.

It is important to use an endotracheal tube that is large enough to provide adequate ventilation but not so large that it will damage the larynx. (See the guidelines in Table 6–2.) A tube that is too large will exert pressure against the mucosa of the subglottic space, resulting in schemic necrosis of the mucosa. This may in turn lead to subglottic stenosis. If the pressure is high enough to block capillary blood flow to the mucosa, mucosal necrosis will ensue if perfusion is not reestablished within a period of several hours. Patients in whom the correct tube size is used may experience a prolonged period of systemic hypotension in subglottic stenosis. While it is difficult to determine precisely the correct tube size in all circumstances, it appears that if there is a leak of air around the tube at a pressure of 25 cm H_2O, the changes of producing mucosal necrosis are relatively small. Therefore, it is important to check for a small leak around the tube at a pressure of 25 cm H_2O and replace the tube if no leak is found.

Some experienced operators may intubate infants without the use of a laryngoscope. This technique, once learned, is quite rapid and useful, particularly for resuscitation of the newborn, although problems may be encountered if the larynx is abnormal. The endotracheal tube is held along the flexor surface of the forefinger, both of which are then inserted into the mouth. The tip of the finger is placed at the orifice of the esophagus immediately posterior to the arytenoid cartilages, giving the operator the necessary landmarks. The tube is then advanced along the finger and into the airway.

NASOTRACHEAL INTUBATION

The endotracheal tube may be passed through the nose, rather than through the mouth. Nasotracheal intubation has several potential advantages, including comfort, stability, and, probably because of the improved stability, a somewhat lower incidence of complications such as accidental extubation. Infants intubated with nasotracheal tubes can suck on a pacifier, which is an important advantage. Nasotracheal intubation also has some disadvantages. In older patients it is usually necessary to use a slightly smaller tube than with orotracheal tubes. It is also technically a more difficult procedure than orotracheal intubation and is definitely a procedure not to be attempted by the novice under less than ideal conditions.

There are two techniques for nasotracheal intubation. The most common technique is to pass the tube through the nose (usually after lubrication with lidocaine jelly) to position the tip of the tube near the glottis. The larynx is then visualized with a laryngoscope, and the tip of the tube grasped with forceps (Magill) and advanced into the airway. Nasotracheal intubation may also be accomplished readily by passing a small flexible bronchoscope through the nose and into the trachea, and then sliding the tube over the bronchoscope to its final position. This technique may be accomplished very rapidly, but requires an operator skilled with the bronchoscope (as well as a small flexible bronchoscope). With the available flexible bronchoscopes, the smallest tube that can usually be used is 4.5 mm (inside diameter), although with a smaller instrument 3.0 mm tubes could be used.

ALTERNATIVES TO INTUBATION.—If the site of airway obstruction is above the larynx (as with hypertrophied adenoids and tonsils or a very large tongue), it may be possible to avoid endotracheal intubation by providing an oral or nasopharyngeal airway. This is only a temporary measure, but it is often associated with fewer complications than direct endotracheal intubation. Nasopharyngeal tubes may be difficult to position properly.

TRACHEOSTOMY

Under most conditions, artificial airway is best established by orotracheal or nasotracheal intubation. However, there are specific indications for tracheostomy as a primary procedure. These include laryngeal trauma, structural disorders of the larynx (such as subglottic stenosis), or the anticipation of prolonged mechanical ventilation. In some patients tracheostomy may be the only method by which an airway can be established. In general, it is preferable to perform a tracheostomy that is removed early than to wait until permanent damage to the larynx has occurred. In patients with subglottic swelling or in whom the endotracheal tube is too tight, mucosal necrosis can occur within hours, leading to subglottic stenosis.

The surgical technique for tracheostomy is in standard surgical textbooks and will not be detailed here. It is important to note, however, that except for in emergencies, a tracheostomy should be performed under the most controlled conditions possible. The trachea should be intubated prior to tracheostomy if at all possible, either with an endotracheal tube or a rigid bronchoscope.

Maintenance of the Artificial Airway

Once the endotracheal tube has been placed into the trachea, it should be advanced until the tip is several centimeters below the glottis, and then its position verified by auscultation of both lungs. Occasionally it is difficult to ascertain whether the tube is actually in the trachea or in the esophagus. If auscultation of the breath sounds leaves any doubt, listen over the end of the tube while the chest is compressed manually. This should produce expulsion of air through the tube; if it does not, the tube is in the esophagus. When it is clear that the tube is in the airway and there is evidence of ventilation to both lungs, the tube should be immobilized with tape and the tube position verified by x-ray film. This is particularly important in infants, in whom auscultation may not reveal that the tube has passed down one mainstem bronchus.

Immobilization of the endotracheal tube is of vital importance. The tube should be prevented from passing too far down the airway, and also from being inadvertently removed from the trachea. Furthermore, excessive movement of the endotracheal tube may traumatize the larynx and airway. There are a number of techniques for immobilizing endotracheal tubes, most of which are satisfactory in experienced hands. Because it is relatively easier to securely immobilize a nasotracheal tube than an orotracheal tube, this may be the preferred technique in patients with potentially life-threatening airway obstruction (e.g., acute epiglottitis).

SUCTIONING

An endotracheal or tracheostomy tube impairs both mucociliary and cough transport of secretions. Therefore, it is necessary to suction the artificial airway in order to maintain airway patency. A number of important principles regarding suctioning are as follows:

1. The duration of suctioning should be relatively short in order not to interfere with ventilation.
2. The suction catheter should be sufficiently large to allow adequate removal of secretions, but not so large as to occlude the tube (and thus deflate the lung). In general, the catheter should be approximately half the diameter of the tube (see Table 6–2).
3. The purpose of suctioning is to remove secretions from the tube (and, if necessary, from the airways) while not damaging the airways. It is relatively easy to traumatize the airway mucosa with a suction catheter. In most clinical situations it should only be necessary to pass the catheter to just beyond the tip of the tube.
4. Suctioning should be performed with technique that minimizes the risk of introducing infection into the lung.
5. Suctioning should not be performed with a high vacuum, in order to avoid hypoxia (by degassing the lung) and trauma to the airway mucosa.

In many patients with artificial airways, excessive amounts of secretion combined with inadequate hydration of the inspired air lead to mucus plugging of the airways. Removal of very thick secretions may be facilitated by lavage with small quantities of sterile normal saline. The addition of 2 to 4% *N*-acetylcysteine may be efficacious, but it may lead to bronchospasm in some patients.

It is often taught that patients should be manually hyperinflated with an anesthesia bag prior to endotracheal suctioning. This procedure tends to stimulate coughing and may move secretions more centrally, but it may also push secretions distally if it is done vigorously prior to clearing secretions from the tube. In general, it is wise to quickly suction the tube before hyperventilating the patient.

In the presence of excessive airway secretions and/or airway obstruction resulting from inflammation and mucosal edema, especially in a patient who does not breathe deeply (sigh), areas of atelectasis may develop beyond obstructed airways. Chest physiotherapy may be very helpful in preventing this problem. If poorly ventilated areas of the lung are hyperventilated with 100% oxygen (as is often practiced during endotracheal suctioning) absorption atelectasis may develop. When hyperventilating a patient, a concentration of oxygen no greater than 10% above the previous level should be used.

Inspissated mucus has the consistency of dried rubber cement, and can lead to fatal occlusion of artificial airways. When it becomes clear that dried secretions have accumulated in the lumen of an endotracheal or tracheostomy tube, the tube should be changed. Tracheostomy tubes are generally changed at least once a week.

Many nonintubated patients with excessive secretions and inadequate cough may require direct suctioning of the airways, both upper and lower. In infants, direct laryngoscopy with a laryngoscope (as for intubation) and passage of a suction catheter into the trachea may be effective. In older patients, a catheter may be passed through the nose and into the trachea. The tip of the catheter is advanced to just above the glottis, and the patient is requested to cough. During the subsequent rapid inspiration the catheter is advanced, and (with a little bit of luck) it will often pass into the trachea. Suctioning is then performed as the catheter is withdrawn from the trachea. These procedures may produce considerable vagal stimulation and are not without potential risk.

A more complicated technique for directly suctioning the airways in patients with extensive airway obstruction involves the use of a bronchoscope, either rigid or flexible. The major advantage of bronchoscopy is that the operator can visually inspect the airways and assess the efficacy of airway cleansing. Open-tube bronchoscopy generally requires general anesthesia, while flexible bronchoscopy is performed with only topical anesthesia (although sedation may be required) and can be repeated several times a day if necessary. In older patients, a flexible bronchoscope can be passed through an endotracheal tube. A 3.5 mm (pediatric) flexible bronchoscope can be used through a tube 5.5 mm in diameter or larger, while the larger (adult) bronchoscopes require proportionately larger tubes in order to allow the patients to breathe during the procedure.

In selected patients it may be useful to place a small (20- or 22-gauge) intravenous catheter through the cricothyroid membrane into the trachea through which saline, mucolytics, and/or antibiotics may be instilled.

HUMIDIFICATION

The artificial airway bypasses the normal mechanisms for humidification and warming of inspired air, and thus considerable care must be taken to provide for these functions. Patients with tracheostomy tubes usually adapt somewhat after a period of weeks to months, so that they will tolerate relatively long periods (up to several hours) without additional humidification (especially if they are also breathing partially through their upper airway). In general, it is a good practice to provide a mist collar for patients with a tracheostomy during those hours when they are sedentary or in bed.

Examination of the Airway

LARYNGOSCOPY

Indirect (mirror) laryngoscopy is a simple technique in principle, but is rather difficult to master in practice. Furthermore, it usually requires a fair degree of cooperation on the part of the patient and is very difficult if not impossible in most infants and children. Indirect laryngoscopy has the advantages of being inexpensive and allowing the demonstration of some physiologic function of the larynx (e.g., phonation) in an unanesthetized patient.

Direct laryngoscopy has been described in the previous section on intubation. The technique is useful for a quick examination, particularly in infants, in order to rule out foreign bodies and to remove secretions and other material from the airway. However, in the unanesthetized awake patient direct laryngoscopy may be very difficult for all but the very experienced operator, and generally anesthesia (and often muscle relaxation) is usually required for a good examination.

Recently, the development of a small flexible fiberoptic bronchoscope has made possible transnasal direct laryngoscopy, even for premature infants. After the administration of a topical anesthesic, a 3.5 mm flexible bronchoscope can be passed through the nose of even the smallest infants with surprising ease. This technique allows examination of the larynx without placing any tension on the laryngeal structures and thus demonstrates the laryngeal dynamics more readily and accurately than direct laryngoscopy.

BRONCHOSCOPY

Endoscopic examination of the trachea and bronchi may be indicated for either diagnostic or therapeutic purposes, some of which are listed in Table 8–1. Two different kinds (i.e., flexible and rigid), of instruments are available for bronchoscopy; the choice depends on the age and size of the patient and the nature of the intended procedure. Any bronchoscope must allow adequate visualization, must be sufficiently maneuverable to reach the desired portion of the airway, and must allow for adequate ventilation of the patient during the procedure.

The open-tube ("rigid") bronchoscope is a hollow metal tube, 3 to 10 mm inside diameter and may be equipped with various types of lenses, telescopes, and mirrors. The open-tube bronchoscope functions as an artificial airway and the patient may be easily ventilated, either by direct positive pressure or with a Venturi device. Open-tube bronchoscopes are indicated for removal of foreign bodies or whenever instrumentation is needed, when the airways are very small (if the procedure requires more than a few seconds), for management of

TABLE 8–1.—INDICATIONS FOR BRONCHOSCOPY

DIAGNOSTIC	THERAPEUTIC
Suspected foreign body	Foreign-body extraction
Congenital anomalies	Airway obstruction
Hemoptysis	Secretions
Airway obstruction	Mass or tumor (endoscopic resection)
Suspected malignancy	Stenosis (dilatation or resection)
Unexplained and persistent cough, wheeze or stridor	Atelectasis
	Massive hemoptysis (bronchial tamponade)
Unexplained and persistent pulmonary infiltrates	
Suspected bronchiectasis (with bronchography)	

massive hemoptysis, and in the presence of airway stenosis. The open-tube bronchoscope is also very useful when there is a great excess of very viscous secretions. The Hopkins-Stortz glass rod telescope system has vastly improved the optical characteristics of open-tube bronchoscopes, and some endoscopists consider this instrument to be indicated for all pediatric procedures. However, our own experience indicates that for the majority of procedures, the flexible instruments are at least as useful and in many cases superior to the rigid instruments.

The flexible bronchoscope has certain advantages and disadvantages in comparison to the open-tube bronchoscope. In general, flexible bronchoscopes are much smaller, but are solid, and the patient must breathe *around* rather than *through* the instrument. Thus, there is an absolute limitation in regard to airway size if the patient is to breathe during the procedure. In very small infants, however, it is usually possible to complete the procedure within 30 to 45 seconds after the bronchoscope enters the trachea, and most infants can tolerate a short apneic period. We have performed a number of therapeutic bronchoscopies (for treatment of massive atelectasis) in infants weighing 700 to 800 g, with a high degree of success.

A major disadvantage in the use of flexible bronchoscopes is the limited capacity for instrumentation. The open-tube bronchoscope is clearly the instrument of choice for removal of foreign bodies. In the management of extremely tenacious secretions or massive hemoptysis, the flexible bronchoscope may have definite limitations.

The major advantages of the flexible instruments include the ability to reach peripheral locations in the airways, especially the upper lobes, and the ability to examine the airway without introducing mechanical distortion. This is particularly important in the evaluation of the upper airway in infants with stridor. Flexible bronchoscopy, in contrast to open-tube bronchoscopy, is much more comfortable for the patients, avoids the necessity of general anesthesia, and is associated with a much lower incidence of complications. Another advantage is that the bronchoscope can be passed through a preexisting endotracheal tube, provided the tube is sufficiently large.

Adequate anesthesia is essential for successful bronchoscopy. Open-tube bronchoscopy is usually performed with general anesthesia, particularly in children; flexible bronchoscopy is more frequently performed with topical anesthesia. Children younger than 10 to 12 years usually require sedation in addition to topical anesthesia of the upper airways and larynx.

The single most common complication of open-tube bronchoscopy is subglottic edema, which may be manifest minutes to hours after the procedure. Epinephrine aerosol is often helpful in treating postbronchoscopy croup. Because a flexible bronchoscope must be sufficiently small for the patient to breathe around it, the subglottic space is unlikely to suffer trauma during flexible bronchoscopy. In more than 2000 patients, we have never seen subglottic edema following flexible bronchoscopy.

The complications of bronchoscopy are determined as much by the nature of the disease process for which the procedure is performed as by the technique used. Bleeding, pneumothorax, bronchial perforation, laryngeal damage, hypoxia, bronchospasm, and cardiac arrhythmias may all occur. Foreign-body extraction has a relatively high complication rate because the procedure is often prolonged and difficult. Flexible bronchoscopy usually is performed for diagnostic purposes and rarely requires more than a few minutes for completion. As noted above, a complete visual inspection of the lower airways can usually be completed in less than 1 minute after entering the trachea. In children the abnormal findings are usually apparent (mucus plugs or anatomic abnormalities). In contrast, the indication for bronchoscopy in adults is frequently suspected malignancy, which requires an exhaustive search. The most common complications of flexible bronchoscopy in infants and children is mild epistaxis (since a transnasal approach is almost always used). Rarely, transient bradycardia is noted, resulting either from vagal stimulation or hypoxia. Infection could possibly result from either open-tube or flexible bronchoscopy, since it is impossible to enter the lung in a completely sterile fashion with a bronchoscope.

RADIOGRAPHIC EXAMINATION OF THE AIRWAYS

The upper airway, including the trachea and mainstem bronchi, can usually be adequately visualized on standard posteroanterior (PA) and lateral chest and neck films. PA and lateral neck films may be particularly helpful in the evaluation of a patient with stridor. In patients with epiglottitis, the swollen epiglottis may often be visualized in lateral films. Subglottic edema is more easily recognized on PA films. Plain tomograms are rarely needed to evaluate the airways in children, but may be helpful in selected circumstances. Computed tomography, a newer technique, is often useful in identifying causes of extrinsic airway compression.

Detailed radiographic examination of the airways requires the deposition of some radiopaque contrast material on the airway mucosa. Indications for bronchography include suspected bronchiectasis and anatomic or structural abnormalities beyond the visual range of a bronchoscope. These abnormalities may be either congenital or acquired. In most situations in which bronchograms are performed, pulmonary surgery is being contemplated.

A bronchogram is usually performed with the patient under anesthesia or sedation, using the smallest amount of contrast material necessary to coat the walls of the airways being studied. Several different contrast materials have been employed, but the most popular is oily Dionosil. In patients with iodide sensitivity, barium sulfate in carboxymethylcellulose may be used. Tantalum powder has been used with great success investigationally, but is not available for routine clinical use. The contrast material should be deposited as close to the area of interest as possible, through an endotracheal tube or tracheal catheter or through a fiberoptic bronchoscope. The deposition of contrast material is observed fluoroscopically, and the injection is stopped when the desired degree of filling has been achieved. Spot films are then made in various projections. Routine chest films may be taken afterward at intervals to assess the rate of clearance of the contrast material from the lung; often this provides very useful information regarding the functional state of the airways.

Bronchography is not without its hazards. Allergic reactions to the contrast material may occur. The deposition of contrast material in the airways may result in airway obstruction, either mechanically or by reflex irritation. In addition, there are the usual risks of placing a catheter or bronchoscope in the airway.

THE CHEST WALL AND PLEURA

THORACENTESIS

Pleural fluid may be removed by thoracentesis for either diagnostic or therapeutic purposes. Thoracentesis is usually performed in the midaxillary or posterior axillary line, in the lowest interspace known to be safely above the diaphragm (usually the 6th to 8th interspace). After preparing the skin with a suitable solution, the selected site should be infiltrated with a local anesthetic, using a small needle (22- or 23-gauge). The needle is slowly advanced, and small volumes of anesthetic are injected. Keep in mind that the intercostal neurovascular bundle lies immediately *beneath* each rib.

Any instrument passed through the intercostal space should be guided to pass just *over* the rib perpendicular to the chest wall or at a slight downward angle. It may be useful to touch the top surface of the rib in order to be certain of the anatomic landmarks. Before each injection, the plunger of the syringe is pulled back; if fluid or air is returned, the depth at which the needle reached the pleura is marked. A larger syringe with a larger needle is then used and the needle passed along the same track to the same depth. Stabilization of the needle (by holding it firmly with the gloved hand braced against the skin) is of crucial importance in preventing deeper penetration than is necessary, with consequent risk of laceration of the underlying lung. It may be helpful to pass a plastic catheter through the needle and into the pleural space; the needle may then be withdrawn, thus eliminating the possibility of damage to the lung. In general, as much fluid is withdrawn as possible. Appropriate specimens should be saved for bacteriologic, chemical, and cytologic analyses. Fluids with a high protein content may clot; it is useful to use a tube containing heparin for collecting chemical and cytologic specimens.

CLOSED THORACOTOMY

For drainage of a pneumothorax, recurrent pleural effusion, or purulent pleural exudates, a chest tube may be needed rather than a simple thoracentesis. Chest tubes are placed by a technique analogous to that used for thoracentesis; however, a skin incision must be made to allow passage of the tube. Because of the possibility of leakage around a large tube, it is good practice to tunnel the tube through several centimeters of skin before entering the intercostal space. The skin incision is made 1 to 2 interspaces lower than the intended site of entry into the thorax. A purse-string suture is then placed around the incision. A subcutaneous tunnel is made with a surgical clamp to reach the site selected for the intercostal penetration, and a hole is made through the intercostal muscles. The chest tube is then passed through the subcutaneous tunnel and into the intrapleural space, using a surgical clamp (or a trocar catheter) to guide the catheter into place. The tube is inserted to the proper depth, and its open end connected to a sterile underwater seal. The tube is anchored in place with the purse-string suture, at least one additional stay suture of heavy material, and adhesive tape. Care msut be taken to ensure that under no circumstances will any material from the water seal bottle flow into the pleural space. Depending on the circumstances, the water seal may either be used alone or connected to constant low suction to help evacuate the pleural contents.

In older children, adolescents, and adults, the diagnosis of pneumothorax is usually fairly straightforward, and these patients usually have sufficient pulmonary reserve that confirmation of the diagnosis may be made radiographically before a tube thoracotomy is performed. The exception to this rule is of course the patient with a tension pneumothorax. If this diagnosis is suspected, a simple needle aspiration for diagnostic purposes may also be therapeutic.

In neonates with respiratory disease, especially respiratory distress syndrome, pulmonary status may suddenly deteriorate for a variety of reasons, and pneumothorax is often difficult to confirm by physical examination. In patients at high risk for pneumothorax, such as infants on mechanical ventilation, diagnostic/therapeutic thoracentesis must sometimes be performed without waiting for radiographic confirmation. In small infants, transillumination of the chest wall with a fiberoptic light source may provide rapid diagnosis of pneumothorax. When the light is held against the chest wall, the surrounding halo will be much larger in the presence of a pleural air collection than over a normally expanded lung.

PLEURAL BIOPSY

Biopsy of the pleura may be indicated for evaluation of chronic infectious processes (including tuberculosis) and to verify suspected pleural malignancy. A special pleural biopsy needle is inserted through the pleura in the same fashion as for a simple thoracentesis and advanced far enough beyond the pleura that the cutting edge of the needle (which points outward) will engage the pleura. The tip of the biopsy needle is usually somewhat blunt, so laceration of the lung is unlikely. The small amount of pleural tissue caught in the cutting edge of the needle is then cut off by advancing the blade through the needle; the process is usually repeated after rotating the needle to obtain three or four specimens before the needle is withdrawn.

THE LUNG PARENCHYMA

Lung Biopsy

When a diagnosis cannot be established by another technique, a lung biopsy often provides a definitive answer. Major indications for lung biopsy include diffuse diseases such as opportunistic infections, interstitial diseases, and pulmonary alveolar proteinosis. Persistent radiographic changes or suspected malignancies are also common indications for biopsy. Lung biopsy may be performed by either closed chest or open procedures, although in general open biopsies are preferable in children.

CLOSED BIOPSY TECHNIQUES

Percutaneous biopsy with a biopsy needle, although frequently performed on adults, is not recommended for children, as the technique has a relatively high incidence of morbidity and even an occasional mortality. Newer techniques have recently been developed in which the biopsy needle is placed under computerized tomographic guidance; it is not clear yet whether these techniques will be realistically applicable to children or how useful they will be. Another technique is a high-speed trephine drill biopsy, which, although successful in adults, is not recommended for pediatric patients. Transbronchial biopsy through a bronchoscope is an acceptable procedure for older pediatric patients, but should be performed with fluoroscopic guidance. Because of the small dimensions of the pediatric patient's lungs, great care must be taken during such procedures to avoid penetration of the pleura and even the abdominal organs by the biopsy forceps.

Closed biopsy techniques are more useful for diffuse disorders than for discrete lesions unless the lesions are located centrally and are thus readily accessible from the larger airways. Complications of closed biopsy techniques include bleeding and pneumothorax. The incidence of complications depends on the type of procedure performed, the nature of the disease process, the age of the patient, and the skill of the operator.

OPEN BIOPSY TECHNIQUES

Open lung biopsy is generally the method of choice for pediatric patients, especially those too young for a transbronchial biopsy with a flexible fiberoptic bronchoscope (pediatric flexible bronchoscopes do not allow use of biopsy forceps). It is also the method of choice when a large amount of lung tissue is needed. In skilled hands, open lung biopsy is a surprisingly benign procedure and can be completed in a few minutes through a very small intercostal incision. Because the duration of anesthesia is short and the amount of tissue taken is relatively small, the procedure can usually be tolerated by seriously ill patients and should not be delayed if a diagnosis is necessary for planning further therapy or for evaluating prognosis.

Percutaneous Lung Puncture

The diagnosis of infectious processes in the lung is often difficult without obtaining material directly from the pulmonary parenchyma. There is no known technique for obtaining specimens from the lung via the trachea without the risk of some contamination from oral or upper airway flora. Percutaneous lung puncture avoids this potential pitfall and may provide very useful diagnostic information. Using a technique very similar to that for thoracentesis, a 1½-in., 20- to 21-gauge short-bevel needle attached to a 10-ml syringe containing 1 ml of sterile saline is very rapidly inserted into the lung. The saline is immediately injected and aspirated, and the needle quickly withdrawn. The procedure usually gains a few drops of ''lung juice'' that may then be submitted for culture and cytologic examination. The lung puncture should be performed at the site indicated by the most involvement on the chest x-ray film, particularly in an area of consolidation, avoiding the heart and other organs. The incidence of pneumothorax following diagnostic percutaneous lung puncture ranges as high as 30% in some series, but the leak is usually small and inconsequential. In patients with decreased pulmonary compliance, pneumothorax may be more likely to occur and is more likely to require a chest tube.

Bronchopulmonary Lavage

Bronchopulmonary lavage is a technique used for the diagnosis and treatment of alveolar filling disorders such as pulmonary alveolar proteinosis and desquamative interstitial pneumonitis. Although lung biopsy is more likely to yield a definitive diagnosis in these conditions, small-volume lavage may be very helpful in diagnosis and in following the course of disease, and has a very low morbidity. Bronchopulmonary lavage is also used to some extent in therapy for extensive airways disease such as refractory status asthmaticus and cystic fibrosis. In the latter case, however, it is of somewhat dubious value because of the extensive parenchymal and airway damage associated with chronic infection.

Several techniques are used for bronchopulmonary lavage. For diagnostic purposes, a flexible bronchoscope is used, and small volumes of saline (50 to 150 ml total) are instilled into and aspirated from a segmental bronchus. In pediatric patients, of course, the volumes are reduced proportionately. The composition of the aspirated lavage fluid depends to a significant extent on the volume of fluid used for the lavage and on the number of washes. For cytologic diagnostic purposes, especially in the evaluation of inflammatory and fibrotic lung diseases, care must be taken to standardize the technique.

Therapeutic lavage usually involves large volumes of saline and requires endotracheal intubation. In adults, a double-lumen tube (Carlens tube or equivalent) is used to ventilate one lung while the other lung is lavaged. The lung is completely filled with saline and may be lavaged with many liters of fluid. Several days later, the other lung may then be lavaged in a similar fashion. In patients too small for a double-lumen tube (the smallest available tube is approximately 11 mm in diameter), a variety of other techniques have been used. A single-lumen endotracheal tube may be used to lavage *both* lungs simultaneously while the patient is maintained on partial cardiopulmonary bypass oxygenation (using the femoral vessels). Alternatively, the patient may be positioned so that one lung is dependent, and saline may be allowed to flow down the endotracheal tube at such a rate that ventilation of the other lung may be maintained. While this technique is reportedly successful, it clearly has many potential problems. In older children, various techniques for regional lavage used a cuffed endotracheal catheter or flexible bronchoscope positioned for lavage of an isolated lobe or segment (or even an entire lung) while the patient maintains spontaneous ventilation.

MISCELLANEOUS TECHNIQUES

Arterial Puncture and Arterial Catheterization

Arterial blood for measurement of blood gases is best obtained by direct arterial puncture. Arterialized capillary blood may be used, but it is subject to error if peripheral perfusion is not well maintained. In the intensive care of seriously ill patients, repeated sampling of arterial blood gases is facilitated by the placement of an indwelling arterial catheter. Furthermore, this also allows continuous direct monitoring of arterial blood pressure by a suitable pressure transducer.

The sites most commonly used for arterial sampling, in order of frequency, are the radial, brachial, temporal, dorsalis pedis, and femoral arteries. The femoral artery is frequently used in adults but should be used only with great caution in children since the complication rate is relatively high. Thrombosis with distal tissue loss and necrosis of the femoral head are well-known complications of femoral artery puncture in children. In most cases the radial or brachial artery will be satisfactory for diagnostic punctures. When using the radial artery, one should always check for collateral circulation in the ulnar artery prior to the procedure.

Under most circumstances the arterial pulse may be located with the first two fingers and the course of the vessel carefully defined. In neonates, the pulse may be difficult to palpate, and transillumination of the wrist with a cold light source is often helpful in identifying the course of the artery.

Many physicians use local anesthesia for arterial puncture to reduce the discomfort to the patient and reduce vasospasm and increase the chance of success of the procedure. A skin bleb is made directly over the intended puncture site with a 25- or 27-gauge needle, and a small skin bleb is raised with 1% lidocaine. The needle is then passed deeper, and approximately 0.5 ml of lidocaine is instilled *alongside* (not into) the artery. This will result in temporary loss of the anatomic landmarks, but massage of the site will not only help restore landmarks, but also spread the anesthetic agent.

Pain and/or the anticipation of pain during arterial puncture usually result in some degree of hyperventilation and consequently a lower P_{CO_2} than would be obtained under completely baseline conditions. Every effort should therefore be made to keep the patient as comfortable and as calm as possible during the procedure (this is also another advantage of the indwelling arterial catheter, in that samples can be taken without any discomfort to the patient). Effective hypnoanalgesia can often be achieved, particularly in children, by simply distracting their attention, or in older children, by actively suggesting that they turn off the sensations from the area involved. Effective surface anesthesia may be obtained for the initial needle prick (to inject local anesthetic) if the skin is stretched very tightly.

When the vessel is located, the overlying skin has been cleansed, and the local anesthetic has been injected, the skin is then entered at approximately a 45-degree angle, using a short-bevel needle, 20 to 22 gauge. The use of a 25- or 26-gauge needle may obviate the need for local anesthesia, but it is more difficult to be certain that the needle is actually in an artery. In infants it is often most convenient to use a scalp vein set, but in older patients a glass syringe previously moistened with heparin solution may be more convenient. The needle is advanced and guided by tactile sensation from the fingers of both hands until the artery is entered and blood flows freely through the needle. It may be necessary in some patients to pass the needle entirely through the artery and obtain blood flow on slow withdrawal of the needle. The site of the arterial puncture must be firmly compressed for at least 5 minutes after the procedure in order to ensure adequate hemostasis.

Care must be taken not to allow air to enter the syringe containing the arterial blood sample, and the syringe should be immediately sealed and transported on ice to the laboratory. The volume of heparin solution in the syringe should be kept to a minimum, since dilution of the blood will result in erroneously low P_{CO_2} and erroneously high pH.

Placement of an intra-arterial catheter is slightly more difficult but can be achieved easily using a plastic catheter placement set. In this case the artery is entered at a more shallow angle, so that the shaft of the needle/catheter is more nearly parallel to the course of the artery. When blood return is noted, the catheter is advanced over the needle and into the artery. Blood return is then impeded by pressure on the artery above the tip of the catheter, and tubing containing heparinized saline is connected. Great care must be taken to avoid the possibility of introducing air into the system, to ensure that there is no possibility of leakage from the catheter and tubing connections, as exsanguination can easily occur. The catheter should be securely taped into position so that no tension on the tubing will dislodge it. Patients with arterial catheters require constant attention and will usually be in an intensive care unit. The patency of the catheter is maintained by constant infusion (at a very low flow rate) of heparinized saline. A variety of continuous flush valves are currently available for such purposes.

It may be difficult or impossible to perform transcutaneous catheterization of a peripheral artery, especially in very small infants (or in patients with poor perfusion). In these cases, the artery may be exposed through a small incision much as for a venous cutdown and then cannulated directly with relative ease. Obviously no ligatures should be placed around the vessel.

The complication rate with indwelling arterial cannulas increases with increasing length of placement. However, in most cases catheters may remain in place 24 to 48 hours with relatively few problems.

Umbilical Arterial Catheterization

The umbilical artery can usually be cannulated during the first week or two of life; this is a most convenient way of sampling multiple blood gases during the intensive care of neonatal disorders. The umbilical stump should be cleaned with a surgical preparation and then cut approximately 1 cm from the abdominal wall. One of the arteries is located and gently grasped with a small, toothed forceps, being careful not to tear the tissue. The lumen of the artery is located with a spreader or a small metal probe and the orifice gently dilated. A 3.5 or 5 French umbilical artery catheter previously filled with heparinized saline is then threaded into the arterial orifice. Some resistance may be met at or just below the abdominal wall, which will usually yield with continued gentle pressure. Occasionally a dilator must be passed, but great care must be taken not to perforate the arterial wall or to create a false tract. When the catheter has been passed far enough so that good arterial blood return is obtained, a purse-string suture is placed around the umbilical stump, and the catheter is secured. The position of the catheter tip is verified by x-ray film and modified as necessary. The most desirable location is just below the aortic bifurcation, although some physicians prefer to place the tip behind the heart shadow. Under no circumstances should the tip of the catheter be left adjacent to the celiac, mesenteric, or renal arteries.

Occasionally great difficulty may be experienced in passing an arterial catheter; novices should be instructed to confine their attempts to only one of the two arteries, so that if they fail, the other vessel is not damaged. In the unusual event that neither artery can be cannulated, a small incision can be made in the abdominal wall just below the umbilical stump. The vessel can be located at that point and cannulated under direct vision. The most common problems associated with umbilical arterial cannulation are selecting the umbilical vein instead of the artery, producing a false tract or perforation of the arterial wall and cannulating a patent urachus.

Ear Oximetry

Recent developments in electronics and fiberoptic technology have made possible a very accurate and useful ear oximeter for the noninvasive measurement of arterial oxygen saturation. This device may be used for spot checking or for continuous monitoring. The principle of ear oximetry involves the spectral analysis of light transmitted through the pinna. Currently available instruments automatically make corrections for skin color and check for sufficient light transmission to ensure adequate regional blood flow for an accurate reading. The blood flow to the ear must be stimulated by either vigorous rubbing or application of a topical vasodilator prior to making a reading. The earpiece of the oximeter is heated to maintain high blood flow. Under normal conditions the oxygen saturation reading obtained by ear oximetry is within 1 to 2% of that calculated from direct arterial puncture. This technique promises to be more useful in the future as instruments designed for pediatric use appear on the market.

Analysis of Expired Gases

Another noninvasive technique that may be used to estimate arterial blood gases is the measurement of end-tidal P_{CO_2}. A CO_2 meter with a sufficiently rapid response time may be used to monitor P_{CO_2}. CO_2 in the expired air, which will approach zero during inspiration and rise rapidly during exhalation to reach a plateau. The plateau value represents mixed alveolar gas, and is an accurate reflection of arterial P_{CO_2}. If there is uneven distribution of ventilation or if the respiratory rate is very rapid, a satisfactory plateau cannot be demonstrated, and this technique becomes much less reliable.

Pulmonary Function and Exercise Testing

CARL F. DOERSHUK, M.D.
DAVID M. ORENSTEIN, M.D.

9

PULMONARY function and exercise testing differs in children and in adults largely because volume changes occur from birth through the period of growth to adulthood, as indicated in Figure 9–1. These differences influence technique, methodology, and interpretation.[12] The pathophysiologic basis for pulmonary function testing has been described.[1, 3, 11, 32] This chapter will provide information primarily relevant to clinical testing.

At any age, the function of the respiratory system, which includes the conducting airways as well as the portions of the lung in which gas exchange occurs, is to provide for oxygenation of the blood and removal of carbon dioxide. A complex neurologic and chemical control system maintains physiologic balance. In addition, the physical characteristics of the respiratory system contribute to the final levels of oxygen and carbon dioxide in the arterial blood that result from breathing.

These physical characteristics can be summarized as follows. Inspired air is warmed and humidified in the nasal airways, trachea, and major bronchi. This conditioned gas then is delivered by the smaller bronchi, bronchioles, and terminal bronchioles to the gas exchange portions of the lung including the respiratory bronchioles, alveolar ducts, alveolar sacs, and alveoli. It is the gas in these spaces that is actively engaged in exchanging oxygen and carbon dioxide across the alveolar membrane. The pulmonary artery distributes blood through its branches, the pulmonary arterioles, to the pulmonary capillaries surrounding the alveoli. As the blood passes along the capillaries, it takes up oxygen from the alveoli and releases carbon dioxide to them. Gas transfer is so rapid that equilibrium between alveolar and capillary gas is nearly complete, even during exercise when the rate of blood flow through the capillaries is greatly increased.

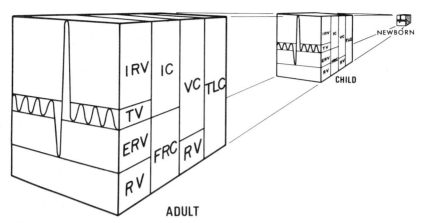

Fig 9–1.—Volume growth of the lung from birth. The tremendous changes that occur with growth must be appreciated in order for the principles of testing and respiratory care developed for the adult to be applied successfully to the child or the infant.

VENTILATION AND PERFUSION OF THE LUNG

The volume of the conducting airways is called the *anatomic dead space* because the gas in this space does not contribute to gas exchange. For example, a 70-kg adult might have a resting tidal volume of 500 ml and a dead space volume of 150 ml (the dead space has a volume of roughly 2 ml/kg body weight). The dead space makes up a relatively large portion of each breath. The remaining 350 ml of inspired air (the alveolar volume) enters the gas exchange portion of the lungs. Each tidal volume is relatively small in proportion to the resting end-expiratory volume of the lungs, the functional residual capacity (FRC), which is about 2,500 ml in the average adult.

The minute volume is the total volume of gas entering through the nose and/ or mouth per minute; for example, tidal volume (500 ml) × breaths/minute (14) = minute volume (7,000 ml/minute). However, the effective alveolar ventilation is reduced by the volume of the anatomic dead space during each breath. Therefore, 500 − 150 = 350 ml × 14 = 4,900 ml/minute is the volume of the resting alveolar ventilation. The corresponding amount of blood delivered to the pulmonary capillaries (cardiac output) would be about 6,000 ml/minute.

Normal Blood Gases

The inspired air at sea level (760 mm Hg) contains almost no carbon dioxide (0.3 mm Hg), its Po_2 is about 160 mm Hg, and it has little water content since the relative atmospheric humidity is usually considerably lower than 100%. The remainder of the pressure (Fig 9–2) is made up almost entirely of nitrogen.

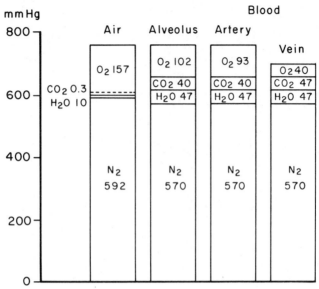

Fig 9–2.—Partial pressures of gas in air and blood at sea level (barometric pressure = 760 mm Hg).

Normal ventilation at sea level results in arterial blood having a partial pressure of oxygen (PaO_2) of 90 to 100 mm Hg and a partial pressure of carbon dioxide ($PaCO_2$) of 37 to 42 mm Hg in normal subjects. Water vapor (47 mm Hg) and nitrogen (about 570 mm Hg) contribute the remaining partial pressure up to 760 mm Hg at sea level in the alveolus.

The large, normally observed difference between the PO_2 of the inspired air and that of the arterial blood is largely a result of diffusion, direct shunt, and ventilation-perfusion imbalance. Diffusion is dependent upon the area and, to some extent, the thickness of the alveolar capillary membrane available for effective gas exchange; it is also dependent on the period of time available for diffusion to occur. The direct shunt of poorly oxygenated venous blood into the arterial blood bypassing the lungs accounts for about a 5 mm Hg PO_2 difference between air and arterial blood. The shunted blood includes venous blood from the heart muscle draining into the left side of the heart, some bronchial venous blood draining into the pulmonary veins, and perhaps some blood from a few normally occurring direct connections between pulmonary arteries and veins in the lungs. The other factor resulting in differences between the PO_2 of the inspired air and that of the arterial blood is the relative imbalance of delivered ventilation to the lung relative to the perfusion of blood through the lung. Both ventilation and blood flow increase in progressive levels from the apex of the upright lung to the base. However, since the blood flow increases at a more rapid rate, high ventilation/perfusion ratios are found in the apical regions, the lower ratios are found at the bases of the lungs, with a mean

ratio of about 0.80. Areas of relatively low ventilation and high perfusion be-
have like shunts, with little oxygen being added to the blood as it passes
through the lungs. In the normal adult, the ventilation-perfusion ratio is repre-
sented by approximately 5 liters/min of alveolar ventilation and 6 liter/min of
total pulmonary blood flow.

Hypoxemia

Diffusion gradient, shunt, and ventilation-perfusion ($\dot{V}/\dot{Q}$) ratio inequality are
normally present in the healthy lung; thus, the arterial Po_2 is less than that of
the inspired air and somewhat less than that of the mean alveolar gas. Exag-
geration of these factors in disease states contributes to arterial Po_2 values
much lower than 90 mm Hg. However, the most important and most common
cause of abnormally lowered PaO_2 (hypoxemia) encountered clinically is further regional imbalance in the distribution of ventilation and perfusion. The
overall effect is to lower the mean $\dot{V}/\dot{Q}$ ratio and thus increase the physiologic
shunt. In the frequently encountered clinical conditions (such as bronchitis,
asthma, bronchiolitis and cystic fibrosis) characterized by severe $\dot{V}/\dot{Q}$ inequal-
ities, the $PaCO_2$ remains normal or even somewhat low until overall alveolar
hypoventilation and CO_2 retention (i.e., respiratory failure) develop.

   Any sudden failure to remove sufficient carbon dioxide from the alveoli and
thus from the blood results in a shift of the $HCO_2{}^-/CO_2$ balance, lowering the
blood pH. When arterial pH levels of less than 7.3 are reached in the presence
of a normal or increased $PaCO_2$, respiratory acidosis is said to be present.
Acute severe CO_2 retention may result in arterial pH levels of 7.10 or less.
However, chronic CO_2 retention can be compensated for by hydrogen excretion
and retention can be compensated for by hydrogen excretion and retention of
bicarbonate by healthy kidneys, so that the pH may be normal or nearly normal
even in the presence of elevated $PaCO_2$ and $HCO_3{}^-$ levels (compensated respiratory acidosis).

   Arterial hypoxemia also can result from general hypoventilation caused by
decreased ventilatory drive (with or without general depression of the central
nervous system, fatigue, or paralysis of the ventilatory muscles,[5, 36] etc.) in the
presence of normal lungs, so that the decrease in PaO_2 is accompanied by an
almost equal increase in $PaCO_2$. The blood gas measurement alone will not
differentiate among the causes of a decreased PaO_2. When general hypoventilation is the cause of a decrease in PaO_2 and an increase in $PaCO_2$, it is apparent that oxygen alone will not correct the condition totally and that ventilatory
assistance is also mandatory to aid in CO_2 removal and correct the blood pH
until the patient has recovered sufficiently to resume adequate alveolar ventilation.

   In a controlled study of 102 patients with cystic fibrosis, the arterial PaO_2
value was found to correlate very well with other parameters of pulmonary
function (such as the vital capacity [VC], forced expiratory volume [FEV] in 1
second, residual volume [RV] to total lung capacity [TLC] ratio, and conduct-

ance) and with the chest x-ray film (Table 9–1). As noted, the $PaCO_2$ remains normal or even a little low until overall alveolar hypoventilation develops.

TABLE 9–1.—MEAN PULMONARY FUNCTION TEST, CHEST ROENTGENOGRAM AND $PaCO_2$
RESULTS GROUPED BY PaO_2 FOR 102 PATIENTS WITH CYSTIC FIBROSIS

PaO_2, mm Hg	90–111*	83–89	76–82	70–75	60–69	50–59
Number of patients	22	21	21	19	11	8
Vital capacity, % predicted	103%	97%	90%	78%	73%	53%
$FEV_{1.0}$†	74%	70%	68%	60%	56%	49%
Conductance,‡ predicted	102%	85%	77%	69%	41%	36%
RV/TLC ratio§	0.27	0.28	0.32	0.41	0.52	0.63
Chest x-ray	Near normal	Slightly abnormal	Moderately abnormal		Markedly abnormal	
$PaCO_2$, mm Hg	36	35	36	34	33	37

*The results in this column are all within normal limits.
†$FEV_{1.0}$, forced expiratory volume in first second expressed as a percentage of the forced vital capacity.
‡Conductance, the reciprocal of airway resistance.
§RV/TLC ratio, residual volume to total lung capacity ratio.

PULMONARY FUNCTION TESTING

There are many different pulmonary function tests and many considerations in carrying out the tests. The tests especially applicable to children will be given the most consideration, and important differences from testing in adults will be included.

It is readily apparent that a variety of pulmonary function parameters are assessed even when spirometry alone is used (Figure 9–3). Spirometry allows assessment of the vital capacity (VC) and its subdivisions, the expiratory reserve volume (ERV) and the inspiratory capacity (IC), along with tidal volume, minute volume and the flow rates, including the FEV in 1 and 3 seconds, maximal expiratory flow rate, and maximal midexpiratory flow. Figure 9–3 shows an idealized tracing from a spirometer and defines the lung volumes and capacities.

PULMONARY FUNCTION TEST DEFINITIONS

A. *Volumes:* There are three primary volumes that do not overlap.

1. *Tidal Volume,* or the depth of breathing, is the volume of gas inspired or expired during each respiratory cycle.

2. *Expiratory Reserve Volume* is the maximal volume of gas that can be expired from the end expiratory level.

3. *Residual Volume* is the volume of gas remaining in the lungs at the end of a maximal expiration.

B. *Capacities:* There are four capacities, each including two or more of the primary volumes.

1. *Total Lung Capacity* is the amount of gas contained in the lung at the end of a maximal inspiration.

2. *Vital Capacity* is the maximal volume of gas that can be expelled from the lungs by forceful effort following a maximal inspiration.
3. *Inspiratory Capacity* is the maximal volume of gas that can be inspired from the resting expiratory level.
4. *Functional Residual Capacity* is the volume of gas remaining in the lungs at the resting expiratory level.

More information about other aspects of lung function becomes available when the FRC is determined by helium, nitrogen, or plethysmographic techniques, and the RV and TLC then calculated. Further data can be obtained when more difficult techniques are used for the measurement of airway resistance, lung compliance, maximal expiratory flow volume curves, closing volume, and diffusion capacity. Procedural details about testing and other information are available.[8, 29, 34, 35] In the remainder of this chapter, it is assumed that the reader already has a basic knowledge of pulmonary function testing.

No single test completely describes the adequacy of pulmonary function in a given patient. In addition, pulmonary function tests do not provide a diagnosis or an etiology except perhaps when there is improvement after the use of a bronchodilator aerosol, suggesting reversible bronchospasm or a decrease in flow rate after exercise or inhaled bronchoprovocation, also suggesting asthma. The tests do distinguish between two major types of disturbances of lung function: the obstructive type and the restrictive type. However, in many patients both types of abnormality may coexist, and the extent of each cannot be determined readily.

Pulmonary function tests are useful in establishing a baseline of information for a patient, and subsequent tests are then useful in quantifying progression of the disease or response to therapy. Testing is especially useful preoperatively in detecting patients with an unsuspected limitation who should have special attention both before and especially after surgery to prevent or minimize res-

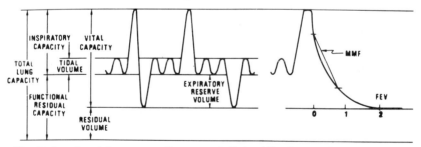

Fig 9–3.—Semidiagrammatic presentation of the lung volumes and a single forced vital capacity. *MMF,* maximal midexpiratory flow rate; i.e., mean flow rate calculated over midportion of forced expiratory curve. *FEV,* forced expiratory volume in a given time, i.e., as 1 second and can be expressed as a percentage of the vital capacity. Maximal expiratory flow rate (liters/min) is abbreviated MEFR. MEFR$_{200-1,200}$, for example, is the flow rate achieved during forced expiration for the liter of expired gas after the first 200 ml have been exhaled.

piratory complications. Pulmonary function tests are also useful in better defining the physiology of respiration and increasing our understanding of altered function, as shown for cystic fibrosis in Figure 9–4.

PREPARATION FOR TESTING

In performing spirometry and other pulmonary testing in children, especially those between 5 and 8 years of age, it is important to explain the test procedure[7] and how the equipment works in order to obtain results that reflect the child's lung function accurately. The child should have an opportunity to turn the equipment on and off and otherwise operate it as well as practice with the mouthpiece and nose clips before trying a test.

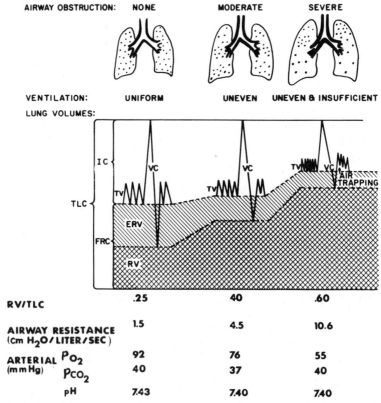

Fig 9–4.—Progression of pulmonary function changes in patients with cystic fibrosis. The rise in *FRC* and the decrease in *ERV* are due to the obstructive disease process that results in an even greater rise in *RV*. The vital capacity and $FEV_{1.0}$/FEV may be reduced to as little as 25 to 30% or less, while the *RV/TLC* ratio may rise to 0.70 to 0.75 or greater in the more severe cases. Although the arterial P_{O_2} decreases quickly when there is uneven ventilation, the P_{CO_2} remains at or below normal levels until the pulmonary disease is far advanced (Table 9–1). (From Matthews, L.W., and Doershuk, C.F.: Measurement of pulmonary function in cystic fibrosis, Mod. Probl. Pediatr. 10:237, 1967.)

Discussion and demonstration of what is meant by the various commands such as "take a deep breath," "blow all the way out," "pant," "breathe naturally," and "hold your breath" are necessary for good testing. The instructions should relate to things the child is accustomed to doing, such as, "blow out as you do the candles on your birthday cake." The best technician will be friendly and understanding as well as firm and somewhat demanding, since good studies require the patient's best effort and do not come with kindness alone. Technicians who get good results frequently "blow out all the way" right along with the child. Some element of competition can be helpful in obtaining a good effort. Praise for a good effort helps ensure a pleasant memory and continued cooperation during future testing. No child should be forced to complete a test that is going poorly. If the technician is calm and unhurried and is able to accept comfortably the occasional bad test, the child usually can accept returning later for another try.

LUNG VOLUMES

Considerable information about pulmonary function can be gained from the history and physical examination, but various testing instruments are used for quantitative measurements. Most commonly these instruments include the spirometer, the pneumotachometer (electronic spirometer), the total body plethysmograph and various gas analyzers. The lung volumes measured are shown schematically and defined in Figure 9–3. The maximal midexpiratory flow rate (MMF) is more frequently called the mean forced expiratory flow (FEF) and is measured during the middle half of the forced vital capacity ($FEF_{25-75\%}$).

Lung volumes are affected by changes in the patient's position. When the subject is supine, the diaphragm shifts upward so that the inspiratory capacity is increased and the functional residual capacity and expiratory reserve volume are decreased. With the patient in the upright position, changes in the opposite direction occur. Diseases of the thoracic cage, neuromuscular and cardiovascular systems, pleura and airways, as well as the lungs may also affect lung volumes.

Lung volumes increase with body growth. In the normal individual they can best be related to body size, particularly to length in the infant and young child when studied supine and to height in older subjects studied in the sitting position. This relationship remains relatively constant from birth through young adulthood. Other factors that correlate with lung volume include sex, age, race, weight and perhaps socioeconomic factors, so a relatively wide range of normal is encountered. An additional variable in these measurements is that repeat test results can vary by as much as 5%.

The vital capacity is normally about three quarters of the total lung capacity and is made up of the inspiratory capacity (⅔) and the expiratory reserve volume (⅓). After a maximal exhalation (the vital capacity), the remaining gas in the lungs is the residual volume (approximately one quarter of the total lung capacity). This portion increases somewhat with the age of the subject. The ratio of residual volume to total lung capacity is frequently calculated since the lung volumes have a wide range of normal. This ratio is usually about 0.25. Some investigators also report ratios of functional residual capacity and the vital capacity to total lung capacity.

SPIROMETRY

Spirometers have been used for over 100 years to measure the volume characteristics of the lungs, and they continue to be in common use. Minimal spirometry standards have been established at a Workshop on Standardization of Spirometry[17] and a conference on Standardization of Lung Function Testing in Children.[9] As concluded by the workshop, diagnostic spirometry requires a graphic recording (tracing) of either volume-time or volume-flow during the entire forced expiration. Spirograms still represent the best method of ensuring that this effort-dependent test is properly performed.

Water-Sealed Spirometers

One of the most commonly used spirometers is the water-sealed type (Fig 9–5). The 9-liter bell capacity can be used effectively in testing patients from about 5 years of age through adolescence. The 13.5-liter bell capacity is more appropriate for adult work. This type of spirometer is ideal for any laboratory doing more than screening examinations. It meets the requirements for a relatively large, permanent record and allows for accurate temperature correction of the gas volume. The expiratory reserve volume and inspiratory capacity can be determined accurately from a well-performed test.

In testing, the subject should be positioned comfortably, seated or standing, and allowed to adjust to the nose clips, mouthpiece and equipment during a few minutes of tidal breathing. The paper is run at slow speed. Several VC and at least one separate ERV measurements should be obtained and interspersed

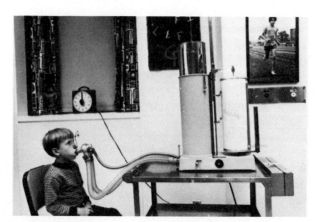

Fig 9–5.—Collins 9-liter spirometer with recording kymograph. This water-sealed spirometer is counterbalanced, ideal for work with children and relatively inexpensive.

with periods of tidal breathing so that a baseline can be established. The paper then is run at a faster speed and several forced expiratory efforts are obtained for determination of the various flow parameters. The temperature in the spirometer is recorded so that the measured volumes can be corrected to body temperature.

Electronic Spirometers

Although the water-sealed spirometer provides a basic unit to which other equipment can be added for the determination of lung volume by the helium or nitrogen method, more recently an increasing number of electronic spirometers are appearing with flowmeters and sophisticated electronic memory equipment. On a single forced exhalation, the forced VC and many aspects of the flow rates can be obtained and either displayed digitally or printed out rapidly. However, there are significant limitations.

An assessment of the problems associated with electronic spirometers contains the recommendation that each laboratory must ensure accurate performance of the device before accepting patient test results.[16, 17] It is important that the laboratory also recalibrate the equipment regularly. The electronic spirometers are limited in that they do not allow division of the vital capacity into the ERV and IC fractions. This means that RV and TLC cannot be calculated even if an FRC reading is available.

Although the Workshop on Standardization of Spirometry recommends that diagnostic spirometry require a graphic recording, the electronic spirometers usually do not provide this capability.[16, 17] The recording is important for the permanent record and it also permits a later inspection to verify that the test was performed properly.

When using most of the electronic equipment, the subject must learn to breathe deeply and then place the lips around the mouthpiece before exhaling. Children frequently have difficulty with this maneuver. When many subjects are to be screened, the electronic units can be useful. However, for diagnostic testing, a permanent record is recommended.[16, 17] In our experience with these units, great variability in testing of children can occur unless considerable care is taken.

DETERMINATION OF FUNCTIONAL RESIDUAL CAPACITY

There are three major methods of determination of FRC, which is the volume of gas remaining in the lung at the end of tidal exhalation. Two of these methods use helium or nitrogen. The other method involves use of a total body plethysmograph. The direct measurement of FRC is preferred to that of RV, since the FRC value is more readily reproducible and represents a more steady-state lung volume than does the RV measurement.

The FRC is added to the inspiratory capacity (IC) to calculate total lung capacity (TLC), i.e., FRC + IC = TLC. Residual volume (RV) is calculated by subtraction of the expiratory reserve volume (ERV) from the FRC, i.e.,

FRC − ERV = RV. The normal values of Helliesen et al.[23] verified in our laboratory, are shown in Tables 10–2 and 10–3 in the next chapter.

The Gas Methods

In the *closed-circuit helium dilution method,* the relatively insoluble helium gas is used. Only the volume of gas in communication with the major airways is measured. A known volume of helium is added to the system, and its concentration (percentage) is measured. The patient's FRC represents the unknown volume and is connected to the helium system at the end of a resting tidal breath. When mixing is complete, the volume of helium is unchanged, the final concentration of helium is read and the volume of gas in the lung can be calculated. In the normal lung, complete mixing and equilibration usually occur within 2 to 3 minutes. However, in patients with severe obstructive disease, equilibration may not occur even after 15 minutes, and the true FRC will be underestimated. The patient must sit quietly erect with nose clips in place and the lips firmly around the mouthpiece for the duration of the test. Any loss of gas from the system will result in a falsely elevated FRC. Duplicate studies should have less than ±5% variation. Children tolerate this test well, and they will return readily for repeat testing.

In the *open-circuit nitrogen washout method,* nitrogen serves as the inert gas. Again, only the air in communication with the major airways is measured. At the end of a resting tidal exhalation, the subject begins to breath 100% oxygen (nitrogen free), and all of the exhaled gases are collected over a 7-minute period, the usual maximal period for which this test is run. The volume of exhaled gas and its concentration of nitrogen are measured and the volume of nitrogen calculated. Since this nitrogen came from the lung, where it existed at an 80% concentration, the FRC is easily calculated. In the normal child, the nitrogen is washed out within a few minutes; however, in patients with severe obstructive pulmonary disease, the nitrogen washout method also will tend to cause underestimation of the FRC, just as the helium method does, because both measure only the gas communicating with the major airways.

An index of the evenness of the distribution of inspired gas can be obtained from the nitrogen method by having the subject exhale forcefully and fully at the end of the 7-minute test to deliver an alveolar sample. If distribution of inspired gas is normal, this gas sample will contain less than 2.5% nitrogen. As with the helium testing, the subject must sit quietly erect with pursed lips, wearing nose clips throughout the test. Any loss of gas from the system will result in a falsely decreased FRC. Children tolerate this test well, and adequate repeat studies yield about ±5% variation.

Total Body Plethysmograph Method

Measurement of thoracic gas volume (VTG) indicates that the plethysmographic method has been used to determine lung volume. This method measures the volume of gas in the thorax whether or not it is in free communication with the airways. This means that the gas in a lung cyst or in a pneumothorax will be included in the measurement of VTG.

The pressure plethysmograph (Fig 9–6) is an airtight box in which the patient is seated and breathes through a heated flowmeter. If the VTG at FRC is desired, the airway is occluded at the end of a tidal exhalation by a shutter at the mouth, and the patient continues to make breathing efforts. Pressure changes in the box reflecting thoracic volume changes, and at the mouth reflecting alveolar pressure changes, are monitored. The changing pressure-volume relationships are described by Boyle's law $(PV = P'V')$ if temperature remains constant. The original pressure (barometric), new pressure, and change in volume are recorded from the pattern observed on the oscilloscope screen. After appropriate calibrations are made, the equation can be solved for the initial volume (VTG), in this example corresponding to FRC. This method is rapid, and repeat determinations can be made in a few minutes once the patient has had a good introduction to breathing against the closed shutter. In patients with obstructive lung disease, a much more accurate measure of the FRC and thus of the TLC is obtained with the plethysmograph method than with either the nitrogen or helium methods. In a patient with obstructive pulmonary disease, the difference in lung volumes are measured by these different methods may provide a quantitation of the volume of trapped gas.[4] Hence, VTG $-$ FRC$_{\text{He}}$ $_{\text{or N2}}$ = volume of trapped gas. In normal children, the difference in volumes between the methods is negligible and within the limits of the testing procedures (see Tables 10–2 and 10–3).

Children aged 7 years or older quickly understand the test procedure; however, extra care must be exercised with younger children so that a true, resting end-tidal expiration is achieved before the shutter is closed. If a rest period is

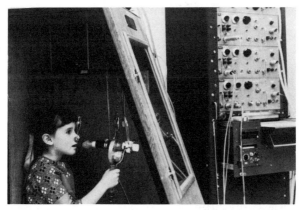

Fig 9–6.—The total body plethysmograph with its recorder. An oscilloscope is also used. This method provides a rapid means of measuring lung volumes and also of determining airway resistance at measured lung volumes. This equipment was assembled in our laboratory to meet our needs; more recently, complete units have become available commercially.

required during the plethysmograph test, the child can remove and later replace the nose clips and the mouthpiece while remaining in the box without interfering with the final results. The testing can be resumed when the child is ready.

Even for the patient with advanced obstructive pulmonary disease, this method is rapid, reproducible and relatively simple. The equipment is more expensive, and a skilled technician is required. If this test is performed daily, the savings in time to the laboratory and to the patient make use of such a unit reasonable.

Most plethysmographs are of the pressure recording type described by DuBois and co-workers;[13] however, occasionally a volume displacement unit is used. The plethysmograph method has been adapted successfully to the study of infants and young children as well. Measurements in these age groups however are substantially more difficult and are very appropriate for a research pediatric pulmonary laboratory. The steady increase in FRC that occurs with increasing body length/height is shown in Figure 9–7.

Maximal Voluntary Ventilation

Measurement of the maximal voluntary ventilation gives the maximal volume of gas that can be exhaled per minute with voluntarily forced breaths while at rest. Maximal voluntary ventilation is determined by a 12- or 15-second effort normalized in liters per minute, with the subject encouraged to breathe as deeply and rapidly as possible. The gas is measured using a spirometer, a collecting bag, or a gas-meter. The results of this test depend strongly upon muscle strength, the compliance of the lung and chest wall, and the motivation of the patient, as well as airway patency, and thus do not provide as direct a reflection of lung function as most of the other tests do.

VENTILATION AND PERFUSION

Several tests are available to assess the distribution of ventilation and perfusion (blood flow) within the lung. Radioactive xenon gas (xenon-133) can be inhaled and its regional distribution into the alveoli determined by counters or a radiation camera. There is greater ventilation per unit volume near the bottom of the lungs than near the top.

Blood flow distribution to the lung can likewise be determined by radiation cameras after a saline solution of xenon-133 is injected into a vein. Since xenon is poorly soluble it evolves into a gas in the lungs and is cleared by ventilation. Further radiation counting over the lungs can therefore also give a measure of xenon clearance, which varies with varying ventilation-perfusion ratios.

Distribution of Ventilation

The single-breath oxygen test and the 7-minute nitrogen test are the two most commonly used measurements of the distribution of ventilation. In the *single-breath oxygen test* (also called the single-breath nitrogen test) the subject in-

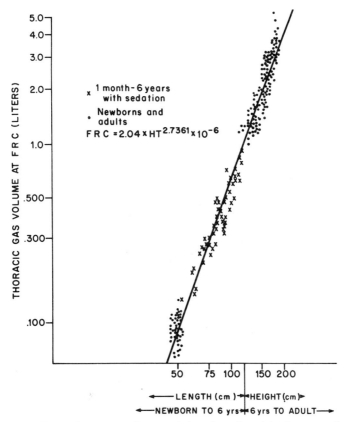

Fig 9–7.—Thoracic gas volume at functional residual capacity versus length/height. The close correlation of the results for functional residual capacity determined by the total body plethysmograph method on newborns, young children to age 6 years, and older children and adults plotted against body length (to age 6 years) or height (beyond 6 years) is shown in this double-log graph. (From Matthews, L.W., and Doershuk, C.F.: Measurement of pulmonary function in cystic fibrosis, Mod. Probl. Pediatr. 10:237, 1967.)

hales a full breath of 100% oxygen and then exhales completely while the nitrogen concentration is monitored at the mouth and the exhaled volume recorded (Fig 9–8). In the normal subject, the percent nitrogen expired will quickly rise to a level that increases only slightly during the remainder of the exhalation. This relative plateau is often called Phase III.

In practice, the percent change in nitrogen concentration that occurs between an expired volume of 750 to 1,250 ml is measured and should not exceed 2%. An increase in nitrogen concentration greater than 2% more than this lung volume suggests there are lung units present that fill and empty asynchronously, resulting in an abnormal distribution of ventilation. The technical procedures used in this test can significantly alter the results. This includes use of

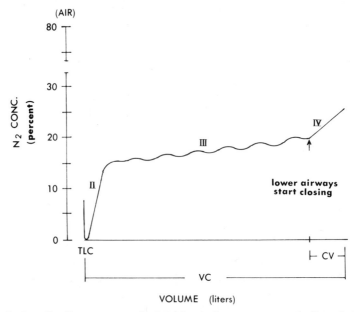

Fig 9–8.—Continuous record of expired nitrogen concentration during exhalation after a full-breath inhalation of oxygen. The slope of Phase III is seen, as well as the onset of Phase IV. Discussion of the breathing maneuver and of Phases III and IV is found in the sections on distribution of ventilation and closing volume.

a controlled, full inspiration and a relatively slow, even and complete exhalation to residual volume. The functional residual capacity is the preferred measurement for the starting point, and there should be minimal delay from full inspiration to the start of exhalation. A well-described study with the appropriate procedural details has been reported.[28]

Although special equipment must be used and the circumstances of the measured breath must be carefully controlled, this simple and useful test is quickly performed and calculated. In adults, increasing attention is being centered on the Phase III portion and Phase IV or closing volume. The volume from the onset of Phase IV to the end of the full exhalation at residual volume has been recognized as having further information of interest (see the later section on closing volume). The single-breath oxygen test has not yet been fully appreciated in pediatric pulmonary research, in part since young children have not yet achieved a vital capacity of 1,250 ml and older children with pulmonary disease may incur a loss of vital capacity to less than 1,250 ml.

The *7-minute nitrogen washout test* is a multibreath test in which the subject breathes 100% oxygen at resting, normal tidal volumes for 7 minutes. The reduction in nitrogen concentration can be recorded breath by breath, and at the end of the test the patient maximally exhales and the peak concentration of nitrogen is recorded at the mouth. Normally, less than 2.5% nitrogen remains in the lung.

In the normal lung, the fraction of nitrogen removed from the lung is nearly equal breath by breath. When plotted on semilog paper, this results in a nearly linear plot. In patients with obstructive lung disease, the nonuniform ventilation results in a curved plot with an early "fast-ventilated space" and a later "slow-ventilated space." Increasing research attention is centered on these breath-by-breath aspects of the test.

Dead Space Ventilation

Physiologic dead space is probably more commonly determined than anatomic dead space because the former measurement is used frequently in the operating room and intensive care areas in patient assessment. Physiologic dead space represents the sum of the anatomic dead space plus the volume of ventilated lung not receiving pulmonary blood flow and thus not participating in gas exchange. The mixed expired carbon dioxide tension ($PECO_2$) in a bag is measured along with the arterial PCO_2 ($PaCO_2$) and the tidal volume (VT). The volume of the physiologic dead space ($VDCO_2$) is calculated from the equation

$$VDCO_2 = \frac{PaCO_2 - PECO_2 \times VT}{PaCO_2}$$

The dead space is frequently reported in relation to the tidal volume; VD/VT is normally less than 0.30. An increase in the ratio suggests pulmonary vascular occlusive disease when the distribution of ventilation is normal, a decrease in blood distribution to ventilated alveoli or a decrease in functioning capillary bed in contact with ventilated alveoli, e.g., significant volumes of lung with high ventilation perfusion ratios (V/Q ratio). This can be used as an indication to increase assisted ventilation to maintain arterial gas tensions.

Closing Volume

The single-breath oxygen test can be used to evaluate the closing volume (Fig 9–8), which is defined as the volume from the onset of Phase IV to the end of the full exhalation (to residual volume). Closing capacity includes both closing volume and residual volume.

At the start of the oxygen breath, dead space gas with its high concentration of nitrogen, goes to the upper portion of the lung. Later in the inspiration, gas (oxygen) is distributed to other portions of the lung. Phase I of expiration (not shown in the figure) will contain only dead space air and therefore only oxygen.

Phase II represents the alveolar gas with its higher nitrogen content being added quickly to dilute the dead space gas. During phase III, as alveoli empty uniformly, there is a relative plateau. Then, as alveoli in the lower lung close, the gas comes mostly from the nitrogen-rich upper lung alveoli, and the expired nitrogen concentration suddenly rises (Phase IV).

An alternative to use of the oxygen breath is found in the use of a bolus of an inert tracer gas such as argon, helium, or xenon-133 early in the inspiration followed by air. A greater amount of the tracer gas will go preferentially to the upper lung as in the oxygen test, and the exhalation pattern will be similar to that observed for exhaled nitrogen in the oxygen test. Closing volume measurement is reported to be a sensitive test for the detection of small airways disease,[30] but it is probably also altered by abnormality at the alveolar level. Measurements of closing volume require great attention to the details of the testing and especially to the performance of the exhalation maneuver by the subject, as with using the single-breath oxygen test for the study of the distribution of ventilation. Closing volume determination remains a research test and is not yet applicable for routine testing or for screening studies in children.

PULMONARY MECHANICS

Pulmonary mechanics deal with the dynamic factors in pulmonary function as compared to the static lung volumes. The major site of pathologic abnormalities in patients with chronic obstructive pulmonary disease is peripheral small airways less than 2 to 3 mm in diameter in excised lungs.[24, 39] The role of increased muscular tone in the airway of living lung tissue has not been evaluated.[39] These changes in the small airways can include inflammation, excess mucus, and bronchial wall narrowing and may be potentially reversible, as opposed to the alveolar wall destruction seen in emphysema victims. Therefore, it is of great interest to determine how small airways influence lung function and to use tests that reflect the structural alterations that occur in small airways in disease processes.[25] However, very few lung function tests are specific for the small airways. Most reflect both the flow-resistive properties of the airways and the elastic properties of the alveoli.

In early disease, at least in adults, routine studies of pulmonary function including FEV_1 and airway resistance may have normal or near-normal results because they do not reflect the peripheral airways that were found to be the site of obstruction in excised lungs.[18] Although individual peripheral airways are tiny, there are so many of them in parallel that their total cross-sectional area is many times that of the more central airways. Current evidence suggests that the peripheral airways normally contribute only 10 to 20% of the total pulmonary resistance, except perhaps in young children, which would indicate that obstructive involvement in the small airways must become marked before airway resistance, forced expiratory volume in 1 second, or other measures can detect it. Therefore, attention has turned to tests that may be more sensitive to this region. These include flow rates obtained at effort-independent lower lung volumes such as the forced expiratory flow over the midportion of the forced expiratory volume (FEF_{25-75}, formerly MMF), use of flow-volume curves (Fig 9–9) and measuring flow at 50% or 25% of vital capacity, frequency dependence of dynamic compliance (C_{dyn}), closing volume, and abnormal gas distribution or exchange. However, the information contained in the first second of timed vital capacity can also be useful.

The maximal expiratory flow-volume (MEFV) curve obtained when a subject

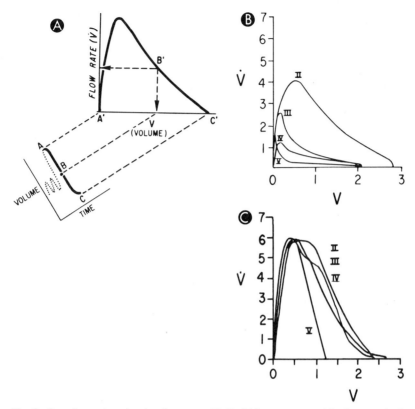

Fig 9–9.—A, a standard spirogram *(A, B, C)* is compared to the expiratory flow-volume (FV) curve in a normal subject. In the FV curve, expiration proceeds from peak lung inflation at *A* along *A-B* to the forced expiratory position, *C.* Flow rate at a given lung volume may be determined by drawing a tangent at any point in the spirogram. Such measurements are subject to error. By contrast, the flow rate at the same lung volume can be read directly at point *B* in the FV curve. $\dot{V}$, flow rate in liters per second; *V,* expiratory volume in liters from the total lung capacity. (From Lord, G.P., et al.: Flow-volume curve in lung disease, Am. J. Med. 46:73, 1969.) **B,** flow-volume curves in patients with obstructive lung disease. Four classes of obstructive disease of increasing severity are shown. The curves in classes III, IV, and V were selected from patients of the same sex and similar height who had roughly the same forced vital capacities. As obstructive disease becomes more severe, the curve becomes more convex to the volume axis. A universal finding in class V is a sudden drop in flow soon after the onset of expiration. This phenomenon occurs even at low intrathoracic driving pressures. $\dot{V}$, flow rate in liters per second; *V,* expiratory volume in liters from the total lung capacity. **C,** the flow-volume curve in patients with pulmonry parenchymal fibrosis is characterized by a high peak flow rate and small forced vital capacity. In class V, with marked decrease in vital capacity, the high, peaked curve is distinctive. $\dot{V}$, flow rate in liters per second; *V,* expiratory volume in liters from the total lung capacity.

is breathing air and subsequently breathing a helium-oxygen mixture can be analyzed in several ways (Fig 9–10).[38] The most commonly used are (1) the increase in flow at 50% of vital capacity breathing He-O$_2$ expressed as a percent of the flow breathing air at the same lung volume ($\Delta \dot{V}$ max 50), where 50 indicates measurement at 50% of the vital capacity, and (2) the volume of exhaled gas that is found when the flow rates are identical for air and He-O$_2$ near the end of the exhaled breath. This latter value, called the *volume of isoflow* (V iso $\dot{V}$), is expressed as a percentage of the forced vital capacity. The finding of an increased V iso $\dot{V}$ cannot indicate whether the underlying mechanism is increased resistance or loss of elastic recoil;[18] however, the $\Delta \dot{V}$ max 50 appears to be relatively specific for the caliber of small airways.

The closing volume test is relatively nonspecific and may reflect the condition of both the airways and the alveoli (lung elastic recoil). However, increasing attention is being centered on the Phase III portion, which reveals a slight slope, referred to as the change in nitrogen per liter of gas exhaled (ΔN_2/liter). This is a measure of the distribution of ventilation and may be relatively specific for the elastic properties of the alveoli.

The frequency dependence of compliance has been used to define individuals with early airway obstruction, and various other tests are compared with it in many reports. Appropriate description of procedures, the basis upon which normal values were derived, and the basis for the interpretation of results are frequently lacking. Omissions of this type in reported studies have resulted in various claims for what the tests or their variations may measure, and for find-

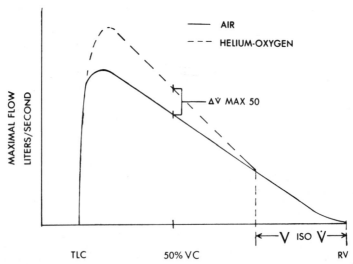

Fig 9–10.—Maximal expiratory flow-volume curves after air and after helium-oxygen breathing. The percent change in the flow at 50% vital capacity after breathing He-O$_2$ is expressed as Δ V max 50%. The volume of isoflow (V iso $\dot{V}$) is determined where the He-O$_2$ and air curves intersect and frequently is expressed as a percent of the vital capacity.

ing a greater sensitivity for one test over another in the early detection of disease.

The efforts to assess the relative merits of the more recent tests of airway obstruction and the many variables that play a role have been discussed.[37] The full significance of finding an early or isolated abnormality by one of these tests remains to be determined in terms of differentiating the site of the abnormality, the reversibility or stage of disease, and the prognostic significance. These tests should remain the subject of research investigation under the most controlled circumstances and are not recommended for screening large populations.

Air Flow Measurements

Use of the spirometer also permits the measurement of various air flow rates. This provides information about the presence or severity of airway obstruction as well as an index of dynamic function. Just as with airway resistance, flow rates are influenced by lung volume. Whichever spirometer system is used, when diagnostic spirometry is performed a permanent record should be made.[17]

The FEV is recorded as the volume of gas expelled from the lungs in a given time, such as 1, 2, or 3 seconds (FEV_1, FEV_2, or FEV_3) or less commonly, in the first ¼, ½, or ¾ second($FEV_{0.25}$, $FEV_{0.50}$, or $FEV_{0.75}$). FEV_1 is the value most frequently reported. It can be expressed as a percentage of the predicted normal VC, the VC achieved during the testing (FEV_1/VC), or the total FEV, also called FVC_1, often expressed as FVC (FEV_1/FEV). Dickman et al. observed that the mean values for FEV_1/FEV were remarkably stable regardless of age, sex, or size.[10] Mean values for boys and girls ranged from 82.9% to 85.8%; however, in view of the relatively large standard deviations observed in normal subjects, it was recommended that a ratio of FEV_1 to FEV of less than 70% be considered abnormal for any age, sex, or height. This ratio is relatively independent of effort except that a maximum FEV is required.

The maximal expiratory flow rate (MEFR) can be determined from the FEV spirogram as another measurement of flow rate. It is also termed *forced expiratory flow* ($FEV_{200-1,200}$). It is defined as the flow rate in liters per minute for the liter of gas that is expired after the first 200 ml has been expired. The maximal midexpiratory flow (MMF) is measured in liters per minute over the middle half of the FEV to avoid some of the variables that occur over the first and last portions of the FEV curve (see Fig 9–3). The MMF is now referred to as the $FEF_{25-75\%}$. In children with an FEV of about 2 liters or less, these latter two measurements are not practical.

Flow-Volume Curves

Maximal expiratory flow-volume (MEFV) curves provide a different means of looking at gas emptying from the lungs from flow-versus-time curves. Specific equipment has been developed so that flow-volume curves can be obtained readily. The reliability of the MEFV curves apparently is improved when the maximum value at a particular portion of the VC is reported, e.g., at 50% or 75% of the VC. There is disagreement as to whether certain flow rates, such as maximum midexpiratory flow rate, are more sensitive than the maximum expiratory flow at stated portions of the VC in children with obstructive pulmonary disease. More specificity probably will be obtained when the MEFV curve and/or the other flow rates are related to the actual lung volume of the subject at that time. Characteristic MEFV patterns are described for obstructive and restrictive types of pulmonary problems (Fig 9–9,B and C).

The timed forced vital capacity and the MEFV curve contain the same information. The flow pattern is better visualized and appreciated from the MEFV curve, however, the curve does not lend itself easily to analysis. Ideally, it would be preferable to utilize the information from the entire curve, including appreciation not only of its slope but also of its curvature. However, this sort of analysis is technically difficult. Consequently, most analyses have been limited simply to the instantaneous flow rate at 50% and/or 25% of the vital capacity. Ligas et al. discuss different approaches to utilize more fully the information available, including a mathematical moment analysis.[27] Inferences about the smaller airways and parenchyma and the distribution of mechanical properties of the lungs are possible using this more complete analysis.

When the curves obtained when the subject is breathing air and helium-oxygen mixtures are compared (Fig 9–10), two single-point measures of the volume of isoflow and the increase in maximum flow at 50% of the vital capacity have been reported (see the earlier section on pulmonary mechanics). These have been reviewed.[18] The increase in $\dot{V}$ max 50 when the subject is breathing helium is thought to be relatively specific for the status of the small airways, whereas the volume of isoflow may be influenced by both the small airways and the alveoli (elastic recoil). These tests are recommended for investigative use and are not yet ready for use in screening programs.[18]

Airway Resistance (Raw)

The body plethysmograph has provided a means for determining airway resistance.[14] Airway resistance = alveolar pressure/air flow. The air flow is measured with a pneumotachometer at the mouth with the subject seated in the plethysmograph. The pressure change in the plethysmograph and the alveolar pressure can be measured as described in the earlier section on functional residual capacity. With appropriate calibrations, airway resistance can be determined repeatedly and rapidly. Technical details and a fuller discussion are available.[34, 35] The lung volume at which the airway resistance is measured also can be determined. The latter aspect is important since flow rates are at least in part dependent upon lung volume and at larger lung volumes the airways will have a greater diameter and less resistance to air flow. Adequate interpretation of flow rates and airway resistance is impaired when the simultaneous lung volume is not measured.

In an individual subject, airway resistance is increased at smaller lung volumes, i.e., approaching RV, and is decreased at larger lung volumes, i.e., approaching TLC. In addition, airway resistance decreases as the lung grows. The newborn infant has a relatively small lung volume and an airway resistance greater than that of the adult. By the age of 6 years, the child's lung volume at FRC has increased to 0.67 L and the airway resistance is about 5 cm $H_2O/$ liter/second. An average adult male FRC is about 2.5 L and the airway resistance has decreased to about 0.5 to 1 cm $H_2O/$liter/second. Thus, both lung volume growth and the degree of lung inflation have an effect on the air flow measurement and its interpretation.

CONDUCTANCE (THE RECIPROCAL OF AIRWAY RESISTANCE, 1/RAW)

When airway resistance is plotted against lung volume, a nonlinear relationship is observed. To overcome this problem, the reciprocal of airway resistance, conductance (Gaw), is used. When conductance is plotted against lung volume, a linear relationship occurs. In our experience, this relationship is improved when the log-log relationship is used, as shown in Figure 9–11, for newborns, younger children, older children and adults. This relationship permits the calculation of a prediction equation for conductance related to lung volume that is applicable to the increase in lung volume with growth or to changes in lung volume with disease.

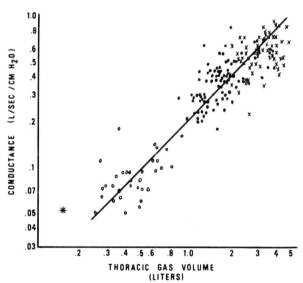

Fig 9–11.—Conductance versus lung volume as measured with the body plethysmograph. Conductance, the reciprocal of airway resistance, has a good correlation with increasing lung volume from the newborn period *(star)* to the larger lung volumes found in young children *(open circles)*, older children *(closed circles)* and adults *(x)*.

SPECIFIC AIRWAY RESISTANCE

The product of lung volume × airway resistance is nearly constant in subjects 6 years of age and older. This product has been termed *specific airway resistance* (SRaw) and is a useful and convenient way to relate airway resistance and lung volume without utilizing the concept of conductance. We determined the SRaw for 74 adult subjects between 19 and 54 years of age and 103 children between 5 and 18 years old. The results, which were quite uniform in both age groups, are summarized in Figure 9–12. An SRaw of greater than 7 sec cm H_2O for males or females 5 to 54 years of age is outside the 95% confidence limit.[12] In children with progressive obstructive pulmonary disease, observed increases in SRaw appear to result from increases in airway resistance or lung volume or both.

Lung Compliance

The measurement of compliance and total pulmonary resistance requires the use of an esophageal balloon for the pressure measurement to reflect intrapleural pressure. Although studies have been carried out to collect data, these tests usually are not performed routinely because of the additional discomfort of the esophageal balloon placement and because the simple tests are usually adequate for clinical work.

Compliance of the lung (C_L) is defined as the volume change per unit of pressure change across the lung (ml/mm Hg). Since the compliance of the lung

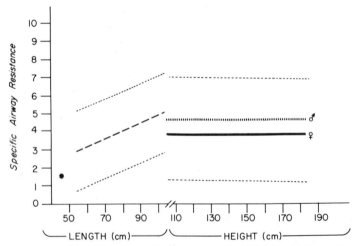

Fig 9–12.—Specific airway resistance versus length/height. Specific airway resistance (SRaw) for newborns *(star)*, young children *(dashed line)*, older females *(solid line)* and males *(dotted line)* are related to length/height. The 95% confidence limits are shown by the *lighter dotted lines.* Beyond age 6 years, the SRaw remained stable through the period of body growth, unlike lung volume and conductance. The females consistently had a lower SRaw.

depends on its size, it is useful to have a measure of the lung volume as well. The compliance per unit of lung volume is called *specific compliance* and is about the same in the infant as in the adult (0.06 liter/cm H_2O/liter).

Static compliance, measured in descending volume steps from above FRC when there is no air flow, allows the creation of a pressure-volume curve. In normal adults the compliance in this range (approximating the normal tidal volume range) is about 0.2 liter/cm H_2O. The static compliance measurement is the only adequate measure of the elastic properties of the lung. In patients with restrictive diseases compliance is decreased, while with an obstructive disorder like emphysema compliance is increased.

When compliance is measured during quiet breathing by taking volume changes between points of no flow (to establish the pressure differential), it is called *dynamic compliance*. In patients with obstructive disease, this method is influenced by altered time constants in areas of partial airway obstruction. Thus dynamic compliance includes both elastic recoil and airway resistance factors. Dynamic compliance will decrease during rapid breathing in patients with obstruction of small airways, whereas other tests may remain within normal limits, and is referred to as frequency dependence of dynamic compliance (C_{dyn}).

Another useful measurement of the elastic properties of the lung is that of maximum recoil pressure, which is stated as the intrapleural pressure at full inspiration (TLC). The intrapleural pressure is usually estimated from the esophageal pressure. The elastic properties of the lungs in younger children seem to be similar to those in older adults as a result of lung growth and aging, which successively influence the elastic behavior of the lung tissue.[22] The transpulmonary pressure at TLC normally decreases with age in the adult and is not influenced by the size of the person or the size of the lung. In a healthy young adult, lung recoil at TLC is about 30 cm H_2O. As with air flow measurements, adequate interpretation of compliance and elastic recoil is improved when the subject's lung volume is measured simultaneously.

DIFFUSION

The measurement of diffusion with carbon monoxide has been used in children. Many factors involved in diffusion, including the thickness of the alveolar membrane, the alveolar and capillary surface area available, red cell factors, and body position, serve to make the interpretation of the diffusion test results difficult. Any process that decreases the capillary bed, increases the distance for diffusion or results in mismatching of ventilation to perfusion may result in lowering the diffusing capacity (DL).

The measurement of diffusing capacity can be performed by either a breath-holding (single-breath) or a steady-state method. In the single-breath method, a dilute mixture of carbon monoxide is maximally inhaled and the breath held for 10 seconds. Helium or argon is included in the inhalation in order to estimate alveolar volume. The rate of disappearance of carbon monoxide is determined from the inspiratory and expiratory measurements.

In the steady-state method, a low concentration (about 0.1%) of carbon monoxide is breathed for about 30 seconds or until a steady state is reached. Exhaled gas is then analyzed for a period of time to determine the uptake of the carbon monoxide. An arterial blood gas sample is required to determine the physiologic dead space. The normal value for D_LCO_2 at rest is about 25 ml/min/mm Hg in adults. It increases twofold to threefold with exercise and is altered by the subject's position.

Since primary membrane diffusion defects are rare in children, and either the breath-holding period or an arterial blood sample is required, this test has not been used frequently in pediatric testing.

EVALUATION OF VENTILATORY MUSCLES

The ventilatory muscles provide the power to run the lung bellows. If they are paralyzed or fatigued, respiratory failure may ensue, no matter how functional the lungs are. The diaphragm is the most important muscle of ventilation, since it dominates inspiratory effort. Expiration is largely passive, but with forced expiration, the abdominal muscles and the intercostals, along with others, assist in generating the necessary force. The ventilatory muscles must have adequate strength and endurance to generate sufficient airflow repeatedly for prolonged periods. It is possible to measure both of these properties.

STRENGTH.—The strength of the ventilatory muscles can be assessed by measuring maximal inspiratory and expiratory pressures that can be generated at the mouth. Most children over 7 years old can master these techniques. The expiratory pressure can provide a quantitation of the effective expulsive strength of the individual's cough effort. A simple manometer or a pressure gauge capable of reading both positively or negatively to about 100 to 150 mm Hg is required. Children achieve the best pressures and reproduce them best if maximal expiratory pressure is exerted after a deep inhalation and if maximal inspiratory pressure is exerted after an exhalation to near residual volume. Most normal children older than 7 or 8 years can exert at least 30 mm Hg pressure on either inspiration or expiration.

ENDURANCE.—The endurance of the ventilatory muscles is more difficult to measure and currently should be considered a research tool.[33] Normal and abnormal structure and function of these muscles have been reviewed.[5, 36]

VENTILATORY DRIVE

The control of ventilation is normally so strict that arterial oxygen and carbon dioxide levels are kept within a few mm Hg and pH is kept within a few hundredths, despite widely varying metabolic demands. In some disease states, the ventilator apparatus is capable of meeting these metabolic demands, yet the appropriate instructions are not relayed from the central nervous system and hypo- and hyperventilation result. These aberrations are all too clear in severe head trauma or encephalitis, but may also occur more subtly in other conditions, including the obesity hypoventilation syndrome, chronic obstructive pulmonary disease, central alveolar hypoventilation ("Ondine's Curse"), etc. Most tests for the adequacy of ventilatory drive are not available in the average clinical lab; however, a relatively simple test can be conducted to give an estimate of the adequacy of the ventilatory response to hypercapnia. The patient breathes into a closed circuit with an anesthesia bag or weather balloon as the main reservoir, while both minute ventilation and PCO_2 of the system are plotted. As the procedure progresses, carbon dioxide levels will rise and ventilation normally also rises as an attempt to "blow off" the carbon dioxide. In some conditions, ventilation will not change as hypercapnia develops, thus indicating an inadequate ventilatory response to carbon dioxide. Equipment for these tests is not standardized, and responses vary over a very wide range in normal people. Consequently, each lab should establish its own reference standards.

INFANT-ADULT COMPARISONS

Although the surface area of the infant lung is equal to that of the adult lung when compared by body surface area or body weight, the oxygen requirements of the infant per kilogram of body weight are nearly twice those of the adult. The pulmonary reserve of the infant thus appears to be much less than that of the adult. Other comparisons are shown in Table 9–2.

The pH, $PaCO_2$, PaO_2 and oxygen saturation of the arterial blood of the infant and young child are very similar to those of the adult. Knowledge of these values alone does not provide information about the size of the lungs, the mechanics of respiration in the individual, or the efficiency of respiration. Figure 9–1 indicates the large increase in lung volume that occurs during the period of growth and maturation.

For example, the FRC increases from a newborn value of 90 ml to an average adult value of about 2,500 ml, while the tidal volume increases from 18 or 20 ml to about 500 ml. It is interesting that the percentage of dead space ventilation with each breath remains about the same despite the overall volume changes that occur with growth. On the other hand, the resting respiratory rate decreases from about 40 breaths/minute in infants to about 14 in the adult, and the airway resistance during mouth breathing, which is estimated to be about 7 cm H_2O/liter/second in the infant, decreases to about 0.5 to 1 cm H_2O/liter/second in the adult. Lung compliance in the normal newborn after 24 hours of life is about 6 ml/cm H_2O, a very low value compared to the approximately 200 ml/cm H_2O of the adult. However, when the lung compliance per unit of lung volume at FRC (called *specific lung compliance*) is calculated, the resulting value of 0.055/liter/cm H_2O/liter lung volume for the infant is quite similar to that for older children and young adults.

TESTING CHILDREN AT RISK FOR APNEA AND SUDDEN INFANT DEATH SYNDROME (SIDS)

Sudden unexpected, unexplained infant death is tragic. An explanation has eluded investigators for decades. In recent years attention has been focused on the possible connection of altered central control of ventilation, upper airway

TABLE 9–2.—COMPARISON OF NORMAL VALUES OF LUNG FUNCTION
IN NEWBORNS AND ADULTS

	NEWBORN	ADULT	FOLD CHANGE
Tidal volume (VT), ml	20 (5–7 ml/kg)	450 (6 ml/kg)	22
Alveolar ventilation ($\dot{V}A$), ml/min	400	4,200	10
ml/sq m/min	2.3	2.3	1
Dead space VD/VT ratio	0.3	0.33	1
Anatomical dead space, ml	7.0	150	20
ml/kg	2.5	2	1
Respiratory quotient	0.8	0.8	1
Ventilatory equivalent (VT/$\dot{V}O_2$)	23	22–25	1
O_2 consumption, ml/min	18	250	14
ml/kg/min	6.0–6.7	3.5	0.5
CO_2 output, ml/kg/min	6	3	0.5
Calories, kg/hr	2.0	1.0	0.5
$\dot{V}O_2/\dot{V}A$	0.067	0.062	1
(VT–VD)/VFRC = VA/VFRC	0.13	0.13	1
Body surface area, sq m	0.21	1.70	8
Body weight, kg	3	70	23
Lung weight, gm	50	800	15
FRC, ml	90	2,400	24
ml/kg	30	34	1
Lung surface area, sq m	2.8	64–75	30
sq m/kg	≈ 1	≈ 1	1
Number of alveoli	24×10^6	296×10^6	12
		375×10^6	15
Alveolar diameter, μm	50	200–300	4–6
Number of respiratory airways	1.5×10^6	14×10^6	10
Respiratory rate	34–36	12–14	2–3

patency, and SIDS.[6] Infants who have experienced "near-SIDS" episodes (cessation of breathing, with color change necessitating resuscitation) frequently have breathing patterns different from their age-matched, low-risk peers. Pneumograms or pneumocardiograms, which are 12- to 24-hour recordings of the respiratory excursions of the chest wall (usually by impedance), and electrocardiograph patterns are being widely employed in attempts to identify children at risk of SIDS. More sophisticated evaluations, often performed during sleep (polysomnography), may employ nasal air-flow sensors, esophageal pH probes, and transcutaneous or ear oximeters.[21] Clinical evaluation of the episode is also important in determining further care recommendations.

BRONCHIAL CHALLENGE

In an occasional child, the diagnosis of asthma or reactive airways disease is suspected, but is not obvious. In these instances, several kinds of bronchial challenge can bring out the abnormality and allow the diagnosis to be established. Inhalation of increasing concentrations of histamine or metacholine is commonly used in adult laboratories, but is reserved more for the research laboratory in investigating children. Exercise challenge, or—what may be its physiologic equivalent[31]—cold air challenge, can be readily and safely applied in children in most pulmonary laboratories. These tests are discussed more fully in the section on exercise testing.

EXERCISE TESTING

Exercise testing provides a new dimension in pediatric pulmonary function testing. Exercise tests can be used to evaluate certain specific symptoms, which will be dealt with later; to detect physiologic abnormalities before they are obvious in the resting state; to quantify abnormalities; to follow disease progression; to pinpoint the factor(s) limiting exercise ability; to make specific diagnoses in some cases, and, perhaps most important, to exclude significant disease in many patients (Table 9–3).

Indications

Any child with a history of exercise limitation—including those whose limitation has been imposed on them by parents or physicians—may be a candidate for exercise testing. Both parents and children are notoriously unreliable in assessing exercise ability; far too many children are restricted from normal activities because of an imagined problem. Innocent cardiac murmurs probably account for more unnecessary restrictions than other conditions. One study that examined parents' assessment of their children's exercise ability and their actual measured exercise ability found no relationship.[19] Many children with normal exercise tolerance were thought by their parents to be severely limited and therefore had been treated as invalids. Exercise testing can serve the important function of freeing children from unnecessary restraints.

Other indications for exercise testing include a history of almost any exercise-associated symptom (Table 9–4). Exercise testing in the laboratory enables the physician to document the symptom and relate its appearance to specific physiologic events.

Contraindications

Patients with cor pulmonale and active right-sided heart failure should not be subjected to vigorous exercise testing because of the danger of increasing hypoxemia and worsening heart failure. Children with acute medical or or-

TABLE 9–3.—USES FOR EXERCISE
TESTING

1. Assess symptoms
2. Quantitate abnormality
3. Follow disease
4. Determine limiting factor
5. Make specific diagnosis
6. Exclude serious disease

TABLE 9–4.—INDICATIONS FOR EXERCISE
TESTING

History of exercise limitation
History of exercise-related symptoms
"Can't exercise"
Pain
Fainting
Cough
Dyspnea
Wheezing

thopedic problems should be excused from exercise testing until they have returned to their usual state of health.

Many limiting factors determine each person's exercise tolerance, especially the conditions of the cardiovascular system, the lungs, and the peripheral musculoskeletal system. These systems form a chain, the weakest link of which will limit exercise. Thus, no matter how strong one's heart and lungs, if the legs are broken—or terribly weak—the individual will not be able to run. Similarly, if the heart cannot pump oxygenated blood to the legs, even someone with the healthiest legs and lungs will not be able to perform. And if the legs and heart are good but the lungs are unable to bring in oxygen and transfer it to the blood, exercise will be limited well before the healthy links in the chain are stressed to their limits.

One of the most important factors influencing the performance of each of these systems, especially the heart and muscles, which are most commonly responsible for limiting exercise, is the amount of exercise a person normally does. Exercise training programs* can increase the performance of the heart and muscles and probably the lungs in most people. Inactivity, as with bed rest, definitely decreases these performance levels.

Equipment

An exercise laboratory must include monitoring equipment and facilities adequate for patients to exercise. For some types of testing this may require no more than a hallway for running and a stethoscope. More sophisticated laboratories will include a treadmill and a cycle ergometer. Each has its advantages and disadvantages. We have found the cycle ergometer generally more suitable than the treadmill for most pediatric testing. Virtually every child knows how to pedal a bike, but treadmill walking and running are awkward and difficult to learn, especially for young children. Falling and injury are more likely, and it is much more difficult to breathe through a stationary mouthpiece during

---

*Exercise programs have proliferated in recent years. The author's exercise philosophy and recommendations are set forth in a booklet, *A Beginner's Guide to Exercise,* which is available on request.

treadmill walking. Finally, in setting up a new laboratory, a good cycle ergometer is substantially less expensive than a sophisticated treadmill.

In selecting a cycle ergometer for pediatric use, one must look for important features. (1) Often overlooked, the cycle must be adjustable so that a small child can comfortably reach the handlebars and pedals while seated. (2) The bike must have small enough stepwise work increments: about 50 kpm/minute* or less. Some bikes (e.g., the Siemans-Elema) are available with continuously adjustable workloads. (3) The bike should have electronic braking—this is better than the friction-braked bikes because the workload on the electronic bike is independent of the pedaling rate over a large range of pedaling frequencies. With the mechanically braked bike, the workload usually depends on pedaling frequency and is thus hard to maintain and measure.

Further equipment should include a cardiotachometer and may include complete ECG-monitoring equipment and blood-pressure cuff. If children with known or suspected heart disease are being studied, the complete ECG system is essential. For more sophisticated testing, special low-resistance respiratory valves, respiratory-volume measuring devices (dry gas meter, pneumotachometer, Douglas bag), and CO_2 and O_2 analyzers may be added. Several suitable models of each are available. For much greater flexibility, respiratory mass spectrometers are available. Finally, to tie everything together and to save technician time, the whole system can be assisted and analyzed by computer.[2, 40] In recent years several excellent but expensive computer-controlled systems have become commercially available.

Specific Tests

There are a number of tests or observations that can be made.

A basic test, *maximum physical working capacity* (PWC_{max}), answers the question: Just how much work can this child do? This test is easy to perform and is well tolerated by children aged 6 years and older. In order for PWC_{max} values to be compared among several children, the children must exercise according to the same protocol. One of the simplest tests is the progressive exercise test.[19] The only equipment needed is a cycle ergometer. The child pedals at the lowest work setting, and the workload is increased every minute by a set amount depending on the child's height. We use increments of 10 watts (W) for children shorter than 125 cm, 15 W for those between 125 and 150 cm, and 20 W for everyone taller than 150 cm. The child is urged to pedal as long as possible. The last workload at which the individual completes a full minute is defined as the PWC_{max}. Most children attain their PWC_{max} in 5 to 10 minutes. PWC_{150} and PWC_{170} tests are common variations on the PWC theme: instead of requiring the subject to exercise to exhaustion, these tests measure

---

*Kilopondmeter (kpm) is the work required to move a 1-kg mass 1 m against the force of gravity. Expressed as power, or work per unit time, this is the kpm/minute. Another power unit is the joule-second or the watt; 1 w is about 6 kpm/minute.

the work level achieved when the subject's heart rate reaches 150 beats/minute to 170 beats/minute. Some patients with severe lung disease may have their exercise limited by their lungs before they have pushed their heart rates as high as 170, or even 150. In these patients, of course, PWC_{150} and PWC_{170} cannot be used.

Minute ventilation ($\dot{V}E$) is the volume of air breathed in 1 minute. $\dot{V}E_{max}$ is a useful measurement in children with lung disease, especially when compared to a resting maximum voluntary ventilation (MVV) value. In children free of lung disease, the $\dot{V}E_{max}$ level during exercise seldom reaches more than 60 to 70% of MVV. However, children with severe obstructive lung disease such as cystic fibrosis, with much less ventilatory reserve than normal subjects, may approach or even surpass their normal MVV levels during exercise. When a child's $\dot{V}E_{max}$ is 110% of the MVV (i.e., when it is more than the supposed *maximum* capacity), it is reasonable to assume that it is the lungs that limit exercise tolerance. $\dot{V}E$ is measured using a pneumotachograph, or a dry gas meter, or can be measured with less accuracy with a Douglas bag.

Maximum oxygen consumption ($\dot{V}_{2max}$) is often used as a direct reflection of fitness, and therefore is a useful measurement. $\dot{V}_{2max}$ is expressed in liters of oxygen per minute and increases with age from about 0.75 liters/min in 6-year-olds to 2 liters/min in 25-year-old nonathletes. In adults older than 25 it decreases with age. In world-class endurance athletes (marathoners, canoers, and cross-country skiers), $\dot{V}_{2max}$ values of 5.5 liters/min or higher are seen. When expressed as ml O_2/kg body weight, maximal oxygen uptake increases from 45 to 50 ml/kg min in 5-year-olds to a peak near 60 ml/kg min in 20-year-olds. A value of 84 ml/kg min has been recorded in a champion cross-country skier.

CO$_2$ production ($\dot{V}_2$) parallels oxygen consumption until the body's ability to supply oxygen is surpassed and anaerobic metabolism begins. At this point, because of accumulation of lactic acid, $\dot{V}CO_2$ values begin to rise much more rapidly than $\dot{V}O_2$. Carbon dioxide production ($\dot{V}CO_2$) is calculated by multiplying the volume of expired air ($\dot{V}E$) and the concentration of CO_2 (Fe_{CO_2}) in that expired air:

$$\dot{V}CO_2 = Fe_{CO_2} \times \dot{V}E$$

Oxygen uptake ($\dot{V}O_2$) is calculated in a similar manner, assuming that the difference between the amounts of inspired and expired O_2 is that which the body has used:

$$\dot{V}O_2 = [(FiO_2) \times (\dot{V}I)] - [(FeO_2) \times (\dot{V}E)]$$

where FiO_2 is the fraction of oxygen in the inspired air, $\dot{V}I$ is the volume of inspired air, FeO_2 is the fraction of oxygen in the expired air and $\dot{V}E$ is the volume of expired air.

The respiratory exchange ratio (R), $\dot{V}CO_2/\dot{V}O_2$, is usually 0.85 at rest. During light exercise it remains less than 1.0, and when anaerobic metabolism begins, R rises to exceed 1.0 R can therefore be a useful tool to see whether anaerobic metabolism has begun and can give a measure of the child's effort.

Blood gas measurements can be obtained from arterialized ear-lobe capillary blood with relative ease and little discomfort to the patient, or from an artery. If an ear-stick is done with a #11 surgical blade 5 to 15 minutes after a vasodilating ointment has been applied to the soft part of the ear lobe, blood flow should be excellent. The blood can then be collected in heparinized capillary tubes and analyzed. Results are virtually identical to those obtained from arterial blood.[20] Oxygen saturation can be measured accurately and noninvasively with an ear oximeter.

Dead space (VD) can be measured during exercise just as at rest.

Cardiac output can be calculated during exercise using the arterialized capillary blood gases and a simple CO_2 rebreathing maneuver. Description of the methodology is beyond the scope of this chapter. Blood pressure should be measured in any child with known or suspected hypertension or primary cardiac disease. Despite the availability of automated electronic cuff methods, the standard manual cuff and stethoscope method is probably the most reliable.

Other tests specific to cardiac patients include careful screening of exercise electrocardiograms for ST-T interval changes in patients who have an abnormal aortic valve (aortic stenosis and/or insufficiency) and for arrhythmia in any patient with a history of arrhythmia or cardiac surgery. Such children should be evaluated by a pediatric cardiologist, who should supervise the exercise tests. Several excellent reviews of the physiology and technology of exercise testing are available.[15, 19, 26]

Exercise and Asthma

Almost every child with asthma has some degree of airway obstruction after exercise. This fact is the basis for one of the most important uses of exercise laboratory, namely, to diagnose asthma in a child with atypical presentation. Many asthmatic children with a history of wheezing never wheeze in the physician's office, and their standard pulmonary function test results may be equivocal. Other children with asthma may never wheeze at all, but instead may have dyspnea or cough, especially with exercise. Most, if not all, of these children can be shown to have asthma by proper exercise testing. The equipment and procedures are quite simple: a spirometer (or any device to measure air flow), a hallway for running, and intermittent measurements of heart rate. The procedure is as follows: (1) obtain a pre-exercise baseline for some measurement of air flow rates (FEV_1 is one of the simplest; others such as peak flow, Gaw, SRaw, and MMEF can also be used); (2) have the child run for 7 minutes at a speed such that the individual's heart rate stays at or above 170 beats/minute; (3) measure air flow rates immediately after exercise and again at 3, 6, 9, 12, 15, and 20 minutes after exercise; (4) finally, give a bronchodilator aerosol (e.g., isoproterenol or isoetharine) before one last measurement of air flow. A difference of 20% or more between the highest and lowest air flow rates is considered diagnostic of asthma. The lowest flow rates are likely to be seen 5 to 15 minutes after exercise. This protocol will result in a decrease in air flow rates in virtually every child with asthma and will induce a frank wheezing attack in many. These induced attacks are readily reversed by inhalation of a bronchodilator aerosol, so these should be immediately available and a physician nearby whenever a test for exercise-induced asthma (EIA) is performed. Any type of exercise can be used for this test, but so-called free-range running, as in a hallway or on a lawn or track, is the most effective in provoking EIA. Treadmill running, cycling, walking, and swimming, in that order, are of decreasing help in demonstrating exercise-induced bronchospasm.[15]

COLD AIR AND ASTHMA

Evidence has accumulated that exercise-induced asthma (EIA) may in large part be caused by the inhalation of a large volume of relatively cool and dry air.[31] This apparently overwhelms the ability of the upper airway to condition the air, and the asthmatic bronchial tree seems to respond with bronchospasm to the delivery of air below body temperature and/or less than fully saturated. EIA can be blocked by inhalation of warm, humidified air during even the most strenuous exercise. More important, it can be produced by breathing large volumes of cold dry air even at rest.[31] Therefore, many pediatric laboratories are now able to test for "exercise-induced" asthma without exercise: subjects breathe cold dry air at a minute volume that duplicates their exercise ventilation. End-tidal P_{CO_2} is kept constant by periodic instillation of CO_2 into the breathing circuitry to prevent hypocapnia. The same measurements of expiratory flow are made as described above, and the results are interpreted the same way. Although the equipment is somewhat more sophisticated (one-way valves, CO_2 monitor, source of dry cold air, method for measuring and displaying "target" ventilation level, etc.), the results have been most satisfactory.[31]

REFERENCES

1. Altose, M.: Pulmonary mechanics, in Fishman A. (ed.): *Pulmonary Diseases and Disorders* (New York: McGraw-Hill, 1980).
2. Bacevice, A.E., Hellerstein, H.K., and Katona, P.G.: An automated system for estimating exercise cardiac output by a rebreathing technique, proceedings of the 29th Annual Conference in Engineering in Medicine and Biology, Boston, Massachusetts, November 6–10, 1976.
3. Bates, D.V., Macklem, P.T., and Christie, R.V. (eds.): *Respiratory Function in Disease* (Philadelphia: W.B. Saunders Co., 1971).
4. Beier, F.R., et al.: Pulmonary pathophysiology in cystic fibrosis, Am. Rev. Respir. Dis. 94:430, 1966.
5. Belman, M.J., Sieck, G.C.: The ventilatory muscles. Fatigue, endurance, and training, Chest 82:761, 1982.
6. Brooks, J.G.: Apnea of infancy and sudden infant death syndrome, Am. J. Dis. Child 136:1012, 1982.
7. Brough, F.K., Schmidt, C., and Dickman, M.: Effect of two instructional procedures on the performance of the spirometry test in children five through seven years of age, Am. Rev. Respir. Dis. 106:604, 1972.

8. Comroe, J.H., Jr., et al.: *The Lung* (Chicago: Year Book Medical Publishers, Inc., 1962).

9. Cystic Fibrosis "GAP" Conference Report: Standardization of lung function testing in children. Vol. 3, No. 1, 1979. Cystic Fibrosis Foundation, Rockville, Maryland.

10. Dickman, M.L., Schmidt, C.D., and Gardner, R.M.: Spirometric standards for normal children and adolescents, Am. Rev. Respir. Dis. 104:680, 1971.

11. Doershuk, C.F., Fisher, B.J., and Matthews, L.W.: Pulmonary Physiology of the Young Child, in Scarpelli, E.M. (ed.): *Pulmonary Physiology of the Fetus, Infant and Child* (Philadelphia: Lea & Febiger, 1975).

12. Doershuk, C.F., Fisher, B.F., and Matthews, L.W.: Specific airway resistance from the perinatal period into adulthood, Am. Rev. Respir. Dis. 109:452, 1974.

13. DuBois, A.B., et al.: A rapid plethysmographic method for measuring thoracic gas volume, J. Clin. Invest. 35:322, 1956.

14. DuBois, A.B., et al.: A new method for measuring airway resistance in man using a body plethysmography, J. Clin. Invest. 35:327, 1956.

15. Fitch, K.D.: Comparative aspects of available exercise systems, Pediatrics 56:904–907, (suppl.), 1975.

16. Fitzgerald, M.X., Smith, A.A., and Gaensler, E.A.: Evaluation of "electronic" spirometers, N. Engl. J. Med. 289:1283, 1973.

17. Gardner, R. (Chairman): Standardization of Spirometry: Report of Snowbird Workshop, Am. Rev. Respir. Dis. 119:1979.

18. Gelb, A.F., and Klein, E.: The volume of isoflow and increase in maximal flow at 50 percent of forced vital capacity during helium-oxygen breathing as tests of small airway dysfunction, Chest 71:396, 1977.

19. Godfrey, S.: *Exercise Testing in Children* (Philadelphia: W.B. Saunders Co., 1974).

20. Godfrey, S., et al.: Ear lobe blood samples for blood gas analysis at rest and during exercise, Br. J. Dis. Chest 65:58–64, 1971.

21. Guilleminault, C., Ariagno, R., Korobkin, R., et al.: Sleep parameters and respiratory variables in "near miss" sudden infant death syndrome infants, Pediatrics 68:354, 1981.

22. Hardt, H., et al.: Static recoil of the lungs and static compliance in healthy children, Respiration 32:325, 1975.

23. Helliesen, P.J., et al.: Studies of respiratory physiology in children. I. Mechanics of respiration of lung volumes in 85 normal children 5–17 years of age, Pediatrics 22:80, 1958.

24. Hogg, J.C., Macklem, P.T., and Thurlbeck, W.M.: Site and nature of airway obstruction in chronic obstructive lung disease, N. Engl. J. Med. 278:1355, 1968.

25. Ingram, R.H., Jr., and McFadden, E.R., Jr.: Localization and mechanisms of airway responses, N. Engl. J. Med. 297:596, 1977.

26. Jones, N.L., and Campbell, E.J.M.: *Clinical Exercise Testing* (Philadelphia: W.B. Saunders Co., 1982).

27. Ligas, J.R., Primiano, F.P., Jr., Saidel, G.M., and Doershuk, C.F.: Comparison of measures of forced expiration, J. Appl. Physiol. 42:607, 1977.

28. Martin, R.R., et al.: The early detection of airway obstruction, Am. Rev. Respir. Dis. 111:119, 1975.

29. McBride J.T., and Wohl, M.E.B.: Pulmonary function tests, Pediatr. Clin. North Am. 26:537, 1979.

30. McCarthy, D.S., et al.: Measurement of "closing volume" as a simple and sensitive test for early detection of small airways disease, Am. J. Med. 52:747, 1972.

31. McFadden, E.R., and Ingram, R.H., Jr.: Exercise-induced asthma. Observations on the initiating stimulus, N. Engl. J. Med. 310:763, 1979.

32. Murray, J.F.: *The Normal Lung* (Philadelphia: W.B. Saunders Co., 1976).

33. Nickerson, B.G., and Keens, T.G.: Measuring ventilatory muscle endurance in humans as sustainable inspiratory pressure, J. Appl. Physiol.: Respir. Environ. Exercise Physiol. 52:768, 1982.

34. Polgar, G., and Promadhat, V.: *Pulmonary Function Testing in Children: Techniques and Standards* (Philadelphia: W.B. Saunders Co., 1971).

35. Primiano, F.P., Jr.: Measurements of the respiratory system, in Webster, J.G. (ed.): *Medical Instrumentation: Application and Design* (Boston: Houghton Mifflin Co., 1978).

36. Roussos, C., and Macklem, P.T.: Medical progress: The respiratory muscles, N. Engl. J. Med. 307:786, 1982.

37. Sobol, B.J.: The early detection of airway obstruction: Another perspective, Am. J. Med. 60:619, 1976.

38. Taussig, L.M.: Maximal expiratory flows at functional residual capacity: A test of lung function for young children, Am. Rev. Respir. Dis. 116:1031, 1977.

39. Thurlbeck, W.M.: Aspects of chronic air flow obstruction, Chest 72:341, 1977.

40. Waterloh, E., and Rittel, H.F.: Computerized ergometry, in Mellerowicz, H., and Smodlada, V.N. (eds.): *Ergometry. Basis of Medical Exercise Testing.* (Baltimore and Munich: Urban and Schwarzenberg, 1981).

Significance of Pulmonary Function and Exercise Tests

ROBERT J. FINK, M.D.
DAVID M. ORENSTEIN, M.D.
CARL F. DOERSHUK, M.D.

10

ADEQUATE INTERPRETATION of pulmonary function and exercise test results requires not only an appropriate selection of tests but also the patient's full cooperation and standardized and valid test results.

SELECTION OF TESTS

Knowledge of pulmonary physiology has expanded greatly in the last 10 years. As a result, numerous new pulmonary function tests have been developed. Each of these tests attempts to quantitatively evaluate a specific facet of lung function. The clinician cannot order ''pulmonary function tests'' without specifying the particular tests the laboratory is to perform.

No one or two tests adequately describe the pulmonary function in most clinical situations. The choice of appropriate pulmonary function tests depends on numerous considerations. Important considerations include the availability of the tests, the ease of testing, and the subject's ability to.perform the tests. The choice of appropriate tests also depends on what is suspected as being the primary pulmonary abnormality and which tests would give the most meaningful data in assessing this abnormality.

Tests that might be appropriate for a diagnostic evaluation may not always be appropriate for follow-up evaluation due to their difficulty in performance, subject discomfort, or cost. For example, in the evaluation of suspected hypersensitivity pneumonitis, assessment of compliance, diffusing capacity for carbon monoxide, ventilation-perfusion relationships using xenon scanning, and a lung biopsy may all be indicated. However, for monitoring the subject's response to therapy and long-term follow-up observations, spirometry to measure lung volumes and flow rates and occasional arterial blood gas readings are adequate.

The two major categories of pulmonary function tests are those that assess *ventilation,* such as the measurement of lung volumes, flow rates, and maximum voluntary ventilation, and those that assess *gas exchange,* such as arterial blood gases, the diffusing capacity of carbon monoxide, and xenon ventilation-perfusion scanning.

QUALITY CONTROL

There are two important aspects of quality control in the pediatric pulmonary function laboratory. First, the technicians conducting the testing procedure must be well trained and supervised. They must be able to explain the testing procedure to the child and allay any fears the child might have about the various pieces of equipment.[6] During the testing procedure, the technician must be able to elicit a maximum effort from the child without making testing so unpleasant that the child will not be willing to return for repeat testing. This aspect of pulmonary function testing is critical in patients in the pediatric age group, particularly if one is attempting to test children between ages 5 and 10 years. Comments recorded by the technician conducting the tests such as "the patient didn't try" or "the patient didn't seem to understand the testing procedure" should be considered in the interpretation of the tests.

The second major aspect of quality control concerns the apparatus used to measure the various pulmonary function parameters. The equipment must be kept in good working order and must be calibrated and standardized on a regular basis. The American Thoracic Society guidelines for spirometric equipment describe minimal standards for equipment used clinically and recommendations for calibration of equipment and record keeping.[21] Standardization of pulmonary function testing procedures and apparatus is necessary if studies performed in different laboratories are to be compared, critically analyzed, or used to interpret the status of lung function in a subject. A conference was held to determine pediatric standards.[14] Criteria for standardization are essential for the establishment of normal values for pulmonary function tests if these tests are to be applied in many different laboratories.[23]

Technical competence and rigorous quality control must be maintained, particularly in a pediatric pulmonary function laboratory. The overall quality and consistency of an individual pulmonary function test can be assessed by examining its internal consistency. For example, repeat measurements of the vital capacity should agree within 10%. The forced vital capacity should approximate the slow vital capacity except in patients with moderate or severe obstructive disease. A retrievable copy of the spirogram is necessary for later evaluation if required as part of the interpretation and for the permanent patient record.[20,21] The spirogram should be examined for a stable baseline and the shape of the forced vital capacity curve should be examined; its time span should show an expiration of at least 5 seconds, indicating an adequate effort.

It is important for the subject to be relaxed so that the baseline breathing is at the subject's usual functional residual capacity. Otherwise the expiratory reserve volume and functional residual capacity will appear falsely increased and the inspiratory capacity decreased. Air leaks at the nose or mouth will result in a variety of faulty results depending on the test.

Test results may be normal or may demonstrate abnormalities suggestive of obstruction or restriction, as detailed later. Thus, diminished forced expiratory flow rates, which are usually associated with obstructive disease, would be consistent with finding on the same test an increase in the airway resistance and the residual volume and a decrease in the vital capacity, conductance, and maximum voluntary ventilation. Total lung capacity is usually normal or moderately increased in patients with obstructive lung disease. Similarly, a decrease in total lung capacity is usually associated with restrictive disease, and one would then expect to find normal forced expiratory flow rates, airway resistance, and conductance and a decreased vital capacity.

ARTERIAL BLOOD GASES

There are many detailed publications about the interpretation of blood gases,[1, 2, 11, 22, 31, 34] therefore, this discussion will be limited to more general comments. The method by which the blood gas measurement is obtained may substantially alter the results. The subject's temperature, inspired oxygen concentration, and ventilatory status (e.g., respiratory rate, CPAP, ventilator) should be recorded. Blood gases obtained from an indwelling arterial catheter or from noninvasive measurements, such as ear oximetry or end-tidal CO_2, will most accurately reflect the subject's baseline respiratory status. Blood gases obtained from a single arterial puncture may demonstrate a variety of artifacts—most commonly the effects of hyperventilation prior to and during the procedure. When the lung disease is mild, hyperventilation will rapidly cause some increase in the PaO_2, decrease in the $PaCO_2$ and concomitant rise in the pH. The finding of a lower than normal $PaCO_2$ (less than 35 mm Hg) with a pH higher than 7.45 is indicative of hyperventilation. Occasionally a subject may breath-hold during the arterial sampling, thus yielding a falsely elevated $PaCO_2$ and lower than normal pH and PaO_2. Identification of breath-holding requires observation during the arterial puncture and should be noted on the record. A common error in the interpretation of blood gases is failure to consider the normal compensatory change in the respiratory drive elicited by a change in the pH. A rise in pH will decrease the respiratory drive, and a fall in pH will increase the respiratory drive. Analysis of the normal compensatory responses to acid-base disturbances is presented in Figure 10–1.[31] The pH and bicarbonate are determined by the acid-base status of the individual and reflect the combined influences of metabolic, renal, and respiratory events. For example, a subject with a metabolic alkalosis (pH greater than 7.45) will often demonstrate an elevated $PaCO_2$, which represents an effort to partially compensate for the elevated pH. Respiratory compensation of a metabolic alkalosis can

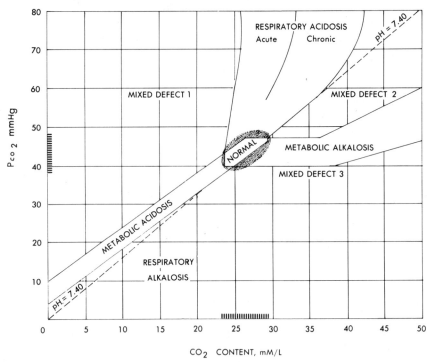

Fig 10–1.—Acid-base pattern analysis diagram showing expected degree of compensation for primary acid-base disturbances. Mixed defects are as follows: (1) metabolic and respiratory acidosis, (2) respiratory acidosis and metabolic alkalosis, and (3) metabolic and respiratory alkalosis. (From Stinebaugh, B. J., and Austin, W. H.: Acid-base balance, Arch. Intern. Med. 119:182, 1967.)

be differentiated from CO_2 retention by examining the pH, which will be greater than 7.40 in patients with uncomplicated metabolic alkalosis and less than 7.40 in those with uncomplicated CO_2 retention.

A subject with a metabolic acidosis (pH less than 7.35) will compensate with an increased ventilatory drive to lower $PaCO_2$ and thus return the pH to a more normal value. Respiratory compensation is a normal physiologic event and should be present in all subjects in whom pH is less than 7.30 because of metabolic acidosis. The increased respiratory effort (hyperpnea) is especially recognized clinically as pH levels approach 7.00. The importance of this concept occurs in the interpretation of the following blood gas: pH 7.27, PaO_2 82 mm Hg, $PaCO_2$ 41 mm Hg, HCO_3^- 18.4 mEq/liter. The failure of respiratory compensation to lower the $PaCO_2$ in the presence of acidosis of moderate severity is indicative of respiratory insufficiency or early respiratory failure even though the PaO_2 and $PaCO_2$ are within the "normal range." This blood gas is therefore respresentative of a mixed metabolic and respiratory acidosis. Infants and children are much more prone to develop metabolic acidosis than are adults or older children,[34] and they are in double jeopardy if respiratory failure is not detected early.

The PaO_2 reflects the gas exchange status of the lungs. Hypoxemia exists when the PaO_2 is less than 80 mm Hg in room air with the subject at rest. The $PaCO_2$ reflects primarily the mechanical ventilatory status of the lungs and changes in response to either generalized hypo- or hyperventilation because the diffusing capacity for CO_2 is approximately 20 times that of oxygen, and because the CO_2 dissociation curve is linear over the physiologic range, in contrast to the O_2 dissociation curve.

The four major physiologic mechanisms of hypoxemia (Table 10–1) are (1) hypoventilation (e.g., epiglottitis, obesity-hypoventilation syndrome, central nervous system lesions); (2) right-to-left shunt (e.g., congenital heart disease, intrapulmonary-arteriovenous malformations); (3) ventilation-perfusion ($\dot{V}/\dot{Q}$) inequality (e.g., asthma, cystic fibrosis, bronchiolitis); and (4) diffusion limitation (e.g., pneumonia, pulmonary edema, interstitial fibrosis). Frequently, more than one of these mechanisms may be present. The four mechanisms of hypoxemia often may be differentiated (see Table 10–1). The arterial blood gases must be obtained with the subject at rest (ideally from an indwelling catheter) both in room air and after breathing 100% oxygen for 20 minutes. The venous admixture represents the percentage of mixed venous blood that when mixed with "ideal" arterial blood (i.e., $PAO_2 = PaO_2$, where PAO_2 equals the alveolar PO_2) will yield the observed PaO_2. The percent venous admixture can be estimated from Figure 10–2 for room air and 100% oxygen with the following assumptions: (1) pH = 7.40; (2) arteriovenous oxygen difference approximately 4.5 vol %; (3) hemoglobin = 13–15 gm/dl and (4) $PAO_2 = 100$ mm Hg in room air and $PAO_2 = 670$ mm Hg in 100% oxygen.[11] The alveolar-arterial oxygen (A-aO_2) gradient can be estimated by subtracting the measured PaO_2 from the "ideal" PAO_2. The PAO_2 equals $PIO_2 - PaCO_2/R$, where PIO_2 is the partial pressure of inspired oxygen (FIO_2 times barometric pressure) and R is the respiratory exchange quotient (approximately 0.8 at rest).[2, 8] Diffusion limitation can be differentiated from $\dot{V}/\dot{Q}$ inequality by retesting after exercise. The PaO_2 will decrease during exercise in patients with diffusion limitation but will remain stable or even increase in patients with $\dot{V}/\dot{Q}$ inequality. Often more than one mechanism will contribute to a subject's hypoxemia. Therefore, the blood gas tests may not clearly indicate a single physiologic mechanism as the cause of hypoxemia.

PREDICTED NORMAL VALUES

A single pulmonary function study is difficult to interpret because of the wide range of normality observed in control subjects. The normal variation may be as much as 20% of predicted on either side of the observed mean values (100% predicted) for each of the lung volumes. To better define the range of normal, height, age, sex, and race frequently have been used alone or in combination to define more precisely the predicted normals for a given subject. The use of

TABLE 10–1.—DIFFERENTIATION OF MECHANISMS OF HYPOXEMIA

	ROOM AIR				100% OXYGEN		
	PaO₂* (<80)	PaCO₂* (>45)	A-aO₂* GRADIENT (<20)	VENOUS ADMIXTURE (<10%)	PaO₂* (>500)	PaCO₂* (>45)	VENOUS ADMIXTURE (<10%)
Hypoventilation	sl $\downarrow$	$\uparrow$	$\rightarrow$	$\rightarrow$	$\rightarrow$	$\uparrow$	$\rightarrow$
Right-to-left shunt	$\downarrow$	$\rightarrow$ to $\downarrow$	$\uparrow$	$\uparrow$	$\uparrow$	$\rightarrow$, $\uparrow$, $\downarrow$	$\uparrow$
V̇/Q inequality	$\downarrow$	$\uparrow$, $\downarrow$, $\rightarrow$	$\uparrow$	$\uparrow$	$\uparrow$	$\rightarrow$	$\uparrow$
Diffusion limitation	$\downarrow$	$\uparrow$ to $\rightarrow$	$\uparrow$	$\uparrow$	$\uparrow$	$\uparrow$	$\uparrow$

* = mm Hg
$\uparrow$ = increased
$\rightarrow$ $\downarrow$ = decreased
$\uparrow$ = normal

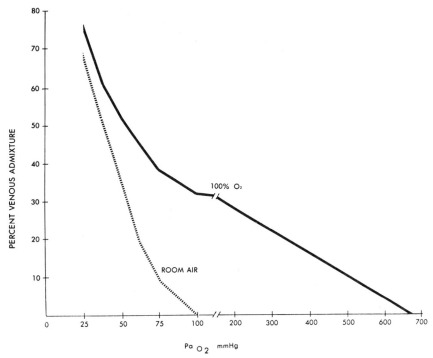

Fig 10–2.—Estimation of percent venous admixture from arterial Po_2 in room air *(dotted line)* and 100% oxygen *(solid line)*. See text for details and assumptions made in deriving these relationships.

standard deviations from the norm to express the variability encountered in a group of control subjects permits a better appreciation of normality. In our laboratory we have relied chiefly on standing height as the predictor of normal values. We verified and have used the regressions of Helliesen et al. for the calculation of predicted lung volumes (Tables 10–2 and 10–3).[16] Plethysmographic and helium dilution functional residual capacity (FRC) are similar in normal controls. Other pediatric normal values are readily available.[20] Every pulmonary function laboratory should obtain its own normal values by utilizing its own equipment and testing procedures.[23]

We recently collected pulmonary function data on more than 300 children aged 6.5 to 16 years from both inner-city and suburban schools. Analysis of the data revealed no difference between the urban and suburban populations. When standing height was used as the predictive variable, a significant difference was observed between the white and the black populations. White subjects had a statistically greater value per unit standing height for TLC, FRC, RV, VC, and FEV_1, but there was no difference observed for FEV_2/FVC, RV/TLC, FVC/MMF, and FEF_{50}/TLC. Inclusion of age, sex, and economic status in the predictive equations did not significantly improve the reliability. The difference

TABLE 10–2—NORMAL LUNG VOLUMES BY HELIUM
DILUTION METHOD VERSUS HEIGHT*

HEIGHT (CM)	VC (LITERS)	FRC (LITERS)	RV (LITERS)	TLC (LITERS)
100	0.896	0.581	0.385	1.194
101	0.922	0.598	0.393	1.228
102	0.948	0.616	0.401	1.262
103	0.975	0.634	0.409	1.297
104	1.002	0.652	0.417	1.333
105	1.030	0.670	0.425	1.369
106	1.059	0.689	0.433	1.406
107	1.088	0.708	0.442	1.443
108	1.117	0.727	0.450	1.482
109	1.147	0.747	0.459	1.520
110	1.178	0.767	0.467	1.560
111	1.209	0.788	0.476	1.600
112	1.240	0.809	0.485	1.640
113	1.272	0.830	0.494	1.682
114	1.305	0.851	0.503	1.724
115	1.338	0.873	0.512	1.766
116	1.371	0.895	0.521	1.810
117	1.406	0.918	0.530	1.854
118	1.440	0.941	0.539	1.898
119	1.476	0.965	0.549	1.944
120	1.512	0.988	0.558	1.990
121	1.548	1.012	0.568	2.037
122	1.585	1.037	0.577	2.084
123	1.623	1.062	0.587	2.132
124	1.661	1.087	0.597	2.181
125	1.699	1.113	0.607	2.231
126	1.739	1.139	0.616	2.281
127	1.779	1.166	0.626	2.332
128	1.819	1.193	0.637	2.384
129	1.860	1.220	0.647	2.437
130	1.902	1.248	0.657	2.490
131	1.944	1.276	0.667	2.544
132	1.987	1.304	0.678	2.599
133	2.031	1.333	0.688	2.654
134	2.075	1.363	0.699	2.710
135	2.120	1.392	0.710	2.767
136	2.165	1.423	0.720	2.825
137	2.211	1.453	0.731	2.884
138	2.258	1.484	0.742	2.943
139	2.305	1.516	0.753	3.003
140	2.353	1.548	0.764	3.064
141	2.401	1.580	0.775	3.126
142	2.451	1.613	0.787	3.188
143	2.500	1.646	0.798	3.251
144	2.551	1.680	0.809	3.315
145	2.602	1.714	0.821	3.380
146	2.654	1.749	0.833	3.446
147	2.706	1.784	0.844	3.512

TABLE 10–2—Continued

HEIGHT (CM)	VC (LITERS)	FRC (LITERS)	RV (LITERS)	TLC (LITERS)
148	2.760	1.819	0.856	3.580
149	2.813	1.855	0.868	3.648
150	2.868	1.892	0.880	3.717
151	2.923	1.929	0.892	3.787
152	2.979	1.966	0.904	3.857
153	3.036	2.004	0.916	3.929
154	3.093	2.043	0.928	4.001
155	3.151	2.081	0.941	4.074
156	3.210	2.121	0.953	4.148
157	3.269	2.160	0.966	4.223
158	3.329	2.201	0.978	4.299
159	3.390	2.242	0.991	4.376
160	3.452	2.283	1.004	4.453
161	3.514	2.325	1.016	4.531
162	3.577	2.367	1.029	4.611
163	3.641	2.410	1.042	4.691
164	3.705	2.453	1.055	4.772
165	3.770	2.497	1.069	4.854
166	3.836	2.541	1.082	4.937
167	3.903	2.586	1.095	5.020
168	3.970	2.631	1.109	5.105
169	4.039	2.677	1.122	5.190
170	4.107	2.723	1.136	5.277
171	4.177	2.770	1.149	5.364
172	4.248	2.818	1.163	5.453
173	4.319	2.865	1.177	5.542
174	4.391	2.914	1.191	5.632
175	4.464	2.963	1.205	5.723
176	4.537	3.012	1.219	5.815
177	4.612	3.063	1.233	5.908
178	4.687	3.113	1.247	6.002
179	4.763	3.164	1.262	6.097
180	4.840	3.216	1.276	6.193

*Calculated from the regressions of Helliesen et al.[16] and verified in our laboratory.

in predicted lung volumes was not observed when sitting height was used as the predictive variable. Lung volumes related most closely to the sitting trunk length when black and white subjects were compared. The predicted normal lung volume values versus sitting height are presented in Table 10–4 and include the 95% confidence intervals to allow a more meaningful analysis of a given person's pulmonary function test results.

Figure 10–3 shows the relation of vital capacity to sitting height with confidence intervals. Plots of this type may be useful in following pulmonary disease during childhood and adolescence in a manner analogous to the use of "growth charts" for linear growth.

TABLE 10–3.—NORMAL PLETHYSMOGRAPH
LUNG VOLUMES AT FRC VERSUS HEIGHT*

HEIGHT (CM)	FRC (LITERS)	HEIGHT (CM)	FRC (LITERS)
100	0.530	141	1.523
101	0.547	142	1.557
102	0.564	143	1.591
103	0.581	144	1.625
104	0.598	145	1.660
105	0.616	146	1.696
106	0.634	147	1.731
107	0.653	148	1.768
108	0.672	149	1.805
109	0.691	150	1.842
110	0.711	151	1.880
111	0.731	152	1.919
112	0.751	153	1.958
113	0.772	154	1.997
114	0.793	155	2.038
115	0.815	156	2.078
116	0.837	157	2.119
117	0.859	158	2.161
118	0.882	159	2.203
119	0.905	160	2.246
120	0.928	161	2.290
121	0.952	162	2.334
122	0.977	163	2.378
123	1.002	164	2.423
124	1.027	165	2.469
125	1.052	166	2.515
126	1.079	167	2.562
127	1.105	168	2.609
128	1.132	169	2.657
129	1.159	170	2.706
130	1.187	171	2.755
131	1.215	172	2.805
132	1.244	173	2.855
133	1.273	174	2.906
134	1.303	175	2.958
135	1.333	176	3.010
136	1.364	177	3.063
137	1.395	178	3.116
138	1.426	179	3.170
139	1.458	180	3.225
140	1.491		

*As determined in our laboratory for subjects 6 years
and older.

TABLE 10–4.—Normal Lung Volumes With 95% Confidence Intervals by Plethysmograph Method Versus Sitting Height*

SITTING HEIGHT (CM)	VC† (LITERS)			FRC† (LITERS)			RV† (LITERS)			TLC† (LITERS)		
58	0.75	0.99	1.32	0.62	0.87	1.21	0.32	0.57	1.02	1.24	1.57	1.99
59	0.79	1.05	1.39	0.65	0.90	1.26	0.33	0.59	1.05	1.30	1.65	2.09
60	0.84	1.11	1.47	0.67	0.94	1.31	0.34	0.60	1.07	1.36	1.72	2.19
61	0.88	1.17	1.55	0.70	0.98	1.37	0.35	0.62	1.10	1.42	1.80	2.29
62	0.93	1.23	1.63	0.73	1.02	1.42	0.36	0.63	1.12	1.48	1.88	2.39
63	0.98	1.30	1.72	0.75	1.05	1.47	0.36	0.65	1.15	1.55	1.97	2.50
64	1.02	1.36	1.80	0.78	1.09	1.53	0.37	0.66	1.18	1.62	2.05	2.61
65	1.08	1.43	1.90	0.81	1.13	1.59	0.38	0.68	1.20	1.69	2.14	2.72
66	1.14	1.50	1.99	0.84	1.17	1.64	0.39	0.69	1.23	1.76	2.23	2.83
67	1.19	1.58	2.09	0.87	1.22	1.70	0.40	0.70	1.26	1.83	2.33	2.95
68	1.25	1.65	2.19	0.90	1.26	1.76	0.41	0.72	1.29	1.91	2.42	3.07
69	1.31	1.73	2.30	0.93	1.30	1.82	0.42	0.74	1.31	1.99	2.52	3.20
70	1.37	1.82	2.40	0.96	1.35	1.88	0.42	0.75	1.34	2.06	2.62	3.32
71	1.43	1.90	2.52	1.00	1.39	1.95	0.43	0.77	1.37	2.15	2.72	3.46
72	1.50	1.99	2.63	1.03	1.44	2.01	0.44	0.79	1.40	2.23	2.83	3.59
73	1.57	2.08	2.75	1.06	1.49	2.08	0.45	0.80	1.43	2.31	2.94	3.73
74	1.64	2.17	2.87	1.10	1.54	2.15	0.46	0.82	1.46	2.40	3.05	3.87
75	1.71	2.26	3.00	1.13	1.58	2.21	0.47	0.83	1.48	2.49	3.16	4.01
76	1.78	2.36	3.13	1.17	1.63	2.28	0.48	0.85	1.51	2.58	3.28	4.16
77	1.86	2.46	3.26	1.20	1.68	2.36	0.49	0.87	1.54	2.67	3.39	4.31
78	1.94	2.57	3.40	1.24	1.74	2.43	0.50	0.88	1.57	2.77	3.52	4.46
79	2.02	2.67	3.54	1.28	1.79	2.50	0.51	0.90	1.60	2.87	3.64	4.62
80	2.10	2.78	3.69	1.32	1.84	2.58	0.52	0.92	1.63	2.97	3.77	4.78
81	2.19	2.90	3.83	1.36	1.90	2.65	0.52	0.93	1.66	3.07	3.90	4.94
82	2.27	3.01	3.99	1.40	1.95	2.73	0.53	0.95	1.69	3.17	4.03	5.11
83	2.36	3.13	4.15	1.44	2.01	2.81	0.54	0.97	1.72	3.28	4.16	5.28
84	2.46	3.25	4.31	1.48	2.06	2.89	0.55	0.98	1.75	3.39	4.30	5.46
85	2.55	3.38	4.47	1.52	2.12	2.97	0.56	1.00	1.78	3.50	4.44	5.63
86	2.65	3.51	4.64	1.56	2.18	3.05	0.57	1.02	1.81	3.61	4.58	5.82
87	2.75	3.64	4.82	1.60	2.24	3.13	0.58	1.04	1.84	3.73	4.73	6.00
88	2.85	3.78	5.00	1.65	2.30	3.22	0.59	1.05	1.88	3.84	4.88	6.19
89	2.96	3.91	5.18	1.69	2.36	3.30	0.60	1.07	1.91	3.96	5.03	6.38
90	3.06	4.06	5.37	1.73	2.43	3.39	0.61	1.09	1.94	4.09	5.19	6.58
91	3.17	4.20	5.57	1.78	2.49	3.48	0.62	1.11	1.97	4.21	5.34	6.78
92	3.29	4.35	5.76	1.83	2.55	3.57	0.63	1.13	2.00	4.34	5.51	6.99
93	3.40	4.51	5.97	1.87	2.62	3.66	0.64	1.14	2.03	4.47	5.67	7.19
94	3.52	4.66	6.17	1.92	2.69	3.75	0.65	1.16	2.07	4.60	5.84	7.41

*Data courtesy of F.P. Primiano, Jr., Ph.D., and J.G. Horowitz, Ph.D. Values derived from data collected from 328 normal, nonsmoking black and white children aged 6 to 16 years.
†Values presented as lower limit of confidence, mean value, and upper limit of confidence.

For patients with kyphoscoliosis or other severe truncal deformity, the vital capacity may be more appropriately predicted by the use of arm span rather than height. The predicted vital capacity in liters for the 328 children studied is 1.237×10^{-5} [arm span (cm)]$^{2.443}$ for white subjects, and 1.025×10^{-5} [arm span (cm)]$^{2.443}$ for black subjects.

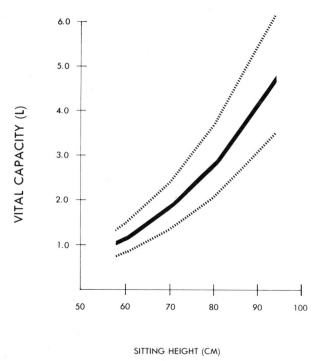

Fig 10–3.—Graph of vital capacity versus sitting height for 328 normal subjects aged 6 to 16 years. Mean values are graphed by the solid line, and the 95% confidence interval is graphed with broken lines. (Courtesy of F.P. Primiano, Jr., Ph.D., and J.G. Horowitz, Ph.D.)

LUNG VOLUMES

The vital capacity (VC) is a measure of the stroke volume of the thoracic bellows. Its subdivisions are the inspiratory capacity (IC), making up about ⅔ of the vital capacity with the subject in the erect position, and the expiratory reserve volume (ERV), contributing the other ⅓. There is normally a small decrease in the VC when the subject is in the supine position. The VC is divided into the IC and ERV by drawing a baseline through the end-tidal points of expiration on the spirogram (Fig 10–4,A). Variations in drawing this baseline will alter the IC and ERV but not the total VC. The vital capacity may be decreased in patients with either obstructive or restrictive disorders (Table 10–5):

By definition, *restrictive disease* is said to exist when both the vital capacity and the total lung capacity are decreased. If only spirometry is available for testing and a decreased VC is observed, the flow rates can be used to help differentiate restrictive from obstructive disease. In patients with pure, mild or moderate restrictive disease, the flow rates should be normal when expressed as a percentage of the vital capacity or the forced vital capacity. In patients with *obstructive disease,* the flow rates should be decreased. The VC may be

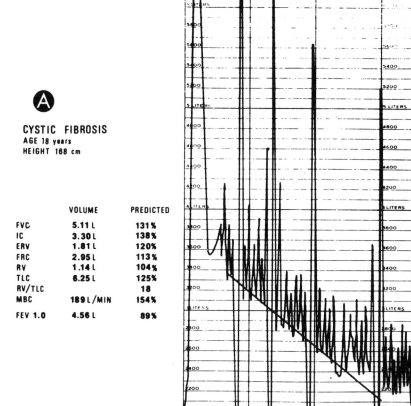

CYSTIC FIBROSIS
AGE 18 years
HEIGHT 168 cm

	VOLUME	PREDICTED
FVC	5.11 L	131%
IC	3.30 L	138%
ERV	1.81 L	120%
FRC	2.95 L	113%
RV	1.14 L	104%
TLC	6.25 L	125%
RV/TLC		18
MBC	189 L/MIN	154%
FEV 1.0	4.56 L	89%

Fig 10–4.—Three patients of approximately the same height (166 to 168 cm) and thus anticipated similar lung volumes (±20%) are compared. **A,** large normal lung volumes in a patient with cystic fibrosis without evidence of overinflation of airway obstruction. *(Continued.)*

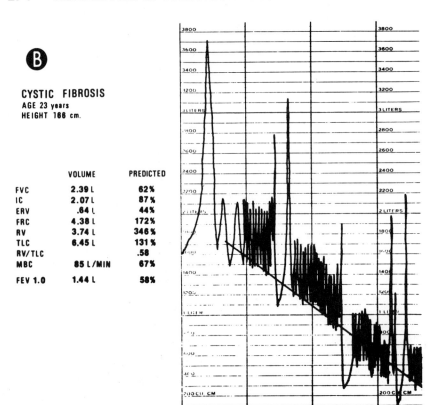

B

CYSTIC FIBROSIS
AGE 23 years
HEIGHT 166 cm.

	VOLUME	PREDICTED
FVC	2.39 L	62%
IC	2.07 L	87%
ERV	.64 L	44%
FRC	4.38 L	172%
RV	3.74 L	346%
TLC	6.45 L	131%
RV/TLC		.58
MBC	85 L/MIN	67%
FEV 1.0	1.44 L	58%

Fig 10–4 (cont.).—B, another patient with cystic fibrosis with evidence of airway obstruction. Although *IC* remains near normal, *ERV* shows a marked decrease in volume and delay in emptying compared to **A.** A reduced *FVC, FEV 1.0* and *MBC (MVV)* along with an increased *FRC, RV* and *RV/TLC* are consistent with moderately severe obstructive pulmonary disease. *(Continued.)*

reduced; however, it also may be normal or even somewhat increased. The latter condition is observed in some patients with bronchial asthma in whom the total lung capacity has increased. During symptom-free periods in such patients, the vital capacity may be in the high normal range.

The vital capacity is an easily obtained and repeated test to evaluate the response to therapy or the progression of a variety of restrictive-type disorders of diverse cause including interstitial lung changes (e.g., pulmonary edema, sarcoidosis, idiopathic fibrosis, or other interstitial disease), neuromuscular diseases (e.g., Guillain-Barré syndrome, muscular dystrophy), anatomic deformities (e.g., scoliosis, kyphosis), or space-occupying conditions (e.g., pneumothorax, hydrothorax, tumors, enlarged heart, massive ascites). In some cases, the VC may be improved by appropriate treatment, while in others it may be permanently or progressively impaired. The VC may become limited in severe

IDIOPATHIC SCOLIOSIS
AGE 18 years
HEIGHT 167 cm.

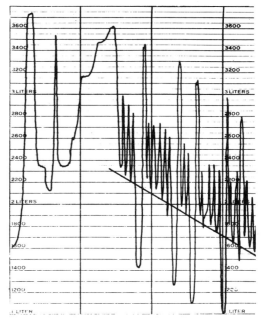

	VOLUME	PREDICTED
FVC	2.37 L	61%
IC	1.47 L	62%
ERV	.85 L	56%
FRC	2.10 L	81%
RV	1.25 L	115%
TLC	3.57 L	72%
RV/TLC	.42	
MBC	70 L/MIN	65%
FEV 1.0	1.98 L	84%

Fig 10-4 (cont.).—C, a patient with idiopathic scoliosis with evidence of restrictive disease. The *FVC* is decreased in the presence of a loss of *TLC,* while the *FEV 1.0* remains normal, and the *MBC (MVV)* is reduced only to the same extent as the *TLC,* consistent with a moderate restrictive type of pulmonary problem. Although the *RV/TLC* ratio appears significantly increased, it does not indicate obstructive pulmonary disease in this case since the *RV* and *RV/TLC* ratio should not be interpreted when there has been a loss of *TLC* as has occurred in this patient.

conditions even down to the level of the tidal volume. The ability to sigh or to cough effectively is then lost.

Functional residual capacity (FRC) is defined as the volume of gas in the lungs at end-tidal expiration. FRC can be measured by plethysmography, nitrogen washout, or helium dilution. The FRC is composed of the ERV and the residual volume (RV). In young children, FRC receives approximately equal contributions from the ERV and the RV. In older children and adults, the FRC consists of approximately ⅔ ERV and ⅓ RV. The FRC is decreased in patients with restrictive disease. The FRC is increased in those with obstructive disease due to air trapping with proportionate or greater increases in the residual volume. In persons with moderate to severe obstructive disease, the FRC may be underestimated if it is measured by the nitrogen washout or helium dilution techniques because "trapped" gas is not measured by the latter two methods.

The total lung capacity (TLC) is the volume of gas in the lungs at the end of a maximal inspiration. It is generally obtained by adding the inspiratory capacity to the functional residual capacity. The TLC is always reduced in patients with restrictive disease. The TLC may be normal or, more commonly,

TABLE 10–5.—SUMMARY OF PULMONARY
FUNCTION PROFILE IN OBSTRUCTIVE
AND RESTRICTIVE DISEASE*

	OBSTRUCTION	RESTRICTION
VC	→ to ↓	↓ to ↓ ↓
FEV$_1$/FVC	↓ to ↓ ↓	→ to ↓
TLC	→ to ↑	↓ to ↓ ↓
FRC	↑ to ↑ ↑	→ to ↓
RV	↑ to ↑ ↑	→ to ↓
RV/TLC	↑ to ↑ ↑	→ to ↑
MBC	↓ to ↓ ↓	→ to ↓
MMF	↓ to ↓ ↓	→ to ↓

*Symbols: → = normal, ↑ = increased and ↓ =
decreased. Typically restriction means ↓ VC and TLC;
normal flow rates. Obstruction means ↓ VC and flow rates;
normal or increased TLC.

increased in those with obstructive disease. An occasional subject may show
evidence of both obstructive and restrictive disease in which the total lung
capacity, vital capacity, and flow rates are all less than normal.

The residual volume (RV) is defined as the volume of gas remaining in the
lungs and the end of a maximal expiration. It is this volume of gas that maintains the stability of the alveoli and provides for continued gas exchange between inspirations. The RV is calculated by subtracting the ERV from the
FRC. Residual volume is the smallest of the lung volumes and will therefore
exhibit the largest changes from test to test when expressed as a percentage of
predicted. The RV is normal or slightly decreased in patients with restrictive
disease. The RV is usually increased in those with obstructive disease, sometimes to values 400 to 500% of normal. Calculation of the RV will be affected
by errors in the determination of FRC (e.g., the failure to measure trapped gas
by nitrogen or helium techniques) or by an incorrectly drawn baseline on the
vital capacity spirogram, which results in an erroneous ERV.

The ratio of residual volume to total lung capacity (RV/TLC ratio) is useful
in following the progression of obstructive disease. The RV/TLC ratio is normally 0.3 or less in the young child and decreases with linear growth to 0.2 or
less in the young adult.[16] The RV/TLC ratio should not be interpreted in subjects with restrictive disease because it will be abnormally elevated (but not
indicative of an obstructive process) due to the loss of total lung capacity while
a normal residual volume is maintained. The RV/TLC ratio tends to increase
with the severity of the obstructive disease. In patients with severe cases of
cystic fibrosis, the RV/TLC ratio may approach values as high as 0.75 to
0.80, but it usually does not reach such high levels in other conditions.
Table 10–6 shows some of the interrelationships encountered with progressively more severe clinical lung involvement in patients with cystic fibrosis.

TABLE 10–6.—Correlation of Clinical Pulmonary Status, Chest X-ray Evaluation, Pulmonary Function Tests and Arterial P_{O_2} in Patients With Cystic Fibrosis

CLINICAL PULMONARY STATUS	NUMBER OF PATIENTS	CHEST X-RAY SCORE*[†]	VC[†]	RV[†]	TLC[†]	RV/TLC[†] RATIO	$\dfrac{FEV_1[†]}{FVC}$	Pa_{O_2}[†] MM Hg
Excellent	35	22	101	93	99	0.25	0.79	85
Mild	32	17	92	119	99	0.31	0.70	81
Moderate	20	10	78	115	100	0.41	0.61	74
Advanced	21	7	67	207	101	0.50	0.57	68
Severe	10	4	63	277	114	0.58	0.49	—

*Based on 25 points maximum for normal x-ray.
†Mean value.
Vital capacity (VC), residual volume (RV) and total lung capacity (TLC) are in percent of predicted normal values.

FLOW RATE PARAMETERS

Flow rate measurements provide information about the status of the airways during dynamic function. Numerous flow parameters such as the forced expired volume in the first second (FEV_1); the maximum expiratory flow rate (MEFR), also known as the forced expiratory flow between 200 ml and 1,200 ml ($FEF_{200-1,200}$); peak flow rate; the maximal midexpiratory flow (MMF or MMEF), also known as the forced expiratory flow measured between 25% and 75% of the forced vital capacity ($FEF_{25-75\%}$); and the forced expiratory flow rate at a given percentage of the forced vital capacity (FVC) such as the $FEF_{50\%}$ have been developed to describe characteristics of the flow. All of these parameters are calculated from the forced vital capacity maneuver in which the patient exhales as rapidly and fully as possible from total lung capacity to residual volume.

The differences in the normal values for various flow parameters relate to the fact that they are measuring the flow over different portions of the FVC curve.[24, 28] Expiratory flow is largely determined by the recoil force generated by the lungs and by the diameters of the conducting airways. Near TLC, the lung will be more distended, providing a larger recoil force, and the airways will be larger, thus yielding higher flow rates. Flow rates measured near TLC depend on effort and are affected by the resistance and dynamic response characteristics of the recording device. Therefore, flow parameters such as FEV_1, peak flow rate, and MEFR depend on effort and yield information mainly on lung recoil forces and the status of the larger conducting airways.

The FEV_1 is the most commonly used of these parameters. It is generally expressed as a percent of the FVC, that is FEV_1/FVC or $FEV_{1\%}$. Dickman et al. suggested that an FEV_1/FVC value of less than 70% be considered abnormal for persons of any age, sex, or height.[9] The FEV_1/FVC is normal in patients with mild and moderate restrictive disease; it is usually abnormal in those with obstructive disease and becomes progressively lower as the disease progresses.

An inhalation of isoproterenol may differentiate between reversible obstruction due to bronchospasm (e.g., bronchial asthma) and more fixed obstruction (e.g., edema, infiltration or fibrosis along the airways) or destruction of tissue with loss of airway support (e.g., emphysema).

The maximal midexpiratory flow (MMF) is the flow rate measured between 25% and 75% of the FVC and is expressed in liters per minute. The MMF measures flow over the portion of the FVC curve during which flow limitation occurs. That is, flow from the periphery of the lung to the large central airways is limited by the size of the peripheral airways (airways approximately 2 mm in diameter). An increase in expiratory effort will not lead to an increase in flow rate in this portion of the FVC curve. The MMF has gained popularity recently because it is relatively independent of effort and is more sensitive to changes in the status of the small peripheral airways.[24, 28] The MMF is usually normal in patients with mild to moderate restrictive disease and abnormally low in those with obstructive disease. The major advantage of the MMF is that it may indicate an abnormality in the small airways at a time when other pulmonary function tests remain within normal limits. In this respect, it is interesting to note that many smokers have abnormal ventilatory function, which can return to normal over a period of time if they stop smoking.[12]

The maximum breathing capacity (MBC) or maximum voluntary ventilation (MVV) is the maximum volume of air a subject can ventilate over a 12–15-second period, expressed in liters per minute. This test is extremely dependent on effort, and its results often show a poor correlation with other pulmonary function parameters. The MVV is usually normal in patients with mild restrictive or obstructive disease and is decreased in patients with the severe forms of both restrictive and obstructive disease. The MVV has been found to be a useful test for adults in the preoperative assessment of surgical risk secondary to pulmonary disease. The MVV may be a good indicator of surgical risk because the test requires understanding, cooperation, motivation, maximal effort, and relatively normal pulmonary function for a good performance. All of these aspects may be important in preventing pulmonary complications in the patient following surgery.

TYPICAL ALTERATIONS

A summary of the typical alterations encountered in lung volumes and flow rate parameters in patients with obstructive and restrictive diseases is presented in Table 10–5. In addition to classifying the test results as being typical of either obstruction or restriction, it is important to give some assessment of the severity of the pulmonary involvement. Our guidelines for the assessment of mild, moderate or severe pulmonary involvement in obstructive or restrictive pulmonary disease are presented in Table 10–7. These represent our assessment as to the severity of the disease based on both clinical observation and pulmonary function test results and are similar to those published by other groups.[18, 19]

TABLE 10–7.—Assessment of Severity for
Obstructive and Restrictive Pulmonary Diseases

	MILD	MODERATE	SEVERE
Obstruction			
VC (% pred)	70–80	50–70	<50
FEV_1/FVC (%)	65–80	50–65	<50
RV/TLC	0.30–0.45	0.45–0.60	>0.60
Restriction			
VC (% pred)	65–80	50–65	<50
TLC (% pred)	70–80	50–70	<50
MBC (% pred)	70–80	50–70	<50

Various aspects of the nature of the spirometer tracing and the results of routine pulmonary function testing are shown in Figure 10–4 for three patients of the same height. The maintenance of normal pulmonary function in an 18-year-old patient with cystic fibrosis is shown in Figure 10–4,A. An increasing number of patients are showing similar results due to earlier diagnosis and therapy, especially measures to delay the progression of the obstructive pulmonary disease. The patient in Figure 10–4,B, also has cystic fibrosis, and the tests results are typical of pulmonary involvement with moderate obstructive disease. The patient in Figure 10–4,C, has idiopathic scoliosis, and the test results are typical of pulmonary involvement with moderate restrictive disease. The decrease in vital capacity, the changes in lung volumes, and the differences in FEV_1/FVC illustrated in Figure 10–4,B and C, are representative changes in pulmonary function encountered in children and adolescents with obstructive and restrictive pulmonary disease.

Longitudinal studies of pulmonary function are valuable in describing the course, prognosis, and response to therapy for patients with various chronic lung disorders. Longitudinal studies have been published describing adults with cystic fibrosis[13] and other obstructive lung diseases.[4, 7, 25]

BRONCHODILATOR EVALUATION

Pulmonary function tests obtained before and after the administration of a bronchodilator are extremely important in the assessment of obstructive lung disease. If a rapidly acting bronchodilator such as aerosolized isoproterenol (usual dose of 1:200 solution, 0.01 ml/kg; maximum dose of 0.3 to 0.5 ml) is administered, the entire testing procedure can be accomplished in less than 1 hour. In this instance, any significant improvement (15% or more) in pulmonary function after bronchodilator aerosol can be attributed to the *rapidly* reversible component of obstructive disease (i.e., predominantly relaxation of bronchial smooth muscle). The complete pulmonary function evaluation of a subject with obstructive disease should include pre- and postbronchodilator pulmonary function tests.

A positive response to the administration of a bronchodilator may be indicated by improvement in the pulmonary function parameters associated with either hyperinflation (air trapping) or airway obstruction, or both. A decrease in hyperinflation is reflected in an increase in the vital capacity and decreases in the functional residual capacity, residual volume, and RV/TLC ratio. A decrease in the airway obstruction is reflected in an increase in the flow rate parameters (e.g., FEV_1, MMF, peak flow) and a decrease in airway resistance (RAW). In general, these pulmonary function parameters should improve by at least 15% compared to the prebronchodilator study in order to be considered a significant response to the bronchodilator.[26, 27] A typical study of a patient with bronchial asthma is illustrated in Figure 10–5. This subject showed significant improvement after receiving an isoproterenol aerosol. Note that residual obstruction is still evident in the study after aerosol. Although the FEV_1/FVC percentage did not appear to change much, the FEV_1 increased from 0.38 to 1.09 liter, an improvement of more than 150%.

Pre- and postbronchodilator studies are also useful in evaluating a subject's response to chronic oral and/or aerosol bronchodilator therapy. A subject who is receiving optimal bronchodilator therapy will show little difference between

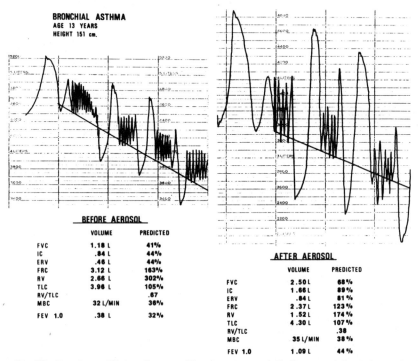

BRONCHIAL ASTHMA
AGE 13 YEARS
HEIGHT 151 cm.

BEFORE AEROSOL

	VOLUME	PREDICTED
FVC	1.18 L	41%
IC	.84 L	44%
ERV	.46 L	44%
FRC	3.12 L	163%
RV	2.66 L	302%
TLC	3.96 L	105%
RV/TLC		.67
MBC	32 L/MIN	36%
FEV 1.0	.38 L	32%

AFTER AEROSOL

	VOLUME	PREDICTED
FVC	2.50 L	68%
IC	1.66 L	89%
ERV	.84 L	81%
FRC	2.37 L	123%
RV	1.52 L	174%
TLC	4.30 L	107%
RV/TLC		.38
MBC	35 L/MIN	38%
FEV 1.0	1.09 L	44%

Fig 10–5.—Bronchial asthma with severe overinflation and impairment of vital capacity and flow rates showing significant improvement after a 10-minute isoproterenol (0.3 ml of 1:200 solution) – 1/8% phenylephrine (1.7 ml) aerosol inhalation (chap. 5). Residual abnormalities persist despite the improvement.

the pre- and postisoproterenol studies. Similarly, a subject who shows a significant improvement in the postbronchodilator study is not receiving maximal chronic bronchodilator effect and may benefit from more vigorous chronic bronchodilator therapy. Occasionally, subject shows a paradoxical response to a bronchodilator. These patients show increased hyperinflation and airway obstruction after bronchodilator treatment due to "excessive" relaxation of bronchial smooth muscles, leading to collapse of these airways on expiration.[3, 35]

Pulmonary function studies are also useful in assessing a subject's response to other therapeutic modalities aimed at relieving bronchial obstruction (e.g., oral or aerosol steroids, antibiotics, bronchial lavage). The "before" and "after" pulmonary function studies in these instances must be separated by several days or weeks. A significant improvement in pulmonary function during or following treatment with one of these therapeutic modalities indicates the presence of *slowly,* reversible bronchial obstruction (i.e., mucus hypersecretion, mucosal edema and hypertrophy, infection and inflammation, mucous plugging of smaller airways).

PREOPERATIVE EVALUATION

Many hospitals perform screening pulmonary function tests on all adults who are scheduled for major elective surgery. These tests will identify patients with abnormal pulmonary function who should be more thoroughly evaluated before surgery and have special attention before, during, and after surgery, depending on the severity of their impairment.

A complete preoperative evaluation of patients with abnormal pulmonary function is important in (1) deciding whether the risk of the surgical procedure outweighs possible benefits; and (2) when surgery is necessary, determining medical management procedures to minimize the risk. There have been few studies in adults and children that relate preoperative pulmonary function status to the occurrence of postoperative pulmonary complications.[17, 32, 33]

In general, patients undergoing thoracic or upper abdominal surgery are at the greatest risk of developing pulmonary complications after surgery. Patients undergoing lung resection should have a thorough preoperative evaluation to ensure that the possible benefits of the surgery justify the risk and to evaluate whether the surgery may leave the patient permanently disabled. Patients who have a marginal or poor cough before surgery can be expected to have postoperative difficulty handling their normal pulmonary secretions. The possible benefit of screening all pediatric patients older than 6 years for abnormal pulmonary function prior to major surgery has not been determined. However, patients with obstructive disease (e.g., cystic fibrosis, asthma) or restrictive disease (e.g., kyphoscoliosis, neuromuscular disease) should have a full evaluation before any surgical procedure. Often, when time and circumstances permit, a period of aggressive pulmonary therapy prior to surgery may improve pulmonary function and lessen the surgical risk. Improvements in anesthesia, surgery, and hospital care have contributed to better surgical outcomes for patients with cystic fibrosis.[10]

The criteria presented in Table 10–8 for the assessment of risk of postoperative pulmonary complicatons are intended to serve only as a rough guideline based upon our experience and that of others. Patients in the low-risk category should not have an increased incidence of pulmonary complications following surgery provided they receive optimal care. Patients who fall into the moderate-risk category will have an increased incidence of postoperative pulmonary complications unless special care and pulmonary support are given before and during the surgical procedure and in the immediate postoperative period. Patients who fall into the high-risk category should be considered only for absolutely essential surgery. Despite optimal pre- and postoperative pulmonary care, high-risk patients can be expected to have an increased incidence of postoperative pulmonary complicatons requiring long-term pulmonary care, support, and observation. Individuals with kyphoscoliosis who have a decreased PaO_2 (less than 70 mm Hg) should be considered at high risk regardless of their other results. It must be stressed that Table 10–8 presents only guidelines, not rigid criteria, for the preoperative evaluation of patients with pulmonary disease. Other factors such as the patient's general condition, cardiac status, type of surgery, and the available facilities are important to consider in making the final decision in regard to surgery.

SLEEP STUDIES IN INFANTS

The significance of sleep studies in infants and the relationship between sudden infant death syndrome (SIDS) and apnea of infancy remain controversial.[5, 29, 30] Nonetheless, many pediatricians perform polysomnograms (1- 4-hour multichannel recordings of parameters such as electrocardiogram (ECG), chest wall movement, nasal air flow, transcutaneous oxygen, etc.) or pneumograms (8- 24-hour recordings of ECG and chest wall movement) to aid in the assessment of infants with apnea, "near miss" events, or a family history of SIDS. Polysomnograms should be analyzed for central apnea, obstructive apnea, periodic breathing, bradycardia, and oxygen desaturation whereas pneumograms can only be analyzed for central apnea, periodic breathing, and bradycardia. In infants under 6 months of age, apneas longer than 15 to 20 seconds or apneas associated with bradycardia or oxygen desaturation are abnormal.[5] Periodic breathing is normally less than 3% of sleep time in term

TABLE 10–8.—General Risk of Developing Postoperative
Pulmonary Complications in Patients
with Abnormal Pulmonary Function

		MODERATE RISK	HIGH RISK
VC (% pred)	>60	40–60	<40
FEV_1/FVC (%)	>55	40–55	<40
MBC (% pred)	>60	40–60	<40
$PaCO_2$ (mm Hg)	<45	45–50	>50
PaO_2 (mm Hg room air)	>60	40–60	<40

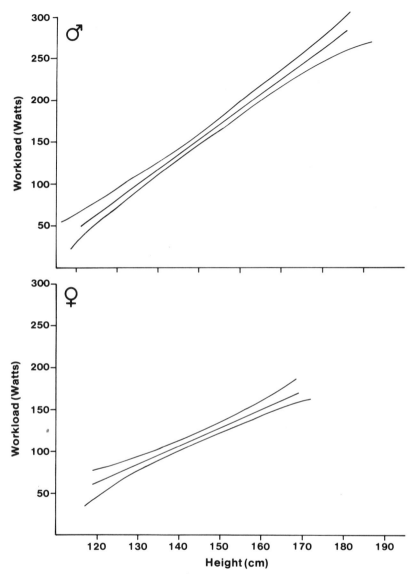

Fig 10–6.—A, maximum work load achieved in simple progressive exercise related to height in boys and girls. The outer lines indicate the 95% confidence limits. *(continued.)*

infants or 5% of sleep time in prematures.[5] The decision to monitor an infant should be based on an assessment of all available data including results of sleep studies and other lab tests,[5] parental observation of "near-miss" events,[5, 15] birth weight (especially if less than 1250 grams),[15] maternal risk factors for SIDS,[15] growth and development, coordination of respiration and sucking dur-

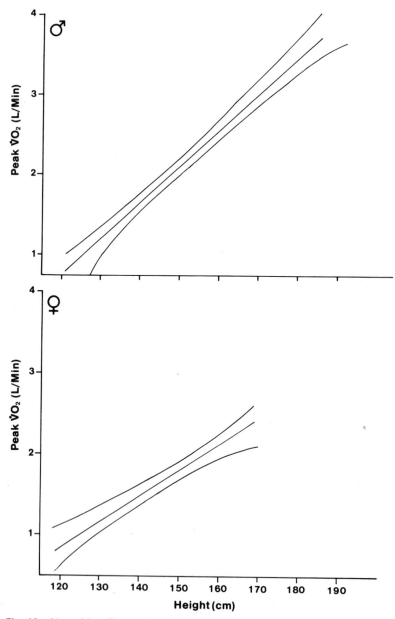

Fig 10–6(cont.).—B, peak oxygen consumption achieved in simple progressive exercise related to height in boys and girls. The outer lines indicate the 95% confidence limits.

ing feeds,[30] and a complete physical examination. The provision of 24-hour-a-day monitor service, psychosocial support, and medical support is necessary for any home monitoring program. The abnormalities of respiratory control associated with apnea of infancy will usually correct themselves by 6 months of age, and monitoring after reevaluation can usually be discontinued.[5] It remains to be determined whether the increased use of home cardiorespiratory monitors will result in a significant decrease in the incidence of SIDS.

EXERCISE TESTING EVALUATION

Interpretation of an exercise test will depend in part on the clinical setting and the purpose of the test. To rule out significant impairment of exercise tolerance, a normal maximum physical working capacity (PWC_{max}) (Fig 10–6, A and B) from the progressive exercise test and maximum oxygen consumption (Peak $\dot{V}O_2$) need to be demonstrated. Similarly, to document exercise intolerance, a low PWC_{max} is all that is required. However, there are pitfalls in interpreting abnormal PWC_{max} results. The most important problem is deciding whether the measured PWC_{max} is truly the best the child can do. In our experience, children are extremely cooperative and eager to do their best; far fewer children than adults will give up without giving their maximum effort.

Several measurements may support the observer's assessment of the child's effort.

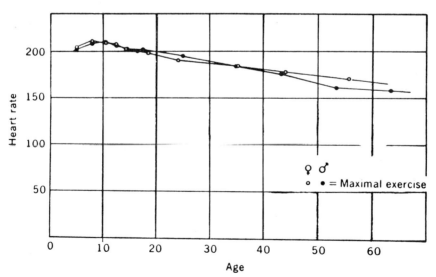

Fig 10–7.—The relationship of maximal heart rate to age in years, and heart rate during a submaximal workload. Mean values from studies on 350 subjects. The standard deviation in maximal heart rate is about ± 10 beats per minute in all age groups. (From Astrand, P. O., and Rodahl, K.: *Textbook of Work Physiology* [New York: McGraw-Hill Book Co., 1970].)

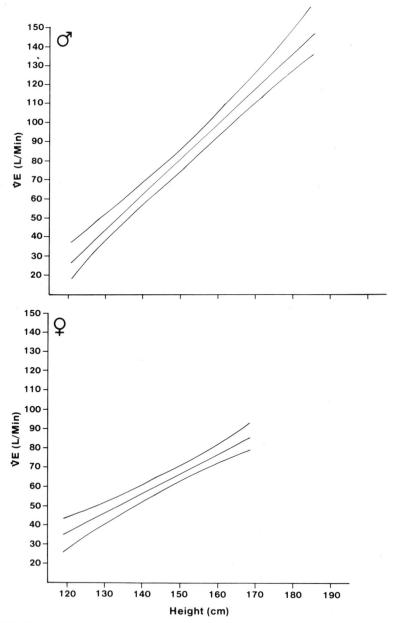

Fig 10–8.—Peak minute ventilation achieved in simple progressive exercise related to height in boys and girls. The outer lines indicate the 95% confidence limits.

HEART RATE.—If a child attains the maximum age-predicted heart rate (Fig 10–7), a good effort probably has been given. It is important to remember that the converse does not hold; if a child has not reached the maximum age-predicted heart rate, it may still be a best effort. A child with a pulmonary, muscular or metabolic problem may reach exercise intolerance before the heart rate reaches its predicted maximum.

RESPIRATORY EXCHANGE RATIO (R), $\dot{V}CO_2/\dot{V}O_2$ (see chap. 9).—Since exhaustion is probably related to the buildup of lactic acid associated with anaerobic metabolism, when R rises above 1.0, indicative of anaerobic metabolism, we assume a good effort has been made. This observation holds true no matter what the exercise-limiting factor.

MINUTE VENTILATION (VE).—As mentioned in Chapter 9, VE seldom reaches more than 60 to 70% of the MBC in children with normal lungs. When the lungs limit exercise, as in patients with cystic fibrosis and other obstructive lung diseases, children approach or even surpass their MBC during exercise. If a child's exercise VE_{max} (Fig 10–8) is greater than 80% of the measured MBC, a good effort is being made.

If the exercise test is being used to find the single factor that most limits a child's exercise ability, we usually ask the child why he or she stopped. If R is greater than 1.0, the test is probably valid. If the heart rate has reached the age-predicted maximum (see Fig 10–7), we usually assume that the cardiovascular system has limited exercise, a common occurrence in normal subjects. If VE is greater than 70% of MBC, the respiratory system has probably been the weak link. If heart rate and VE are low at PWC_{max}, the child often volunteers that leg fatigue made it impossible to continue. Deconditioned legs are often the limiting factor in children kept inactive because of real or imagined disease. Finally, if exercise testing is being done to investigate the possibility of exercise-induced asthma, a 20% or greater difference between the best and worst flow rates will confirm the presence of exercise-induced asthma.

REFERENCES

1. Ayers, L.N., Whipp, B.J., and Ziment, I.: Guide to the interpretation of pulmonary function tests, Projects in Health Inc., New York, N.Y.
2. Bates, D.V., Macklem, P.T., and Christie, R.V.: *Respiratory Function in Disease* (Philadelphia: W.B. Saunders Co., 1971).
3. Bouhuys, A., and van de Woestiune, K.P.: Mechanical consequences of airway smooth muscle relaxation, J. Appl. Physiol. 30:670, 1971.
4. Boushy, S.F., et al.: Prognosis in chronic obstructive pulmonary disease, Am. Rev. Respir. Dis. 108:1373, 1973.
5. Brooks, J.G.: Apnea of infancy and sudden infant death syndrome, Am. J. Dis. Child 136:1012, 1982.
6. Brough, F.K., Schmidt, C., and Dickman, M.: Effect of two instructional procedures on the performance of the spirometry test in children five through seven years of age, Am. Rev. Respir. Dis. 106:604, 1972.
7. Burrows, B., and Earl, R.H.: Course and prognosis of chronic obstructive lung disease, N. Engl. J. Med. 280:397, 1969.

8. Cherniack, R.M.: *Pulmonary Function Testing* (Philadelphia: W.B. Saunders Co., 1977).

9. Dickman, M.L., Schmidt, C., and Gardner, R.M.: Spirometric standards for normal children and adolescents, Am. Rev. Respir. Dis. 104:680, 1971.

10. Doershuk, C.F., Reyes, A.L., Regan, A.G., and Matthews, L.W.: Anesthesia and surgery in cystic fibrosis, Anesth. Analg. 51:413, 1972.

11. Druger, G.L., Simmons, D.H., and Levy, S.E.: The determination of shunt-like effects and its use in clinical practice. Am. Rev. Respir. Dis. 108:1261, 1973.

12. The effects of smoking on health, Morbidity and Mortality Weekly Report 26:18, 1977.

13. Fink, R.J., et al.: Pulmonary function and morbidity during adulthood in forty patients with cystic fibrosis, Chest 74:643, 1978.

14. GAP Conference on Standards for Pediatric Pulmonary Function Testing, Cystic Fibrosis Foundation, Rockville, Maryland, December, 1978.

15. Guntheroth, W.G.: *Crib Death: The Sudden Infant Death Syndrome* (New York: Futura Publishing Co., 1982).

16. Helliesen, P.J., et al.: Studies of respiratory physiology in children. I. Mechanics of respiration and lung volumes in 85 normal children 5 to 17 years of age. Pediatrics 22:80, 1958.

17. Hodgkin, J.E., Dines, D.E., and Didier, E.P.: Preoperative evaluation of the patient with pulmonary disease, Mayo Clin. Proc. pp. 114–18, February 1973.

18. Horvath, E.P.: Pulmonary function testing in occupational medicine, Department of Navy Technical Manual 77–1, 1977.

19. Kanner, R.E., and Mories, A.H. (eds.): *Clinical Pulmonary Function Testing* (Salt Lake City: Intermountain Thoracic Society, 1975).

20. Polgar, G., and Promadhat, V.: *Pulmonary Function Testing in Children* (Philadelphia: W.B. Saunders Co., 1971).

21. Report of Snowbird Workshop on Standardization of Spirometry, American Thoracic Society, News 3 (no. 3):20, 1977.

22. Shapiro, B.A., Harrison, R.A., and Walton, J.R.: *Clinical Applications of Blood Gases* (2d ed.; Chicago: Year Book Medical Publishers, Inc., 1977).

23. Sobol, B.J.: Assessment of airway obstruction: Which test is best? Proc. R. Soc. Med. 64:1246, 1971.

24. Sobol, B.J.: The early detection of airway obstruction: Another perspective, Am. J. Med. 60:619, 1976.

25. Sobol, B.J., and Emirgil, C.: The first second timed vital capacity and the course of obstructive lung disease, Chest 72:81, 1977.

26. Sobol, B.J., and Emirgil, C.: Pulmonary function tests and the diagnosis of bronchial asthma, Ann. Allergy 37:340, 1976.

27. Sobol, B.J., Emirgil, C., Waldir, J.R., and Reed, A.: The response to isoproterenol in normal subjects and subjects with asthma, Am. Rev. Respir. Dis. 109:290, 1974.

28. Sobol, B.J., Park, S.S., and Emirgil, C.: Relative value of various spirometric tests in the early detection of COPD, Am. Rev. Respir. Dis. 107:753, 1973.

29. Southall, D.P.: Prolonged apnea and cardiac arrhythmias in infants discharged from neonatal intensive care units: Failure to predict an increased risk for SIDS, Pediatrics 70:844, 1982.

30. Steinschneider, A., et al.: The sudden infant death syndrome and apnea/obstruction during neonatal sleep and feeding, Pediatrics 70:858, 1982.

31. Stinebaugh, B.J., and Austin, W.H.: Acid-base balance, Arch. Intern. Med. 119:182, 1967.

32. Tisi, G.M.: State of the art: Preoperative evaluation of pulmonary function. Am. Rev. Respir. Dis. 119:293, 1979.

33. Williams, C.D., and Brenowitz, J.B.: "Prohibitive" lung function and major surgical procedures, Am. J. Surg. 132:763, 1976.
34. Winters, R.W. (ed.): *The Body Fluids in Pediatrics* (Boston: Little, Brown and Co., 1973).
35. Zapletal, A., Motoyama, E.K., Gibson, L.E., and Bouhuys, A.: Pulmonary mechanics in asthma and cystic fibrosis, Pediatrics 48:64, 1971.

Index